PRAISE FOR
THE pH MIRACLE

D0052824

"I am convinced that we must all become more alkaline and Dr. Robert and Shelley Young's books provide much insight about how to do this most effectively. Remember, most illnesses occur when you are too acid. If you cannot do it all, do what you can. Your body will know you are trying."

—Doris J. Rapp, MD, author of *Our Toxic World, a Wake Up Call*, www.drrapp.com

"Dr. Young may be on the threshold of a new biology whose principles could revolutionize biology and medicine and potentially help people worldwide. Additional research is desperately needed."

—Neil Solomon, MD, PhD, director, International Council for Caring Communities' Health Advisory Board, Non-Governmental Organizations, United Nations

"In THE pH MIRACLE, Dr. Young may have discovered the true key to long life and health. It is simple and even spiritual in its approach, and is founded on the truth your mother tried to give you: Eat your vegetables! Ask your doctor to seriously check out this program."

—James Redfield, author of *The Celestine Prophecy*

"Filled with sensible science in an easy-to-read format, flexible guidelines, and delicious recipes . . . a must-read!"

—Verne Varona, author of *Nature's Cancer-Fighting Foods*

more . . .

"Dr. Robert O. Young and his wife, Shelley Redford Young, have established themselves as the preeminent scientific researchers on how to balance the body's chemistry and achieve one's ideal weight. Every African American and African Caribbean, every person suffering from type I and type II diabetes, hypertension, cancer, AIDS, heart disease, and youth obesity, and every person reared on 'soul food' needs to discover *The pH Miracle* and the rejuvenating recipes that alkalize and energize an over-acidified diet. This revolutionary dietary paradigm shift reduced my weight by fifty pounds in less than two months, eliminated my acid reflux without prescriptions and greatly speeded reduction of my PSA level after treatment for low-grade prostate cancer. Dr. Young's new biology and nutrition program rediscover the miraculous link between nutrition, health, and spirituality."

—The Reverend Dean Lawrence Edward Carter Sr., PhD, Martin Luther King Jr. International Chapel, Gandhi Institute for Reconciliation, Morehouse College, Atlanta, Georgia

"Dr. Young will change not just your understanding of how the human body works but also your outlook—your spirit. Diet affects your mind as well as your body and is intricately connected to the soul. This is a completely new way of living and being. You don't have to accept poor health as a regular part of life. With its serious changes, the program can seem drastic, but when you realize how much better you feel and how far the benefits go, the choice is easy."

—Jane Clayson Johnson, former anchor of *The Early Show* and author of *I Am a Mother!*

THE pH MIRACLE

Balance Your Diet, Reclaim Your Health

Robert O. Young, PhD
and Shelley Redford Young

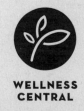

**WELLNESS
CENTRAL**

NEW YORK   BOSTON

This book is not intended as a substitute for medical advice of physicians. The reader should regularly consult a physician in all matters relating to his or her health, and particularly in respect of any symptoms that may require diagnosis or medical attention.

Copyright © 2002, 2010 by Robert Young, PhD
All rights reserved. Except as permitted under the U.S. Copyright Act of 1976, no part of this publication may be reproduced, distributed, or transmitted in any form or by any means, or stored in a database or retrieval system, without the prior written permission of the publisher.

Wellness Central
Hachette Book Group
237 Park Avenue
New York, NY 10017

www.HachetteBookGroup.com

Printed in the United States of America

Originally printed in hardcover by Hachette Book Group.

First Revised Edition: July 2010
10 9 8 7 6 5 4 3 2 1

Wellness Central is an imprint of Grand Central Publishing.
The Wellness Central name and logo are trademarks of Hachette Book Group, Inc.

Library of Congress Cataloging-in-Publication Data

Young, Robert O.
    The pH miracle : balance your diet, reclaim your health / Robert O. Young PhD, and Shelley Redford Young.—1st rev. ed.
       p. cm.
    Includes index.
    ISBN 978-0-446-55618-7
    1. Nutrition. 2. Health. 3. Acid-base imbalances. 4. Acid-base equilibrium.
    I. Young, Shelley Redford. II. Title.
    RA784 .Y68 2010
    613.2—dc22   2009037518

Book design by Charles Sutherland

To Antoine Béchamp. If his profound voice and science had not been silenced, much of humankind may have been spared the worst aspects of the so-called infectious and degenerative dis-eases and diseases of the twentieth and twenty-first centuries.

To our four wonderful and beautiful children: Adam, Ashley Rose, Andrew, and Alex. And to our son-in-law, Matthew, and new daughter-in-law, Arica. And to our pH Miracle grandchildren, CharLee, Isabeau, and Andilyn.

And finally to our future—the children who are at the forefront of an ever-changing and challenging acidic world. It is our hope that the message of the pH Miracle, the New Biology, and the Science of Alkaline Living for health will be received within their minds and hearts and become the foundation for an alkaline world that is healthier and happier.

If any man can convince me and bring home to me that I do not think or act aright, gladly will I change; for I search after truth, by which man never yet was harmed. But he is harmed who abideth on still in his deception and ignorance.

—Marcus Aurelius Antoninus

Contents

Acknowledgments   ix

Foreword by Gabriel Cousens, MD   xiii

Part I: A New Theory

1. The New Biology of Health   3
2. It's All About Alkalinity   11
3. Confusing Symptoms and Disease   29
4. Digestion—and Disease   50

Part II: Eating (and Drinking) Alkaline

5. Eat Vegetarian—Eat COWS   65
6. What to Eat, What to Avoid   86
7. You Are What You Drink: Water, Juice, and Green Drink   120
8. Food Combining   134

Part III: The pH Miracle Program

9. Transitioning   147
10. Putting It Together   158
11. The pH Miracle Whole Body Cleanse   168
12. Alkalizing Nutritional Supplements   181
13. Alkaline Exercise   215
14. Motivation—How to Get It, How to Keep It   230

Part IV: pH Miracle Recipes

Choosing the Right Recipe   245
Recipe Index   255
Juices, Shakes, and Milks   261
Soups   270
Salads   285
Dressings, Dips, Pâtés, Spreads, Toppings, Fillings, and Sauces   295
Entrées   325
Side Dishes   360
Snacks   371
Desserts   377
Recipe Substitutions   379

Resources   381
References   387
About the Authors   405
Index   407

Acknowledgments

Dr. Robert O. Young

If I have seen further it is by standing on the shoulders of Giants.
—Sir Isaac Newton

This quote reflects how I personally feel about the men and women who have had a powerful impact on my life's work and mission. Their gifts of wisdom, knowledge, inspiration, and encouragement have led me to the pH Miracle Lifestyle and Diet, the New Biology, and the Science of Alkaline Living for Health.

The life and research of French scientist and doctor Antoine Béchamp (1816–1908) set the foundation of my understanding on how matter can take on different forms and functions, a doctrine he referred to as pleomorphism. If it had been given the chance, his biological work might have revolutionized medicine with its profound insight into the nature of life, thus providing the cures for many sicknesses and diseases that science is still diligently seeking. His life's work opened my eyes and my heart and set me on my path of scientific research and discovery of the nature of sickness and disease and health and wellness. For this I am eternally grateful.

Modern Western medicine teaches and practices the doctrine of French chemist Louis Pasteur (1822–1895). The concept of specific, unchanging types of bacteria causing specific diseases made perfect sense at the time in my early training. Even though I no longer embrace the doctrine of monophorism, I am grateful to Pasteur for providing the basis of contemporary microbiological thought, which inspired me in my research on the nature of the germ and my quest for the truth of the "how and why" matter organizes and disorganizes.

I am richly blessed with a wonderful heritage of great men and women who in many ways make up who I am. My great-great-grandfather Brigham Young helped me understand the nature of matter, when he said that "matter cannot be created nor can it be destroyed." This very profound statement has echoed in my mind, as I realize that matter is eternal and can only take on different forms and functions.

My eternal companion, friend, and love of my life, Shelley, has been my river of inspiration and light. Through her love of people, especially children, and her creativity and intelligence, she has embraced the pH Miracle diet and lifestyle and made it possible for everyone to learn, understand, and live this New Biology and the Science of Alkaline Living for health in this very acidic world.

Several years ago, Dr. Neil Solomon and his wife, Frema, came to our home in Alpine, Utah, to evaluate the efficacy of my life's work. I was nervous and excited at the same time, because I knew he was a great scientist and researcher at Johns Hopkins University. Since their visit they have become good friends, as well as supporters of my work. In a world where scientific change is not necessarily received with open arms, I am grateful to this medical researcher who has had the courage to express openly the importance of this work and the need for continued scientific investigation.

I will never forget the day I received a call from bestselling author James Redfield, telling me he had given a copy of one of my previous books to Diana Baroni, an editor at Grand Central Publishing, then Warner Books. He told her that she needed to read the book and consider publishing the author. Without the help of James and his belief in, and personal experience with, the pH Miracle, you would not be reading this now.

We then had the wonderful blessing of meeting Diana Baroni. We traveled to New York City, believing we were going into a meeting with a real corporate type. What we found was a very personal, caring, knowledgeable, and delightful person to work with.

Diana then introduced us to Colleen Kapklein, who became our partner in tailoring the pH Miracle into a beautifully simplistic gift to the world. Our thanks and gratitude to Colleen for her many hours of dedicated work.

And finally and foremost to my Creator, who is the giver of all good gifts, the breath of all that is living, and who gives meaning and purpose to my life and mission. And who has also taught me the true nature and meaning of the blood and the anatomical living beings that make up all organized matter. In his words, "Life and death are in the blood and from dust you are and from dust you will return."

Albert Einstein said, "There are only two ways to live your life. One, is as though there are no miracles. The other is as though everything is a miracle." Every day I choose to live my life as if everything is a pH Miracle.

Shelley Redford Young

It has been an incredible journey for me to ride alongside such a gifted and giving messenger. There is no way I can adequately express my gratitude to Robert, for his support and his dedication and perseverance in courageously bringing this truth and light to a suffering world. He is a true servant. His contribution to mankind has made it possible for me to live out my most heartfelt desires—for people to be well, whole, and happy. It has been a rich blessing to share this healing wisdom all over the world with Robert.

I want to express my deepest appreciation for our sons, Adam, Andrew, and Alex, and our beautiful daughter, Ashley Rose. They have been understanding, supportive, and patient in our absence, and have become devoted students and examples of the New Biology and the Science of Alkaline Living for Health. Thank you for the immense joy you have brought to our lives!

Among dear friends whose support has been especially meaningful to this work, I want to include extended family members on both the Young and Redford sides who have encouraged me to produce recipes and get them "out there" into the hands of the public. You know who you are, and I love you!

I am most grateful for the recipe contributions from many creative and inspired chefs who have entered our recipe contests or mailed their recipes in. Thank you for creating recipes that heal from the inside out.

Finally, to our good true friends and pH Miracles around the world, who are now in the hundreds of thousands. Thank you for your conviction, your commitment to change, your never-ending love, encouragement, and support through this great roller coaster called life.

In love and InnerLight, and the Healing love and light of our Creator, who feeds us all,

Dr. Robert O. Young and Shelley Redford Young

"Miracles happen not in opposition to nature,
but in opposition to what we know of nature."
—St. Augustine

Foreword

By Gabriel Cousens, MD

The pH Miracle is a historically and profoundly significant conceptual medical breakthrough in the functional understanding of the basic cause of disease. The focus of Dr. Young on the pH is a major conceptual insight and contribution to natural healing. It reflects a brilliant continuum from the work of medical doctors like Antoine Béchamp and Claude Bernard, who taught that the biological terrain (a person's basic psycho-physical-biochemical balance as reflected in the immune system) was the most important factor in whether a person remained healthy or developed acute or chronic disease. As Florence Nightingale described in the 1850s, the swamp breeds the mosquitoes; the mosquitoes do not create the swamp. As Dr. Young beautifully clarifies, "Germs are really just the expression of the underlying disease condition (overacidity and microform overgrowth)."

This way of understanding disease is distinctly different from the current allopathic model, which is based on the theory of Louis Pasteur of one pathogenic organism—one disease approach. Even Pasteur himself refuted it on his deathbed, when he stated that Claude Bernard was right, the terrain is everything. Today this represents the core of the debate between the holistic approach to disease, which reflects a body-mind-spirit pleomorphic approach to preventing and healing disease, and the allopathic-symptom-focused approach to disease.

The pH Miracle is sharing a new and fundamental view of health and the prevention of disease. It is BASE-ic. When you create a healthy pH, you create a significantly more disease-resistant body. With this book Dr.

Young has established himself as a visionary pioneer in bringing forth this elegant yet profoundly simple approach to maintaining high-level health and healing disease. At the Tree of Life, a clinical study of more than a thousand people found that those who were healthiest had a venous blood pH of approximately 7.46—distinctly more alkaline than the traditional teaching of 7.35 as a healthy blood pH. Research done at UCLA by Dr. Watson produced similar findings; in a study of more than three hundred people, the venous blood pH associated with healthiest brain and emotional functioning was 7.46.

The optimal alkalinizing dietary approach for creating and maintaining optimal well-being is organic, plant source only, 80 percent live food, and low glycemic. Dr. Young's revolutionary teaching about minimizing fruit in the diet, especially sweet fruits, is both courageous and one that I share with him. The other components of the healthy alkalizing diet are good hydration, high oxygen intake, and highly mineralized food intake. In addition, this revised version has made a significant and healthy step away from recommending all forms of soy as part of the diet. The decrease in emphasis on soy shows the evolution of thinking as new information has emerged since the first edition.

After thirty-six years of clinical experience, these are the basics of what I consider the optimal dietary way of life. I would add one additional emphasis, which is to eat moderately, as excessive eating, even of the most alkalinizing food, can also create acidity because it overloads the digestive system.

In sum, this is a powerful approach. As we expand our understanding of the implications of *The pH Miracle,* we begin to look at our whole acidic, high-stress lifestyle as a source of illness. It takes us beyond diet to a whole alkalinizing way of life.

This book is great theoretically, yet also offers a well-balanced practical side. *The pH Miracle* shows how to transition to this lifestyle step by step. Remember that although it may appear difficult to live an alkalinizing, plant-source-only, organic, live-food lifestyle, it is profoundly worth it. From my own experience of living this way since 1983, I know it creates extraordinary vitality, strength, health, and a most delicious sense of well-being. For example, at the age of twenty-one as the captain of an undefeated college football team, I was able to do 70 push-ups more than anyone else on the team could do. That was before I went alkaline. Almost forty years later, having lived for years on an alkalizing diet and lifestyle, I was able to do 601 consecutive push-ups. It is interesting to note that in more than ten studies, nonathletic vegetarians had two to three times more endurance than meat-eating athletes. Research by Dr. Brekman in Russia showed that the same mice eating the exact same amount of cooked and raw food had three times more endurance when eating the raw food. A properly alkalinized person optimizes all mental and physical functions.

A visionary breakthrough, this book is already a classic in natural healing literature. It makes a great contribution to the emerging culture-of-life world in which we choose to return to the natural healing ways of the Divine.

Sir Gabriel Cousens, MD, MD(H), DD is a diplomat of the American Board of Holistic Medicine, director of the Tree of Life Rejuvenation Center and Foundation, and author of Rainbow Green Live Food Cuisine, Conscious Eating, *and* Spiritual Nutrition.

Part I

A New Theory

Chapter 1

•

The New Biology of Health

A new day is dawning. A day of truly holistic health, vitality, and well-being. A time of energizing our very cells, maximizing the life force of our bodies. An era of naturally lean and strong physiques! An era of focusing on right food instead of wrong drugs. This book, based on the microscopic evaluation of blood leading to correct nutrition, will light this path for you. It will help you understand the revolutionary science I (Rob) call the New Biology, and explains practical ways to change your diet and unleash the full power of your body to heal itself.

In truth, the light came over the horizon more than a hundred years ago. Unfortunately, the radical work of some great pioneering scientists has been overlooked by a mainstream medical model so deeply involved with its own myths that it was blind to larger truths. Until now. We are in a process of peeling off the blinders and looking at an entirely new model of human health while correcting the old model of disease. Working from decades of exhaustive research—my own as well as the work of those early (ignored) pioneers—we'll discover the basic pathways to illness and wellness. You'll get the science, of course, but also the practical applications that will allow you to put the science to work.

It's all about balance—pH balance. The universe operates by keeping opposites in balance, and the universe contained within your body is no exception. When imbalance occurs, we get the signs of disease (or *dis-ease*): low energy, fatigue, poor digestion, excess weight, foggy thinking, aches and pains, as well as major disorders. This book is about reclaiming balance: energy; mental clarity; smooth operation of all body systems; clear, bright eyes and skin; and a lean, trim body. By following the program in this book, all that can be yours within weeks.

All you have to do is take a look around you to see that most people with our modern lifestyles are suffering from imbalance. They are obese. Tired. Prematurely aging. Perhaps you are, too. Chances are at least one person you love is suffering from one of the top three killers in the United States—heart disease, cancer, or diabetes. When I asked the audience at one of my lectures how many of them had a family member with one of these big bad three, 80 to 90 percent raised their hands. The fact is, half of us will die from heart disease or diabetes. A third will die from cancer.

If you're like many people in our culture, at this point you're thinking, *Well, you have to die of something.* We've forgotten that it is natural to die—and to live—healthy! In fact, it is your birthright to live healthy, right up until the day you die. Making that vision a reality is the great gift of this program. And believe me, it has nothing to do with mapping the human genome, cutting-edge medical technologies, or even more powerful—and dangerous—pharmaceuticals. The good news is, the answer is much, much simpler than all that. And available right here and now. Today.

One of the most obvious clues is right there in the top three killers—cancer, heart disease, and diabetes. All are directly linked to diet. In fact, eight of the top ten causes of death in America today are—not to mention that diet is obviously the cause of the obesity of 60 percent of Americans. (I have no doubt that if and when we devote enough energy to studying the less common "diseases" and health challenges, we will prove that they are also related to your diet.) Eating the proper foods and getting the best nutrients, in balance, will help you avoid all that—along with the misery and poor quality of life that so often precede death, sometimes by decades. The simple secrets to finding the right combinations are what *The pH Miracle* is all about.

Even mainstream medicine agrees: "Foods contain nutrients essential for normal metabolic function, and when problems arise, they result from imbalances in nutrient intake and from harmful interaction with other factors. For . . . adult Americans who do not smoke and do not drink excessively, *one personal choice seems to influence long-term health prospects more than any other—What We Eat*" (from the 1988 "Surgeon General's Report on Health and Nutrition," emphasis added).

Since that landmark report from C. Everett Koop (and even before, depending on the circles you run in), Americans have been following one diet craze after another, not only in an attempt to drop the excess baggage most of us are carrying around but also as a way to find our way back to good health. Further, since that report, America's agribusiness industry and the advertising world have dramatically and disingenuously increased the false, distorted, misleading, and nonsensical information about the food sold in our grocery stores and served up in our fast-food restaurants. The result? We, as a country, are fatter than ever. And we're certainly no healthier.

The problem is that while diet is the key not only to slimness but also to overall health and well-being, it has to be a diet that properly balances our body chemistry. But every one of the diets Americans have tried—including not just the "average American diet" but also such supposedly healthful regimens as low-fat diets, the food pyramid, the macrobiotic diet, the blood type diet, the metabolic type diet, high-protein and low-carbohydrate diets, the raw food diet, and vegetarianism—creates wildly imbalanced body chemistry. Even if one way of eating does get rid of extra pounds (usually temporarily) or lower cholesterol levels or lessen digestive troubles for some people, it does not fulfill the promise of simple good health. We're so used to our modern medical machinery, in fact, that good health seems anything but simple. I'm here to tell you: It *is* simple.

Forget cholesterol and carbohydrate counts. Forget calories and fat grams. Forget blood pressure, blood sugar, hormone levels, or any of the other markers of health you're used to at the doctor's office. It turns out that the single measurement most important to your health is the pH of your blood and tissues—how acidic or alkaline it is. Different areas of the body have different ideal pH levels, but blood-and-tissue pH is the most telling of all. Just as your body temperature is rigidly regulated, the blood and tissues must be kept in a very narrow pH range—mildly basic or alkaline. The body will go to great lengths to preserve that, including wreaking havoc on other tissues or systems.

The pH level of our internal fluids affects every cell in our bodies. The entire metabolic process depends on an alkaline environment. Chronic overacidity corrodes body tissue, and if left unchecked will interrupt all cellular activities and functions, from the beating of your heart to the neural firing of your brain. In other words, overacidity interferes with life itself. It is (as we'll see in more detail in the next chapter) at the root of all sickness, dis-ease, and disease.

If that's not enough to get you interested in balancing your body pH naturally, nondestructively, keep this in mind: Overacidity is also what's keeping you fat. (More about that later.)

The goal, then—and what this program allows you to do—is to create the proper alkaline balance within your body. The way to do that is by eating the proper balance of alkaline and acid foods. That means 80 percent of your diet must be alkalizing foods such as green vegetables. (This percentage will go down somewhat once you've successfully rebalanced yourself. And if you're very sick, the percentage should go up for some period of time.) That leaves much smaller portions of acid foods (such as meat and grains) on our plates. In addition, carefully chosen, high-quality alkalizing supplements will help you achieve and maintain pH balance. You'll learn more about all this in detail in later chapters. You'll also need to exercise properly (see chapter 13) and adopt other alkaline lifestyle practices, like learning to manage stress (see chapter 14).

That's it. That's all there is to it. Get at least three-quarters of your plate covered with alkalizing food, use the alkalizing supplements as explained in this book, and you'll be good to go.

The following chapters explore the details of why, and the remainder of the book shows you specifically what and how. You'll get the benefit of my own exhaustive research and the work of the great minds that have gone this road before me, and you'll also get Shelley's real-life, practical expertise in how to make all this happen for you.

Bottom line: This program will bring you increased quality and quantity of life. I guarantee you'll see immediate improvement. Your energy will increase, you'll find new mental clarity and powers of concentration, you'll build strength and stamina, and you'll lose excess body fat while increasing muscle mass. You'll have bright eyes and clear skin. You'll look better. You'll improve your athletic performance. Your entire body will function more efficiently. Whatever health challenges you've been facing will improve and most likely evaporate altogether. In short, you'll regain all the effortless, sustainable energy and wellness you thought was lost with your childhood. With the healing, wholeness, and rejuvenation that this program brings, you'll experience, possibly for the first time in your life, vibrant, energetic personal health.

Over and over again, we've witnessed joy, relief, and renewed peace of mind in those who have turned a serious or chronic illness around, those who lost weight that they had been battling for years, those whose cholesterol levels dropped, blood sugars normalized, blood pressure improved, skin cleared up, itching stopped, energy returned. I've seen people who no longer required insulin injections for their diabetes. People whose aches and pains disappeared. Even people who had been diagnosed with cancer whose tumors vanished and who were pronounced cancer-free. We hear frequently from people who haven't been able to work for months or years who are returning to work, people whose allergies are letting up, people whose infections clear. People who are well, whole, and energetic again. People like Sharon and her husband. We'll let her tell their story:

I was up to a record 192 pounds. I was depressed and tired and had attempted almost every diet known to humankind. I would lose weight and then gain it right back when I returned to my old eating habits. I became more and more discouraged. I was sick and tired of being sick and tired—and fat! I knew it was time to make some major lifestyle changes.

So, once again I stepped onto the diet roller coaster by going to a local weight loss organization. It worked for the first few months. I lost thirty-two pounds, traded in my diet sodas for water, and started to exercise. I thought I might really have the problem licked this time.

At this same time, my husband applied for a life insurance policy. The findings of the company's physical exam scared us to death. His cholesterol was practically off the charts at 340. He had fatty growths in his shoulder. He was at his heaviest ever, too: 227 pounds. For someone who is five-foot-nine, that's quite a load to carry around. The report made him out to be a walking time bomb. An accident waiting to happen. Just like me, he realized he needed to make some serious changes. But he was confused about what and how.

Before he could take action, we moved into a new house and went on a vacation. I went back to my old eating habits, stopped exercising, and regained twenty of the thirty-two pounds I had lost. When things settled down again and we realized we had to take action, that's when the pH Miracle came into our lives.

We shared the same first thought: How on earth could we change our lifestyle so drastically? And the same second thought: We had to try. That night we committed to the program—and immediately headed over to a favorite local restaurant to pig out on our last barbecued pork ribs and mud pie. The next morning we changed our diets—and changed our lives. We've never looked back.

My husband's cholesterol dropped to 242 in six weeks, and is now under 200. He had been experiencing arthritis in the hips and had been thinking about surgery. But the pain has disappeared! For the first time in my life, I'm not depressed. I'm no longer a compulsive eater; no longer do I eat until I get sick—and then eat some more. I'm not a slave to my addiction to sugar and breads. Now the foods I crave are avocados and soybeans. We both would still like to lose a few more pounds, but we don't worry about it anymore. We know our bodies will reach an optimum weight. And we'll never regain it because we no longer crave the foods that made us sick, tired, and fat in the first place.

It turns out the weight loss is almost a side benefit. What we've really gotten out of this is feeling better. Our minds and bodies are stronger. We no longer feel sick and tired all the time. Even our relationship has benefited. We have a more fulfilling life. We can more fully enjoy the best things in life—mainly, our kids.

Speaking of our kids, we are now gradually working them into the program, too. They've been raised on fast food and pizza, candy bars and soda pop. And they've been addicted to sugar, bread, and meat— and been tired, obese, and depressed as a result, just like so much of their generation. Who would have thought they would ever be drinking green vegetable juice for breakfast? We feed them healthy meals, and they take supplements as well. They still have some sugar now and then, but we know this is not an overnight process. The whole family is headed in the right direction.

Robert Louis Stevenson wrote: "There will come a time when we will sit down to the banquet of our consequences."

We were. And we are. I like this way much better.

Besides the huge volume of tales like this one—which I'll share more of throughout the book—I've seen the scientific proof of such transformations with my own eyes, though nothing is more persuasive than the radical changes in people's everyday lives. I've observed many thousands of blood samples, including pH levels, from people all over the world, and seen the transformation that occurs—right down to the individual cells—when people change the way they eat, the way they drink, and the way they think.

HOW WE CAME TO EAT THIS WAY

All this healing occurs because people are willing to take responsibility for their own health and make the necessary changes. That was a mission Shelley and I were on for ourselves starting more than thirty years ago. But it took quite a while to realize that what seemed to be optimal in popular thought was still leaving us tired, seemingly prone to every passing cold, and just not able to get the very best out of life. Eventually, through trial and error— experimenting on ourselves—we developed the pH Miracle diet and lifestyle program, and found, finally, the way to get fully, permanently, holistically healthy—physically prepared to live life to its fullest.

We had always been active and on the lookout for ways to improve our health. By 1980, we were on what we thought was an ideal strictly vegetarian regime—mostly complex carbohydrates, along with some simple carbs (sugars), proteins, and fats. We were conforming to what seemed to be the best possible nutrition for our bodies, and we raised our children this way.

We ate the best of all foods sold in our favorite health food stores. Yet still we felt that afternoon fatigue. Our athletic endurance seemed to have plateaued, and we weren't getting any further improvements. We didn't have the strength and stamina we wanted. We were slowly but surely getting one common sign of aging after another. And it all seemed to be getting worse as we grew older.

What we didn't know then was what havoc all this was wreaking on our body chemistry, how it dangerously acidified our bodies, inviting all the disastrous consequences explained in upcoming chapters. Thank goodness the whole family had stayed generally healthy, but with what we know now we can see we were lucky. We were setting ourselves up for a lot of potential trouble.

It took a long time to realize what was going on—and what we could do about it. When we did figure it all out, what a dramatic difference! For one thing, though neither of us was overweight to begin with, we both shed pounds. I lost about twenty pounds—and four inches around my waist. Shelley dropped about fifteen pounds, and is now the same size she was in high school (nine). More important, we felt much better. Not only that, but I also could see astounding changes in our blood, including the pH levels. One good thing about the roughly fourteen-year journey we went through in developing this program was that it gave me time to come to some new (to me) laboratory techniques with which I could chart our progress (which I'll describe more fully later in the book).

Since we were essentially healthy to start out with, I was eager to test the effects of the dietary changes we were making on people facing serious health challenges such as diabetes, cancer, obesity, heart disease, lupus, gout, MS, Parkinson's, and arthritis. Sure enough, in my studies I could see the same sweeping improvements in their blood and the pH of their saliva and urine. They all reported feeling better and losing weight. And in many cases, even the dire conditions healed or disappeared! Witnessing these amazing results, I knew we'd stumbled upon more than a way of eating that just happened to be right for us and our family. We'd found something we wanted to share.

We've been fully on the pH Miracle diet and lifestyle program for more than ten years now, and there's no doubt in our minds: We'll never go back. We've gained too much we'd never want to give up. Even as we get older, we keep feeling better. And we know we're protecting ourselves from the ravages of the diseases that claim so many of our fellow Americans. We've found a way to ensure that we'll be there for each other, for our work, and most of all for our children, over the long haul. And we'll be able to truly enjoy every minute of it.

Good health should be second nature to us, but for many people it seems very difficult to maintain. The pH Miracle plan changes that forever. It will empower you to regain what is rightfully yours, encourage you to take responsibility for your own well-being, and restore the great gift of wellness to you.

I know that there are lots of formulas out there for getting well. And many of them have good track records and positive reputations. Often, that's because they deal partially (perhaps unknowingly) with what you're going to learn here. Also, you can get a lot better without getting completely well, so you might think the job is done without ever reaping the greatest rewards. Once you experience the full, vibrant wellness that comes with this basic change to your diet and lifestyle, however, you'll know just how tremendous the difference can be. So we invite you to begin this journey and experience the results for yourself. Awaken to the light of a new day!

Chapter 2

•

It's All About Alkalinity

Before we get to the specific steps for transforming the way you eat—and the way you feel—I (Rob) want to give you a little background in the science supporting those steps. Think of it this way: I have good news and bad news—and I'm going to give you the bad news first. We'll get to the good news soon enough—the ways you can protect yourself from all this bad news, and the delicious food you can eat in the process—but for now I want you to understand some of the scientific foundation upon which we have built the pH Miracle diet and lifestyle program. Once you do, I think you'll see clearly why following the program is so important and can make such a profound difference in your life.

ACID

We're starting from the premise that of all the balances the human body strives to maintain, the most crucial is the one between acid and base (or alkaline). Mainstream medical texts are all in agreement: The pH balance of the human bloodstream is one of the most important biochemical balances in all of human body chemistry. But mainstream medicine does not understand—and is not yet seriously researching—how the body turns itself inside out and upside down in order to keep that balance. The human body is meant to be alkaline, and the body will go to great lengths to maintain the appropriate, slightly basic, nature of its blood and tissues. But all body functions produce acidic effects; it is all too easy and far too common for blood and tissues to become acidic. That is: The human body is alkaline by design, and acidic by function. What that means in practice is that the body needs alkaline fuel, and that acids are created as a by-product of all human activity. Add to this activity a huge acidic dietary imbalance, and you have massive overacidification of cells, tissues, organs, and eventually blood. Such an imbalance sets the stage for chaos, opening the door to sickness and disease. Overacidification of body fluids and tissues underlies all disease, and general dis-ease as well. For one thing, it's only when it is acidic that the body is vulnerable to germs—in healthy base balance, germs can't get a foothold. Furthermore, acids are the expression of all sickness and disease, as well as of dis-ease. In short, good health requires a body in proper acid–base balance. Proper diet and lifestyle choices (like the ones laid out in this book) are the only way to ensure that.

The relationship between acid and base is scientifically quantified on a scale of 0 to 14 known as pH—pronounced like the two letters—which stand for "potential hydrogen." On that scale, 7 is neutral. Below 7 is acid and above it basic, or alkaline. Technically, pH reflects the concentration of hydrogen ions (positively charged molecules) in any substance or solution. And it is measured on a logarithmic scale, meaning that each number up (or down) the scale represents a tenfold difference in value. A pH 5 acid is ten times as acidic as something with a pH of 6; a pH of 8 is ten times as alkaline as a pH of 7. Higher numbers—more alkaline numbers—mean there's a greater potential for absorbing more hydrogen ions or acids. Lower numbers indicate less potential.

But you don't need to understand the details of the chemistry here. Just know that these two kinds of chemicals—acids and bases—are opposites, and when they meet in certain ratios, they cancel each other out, creating a neutral pH. In the blood and other fluids in body tissue, however, it takes about twenty times as much base to neutralize any given amount of acid, so it's better and easier to maintain balance than it is to regain balance when the body gets seriously out of whack!

BLOOD

Just as our body temperature must be maintained at 98.6 degrees Fahrenheit, our blood is ideally maintained at 7.365 pH—very mildly basic. (A mainstream doctor would accept up to 7.4, but that's problematic, as we'll see later.) Different areas of the body have different specific pH requirements, but the blood needs to stay within a pretty tight range. It is a reliable indicator of internal conditions in general. Maintaining the alkaline pH of the body's fluids, including blood, urine, and saliva (and even, though you don't generally measure these, tears and sweat), is critical for good health. Prime among these is the blood.

Physiological disease and dis-ease are almost always the result of too much acid stressing the body's pH balance, to the point where it provokes the body into producing the symptoms that we call disease. (More about this confusion later.) Disease can also be simply the toxic effects of an external source, such as exposure to air pollution from smoke, cars, or planes, or poisons from a toxic dump site, but that is much more rare. Symptoms can be the expression of that stress, but they can also be a sign of the body's effort to balance it. Depending on the level and extent of the stress, symptoms may not be obvious or even noticeable. The kicker is that excess acid is something we do to ourselves, thanks to the choices we make. The good news, then, is that once we recognize that fact, we can make different choices. But we must be ready to take responsibility for our acidic lifestyle and dietary choices before we'll be able to make the healthy changes.

All of the body's regulatory mechanisms (including breathing, circulation, digestion, and glandular function) work to balance the delicate internal acid–base balance. Our bodies cannot tolerate extended acid imbalances. Acidity reveals itself in our bodies in seven stages:

- Loss of energy.
- Sensitivity and irritation (as in IBS).
- Mucus and congestion.
- Inflammation.
- Hardening of soft tissue ("induration," including lupus, lyme, fibromyalgia, hardening of the arteries, plaque).
- Ulceration.
- Degeneration (cancer, heart disease, stroke, AIDS, ALS, MS, diabetes).

In the early stages of the imbalance, the symptoms may not be very intense and could include such things as skin eruptions, headaches, allergies, colds and flu, and sinus problems. As things get farther out of whack, more serious situations arise. Weakened organs and systems start to give way, resulting in dysfunctional thyroid glands, adrenals, liver, and so on. If tissue pH deviates too far to the acid side, oxygen levels decrease and cellular metabolism will stop. In other words, cells die. You die.

So a declining pH just can't be allowed. To prevent it, when faced with a lot of incoming acid, the blood begins to pull alkaline minerals out of our tissues to compensate. There is a family of base minerals particularly suited to neutralizing, or detoxifying, strong acids, including sodium, potassium, calcium, and magnesium. When these minerals react with acids, they create much less detrimental substances, which are then eliminated by the body.

Now, a healthy body maintains a reserve supply of these alkaline minerals to meet emergency demands. But if there are insufficient amounts in the diet or in the reserves, they are recruited elsewhere, and may be leached from the blood (as with sodium or potassium), the bone or cartilage (as with calcium), or muscles (as with magnesium)—where they are, of course, needed. This can easily lead to deficiencies—and the many and varied symptoms that come with them.

That's just the tip of the iceberg. If the acid overload gets too great for the blood to balance, excess acid is dumped into the tissues for storage. Then the lymphatic (immune) system must neutralize what it can—and try to get rid of everything else. Unfortunately, "getting rid of" acid from the tissues turns out to mean dumping it right back into the blood, creating a vicious cycle of drawing still more basic minerals away from their ordinary functions and stressing the liver and kidneys besides. Furthermore, if the lymphatic system is overloaded, or its vessels are not functioning properly (a condition often caused by lack of exercise), acid builds up in the connective tissues.

This imbalance in the blood and tissue pH leads to irritation and inflammation and sets the stage for sickness and disease. Acute or recurrent illnesses result from either the body trying to mobilize mineral reserves to prevent cellular breakdown or emergency attempts to detoxify the body. For example, the body may throw off acids through the skin, producing symptoms such as eczema, acne, boils, headaches, muscle cramps, soreness, swelling, irritation, inflammation, and general aches and pains. Chronic symptoms show up when all possibilities of neutralizing or eliminating acids have been exhausted.

When acid wastes build up in the body and enter the bloodstream, the circulatory system will try to get rid of them in gas or liquid form, through the lungs or the kidneys. If there is too much waste to handle, they are deposited in various organ systems, including the heart, pancreas, liver, and colon, or stored in fatty tissue, including the breasts, hips, thighs, belly—and brain. We know these "deposits" by names such as polyps, fluids, cysts, acid crystals, tumors, warts, bumps, growths, masses, blemishes, moles, blisters, sacs, and so on.

This process of acid waste breakdown and disposal could also be called the aging process. Ultimately, it will lead (in the seventh of the seven stages of acidity) to degenerative disease, including cancers.

And all this caused by dietary, metabolic, and environmental acids. (Dietary acids are from what you eat and drink; metabolic acids are created as your body processes what you eat and drink, and turns it into energy; environmental acids come from your surroundings, things like the synthetic pillow you may be sleeping on or the smoke you breathe in from the factory a mile or two from your home.)

On the other hand, healthy alkaline blood and tissues create a healthy body.

MICROFORMS

One of the nastiest consequences of an overly acidic body is the beasties that thrive therein, including bacteria, yeasts (or fungi), and molds. (They can be seen very clearly in live blood.) Dietary and metabolic acid waste also set the stage for the potentially devastating development of a host of microscopic organisms in your body, starting with Candida. *Candida* is the Latin name for what is commonly known as a yeast in the human body but is really a kind of fungus. Yeast and fungus (and the closely related mold) are single-celled forms born out of plant, animal, and human matter. They are absolutely everywhere—earth, air, water. For example, Candida is normally found in the gastrointestinal tract due to the breakdown of food matter. (We'd actually die without it.) However, it can easily become drastically overgrown, causing a wide variety of symptoms, from annoying to chronic to fatal. This is the bug all too many women are familiar with as a yeast infection, and parents may have experience with if their infants ever had thrush (which is just Candida growing in the throat).

While mainstream medicine recognizes these and a handful of other medical problems stemming from bacteria, yeast, and fungus, the truth is that on the typical American diet the vast majority of people develop out-of-control growths within their bodies—and the effects are disastrous. Further, mainstream medicine has no solution for these acidic conditions other than toxic drugs. Actually, excess Candida is just one of the villains. We are living in a plague of evolving microforms, including bacteria, yeasts/fungi, and molds, as well as all of their metabolic waste products. We are victimized not only by the microforms themselves, but also by their poisonous excretions, or mycotoxins and exotoxins (from *myco*, meaning "fungus," *exo*, meaning "bacterial," and *toxin*, meaning, of course, "poison"). The microforms produce these acidic wastes when they ingest and digest (ferment, really) energy in the form of electrons from carbohydrates, proteins, and fats—the same substances our bodies are looking to use for energy.

Candida and other microforms take advantage of the body's weaker areas, poisoning and overworking them. In an acidic environment, they basically get free rein to break down tissues and bodily processes. They live on our body's energy, or electrons, and use our fats and proteins (even our genetic matter, nucleic acids) for development and growth. These organisms are literally eating us alive! They then send their waste products (acids) out into the bloodstream, as well as inside the cells, further polluting the system.

To give you a little perspective on just how daunting the potential damage is, consider that over the hundreds of millions of years that bacteria, yeast, fungus, and mold have been on earth, they have developed into more than five hundred thousand different identifiable forms. And they've undergone little genetic change. Apparently, they haven't needed to, because they are great opportunists and survivalists, perfectly suited to what they do. They can go from explosive growth to thousands of years of dormancy. (Living spores have been found in ancient Egyptian tombs only recently excavated.) Furthermore, there are more than a thousand toxins produced by bacteria, yeast, fungus, and mold.

Bacteria, yeast, fungus, and mold do not themselves produce symptoms in the body—their toxic wastes do. Nor do they initiate disease or dis-ease. They only show up because of a compromised internal environment that causes body cells to transform into bacteria, then yeast, and finally mold. As Rudolph Virchow wrote, "Mosquitoes seek the stagnant water, but do not cause the pool to become stagnant."

These organisms—biological transformations from your own body cells—and their wastes contribute directly or indirectly to a huge list of symptoms. Most dis-ease and diseases, especially chronic and degenerative ones from chronic acidity, give rise to microform transformation and then overgrowth. Between the extremes of athlete's foot and AIDS are the underlying symptoms such as diabetes, cancer, atherosclerosis (clogged arteries), osteoporosis, chronic fatigue, and more—including infections that appear to be transmitted person-to-person. The general signs of overacid that lead to transformation of body cells and then overgrowth include pain, infection, fatigue, and body malfunctions such as adrenal/thyroid failure, indigestion, diarrhea, food cravings, intestinal pain, depression, hyperactivity, antisocial behavior, asthma, hemorrhoids, colds and flu, respiratory problems, endometriosis, dry skin and itching, thrush, receding gums, finger/toenail fungus, dizziness, joint pain, bad breath, ulcers, colitis, heartburn, dry mouth, PMS and menstrual problems, irritability, puffy eyes, lack of sex drive, skin rash and hives, lupus, mood swings, hormonal imbalance, vaginal yeast infection, cysts and tumors, rheumatoid arthritis, numbness, hay fever, acne, gas/bloating, bowel stasis, low blood sugar, hiatal hernia, headaches, lethargy/laziness, insomnia, suicidal tendencies, coldness/ shakiness, infections, over- and underweight conditions, chemical sensitivity, poor memory, muscle aches, allergies (airborne or food), burning eyes, multiple sclerosis, malabsorption, and bladder infections. Whew! And that's not even including that general, just overall bad feeling so common these days. You can blame that on out-of-control evolving microforms from body cells and their toxic acid wastes as well.

Microforms are biological transformations of you and live and thrive in . . . acidity! They love to swim in their own waste products. They also love the low oxygen levels that come with acidity. On top of that, the wastes they produce are strong acids themselves. So just in case you needed further convincing about the importance of getting your body back to basics, try the mental image of your body cells swimming in a pool of acid swarming with bacteria, fungus, and mold.

Still, the good news is that eating properly and using alkaline supplements wisely is all you need to do to let your body use and control the dietary and metabolic acids that cause body cells to transform, giving birth to microforms, without risking the development of overgrowths or their dangerous negative forms. Maintaining your acid–base balance through lifestyle and diet provides the optimal environment for the exclusive growth of vibrant body cells and a decrease or elimination of all levels of microforms. The pH of the blood and urine is the most important factor in determining the state of microorganisms in the blood.

Everyone needs to be concerned about excess acidity leading to the development of microforms, even if they are not (yet) experiencing outward signs of overgrowth. That's because overgrowth happens in two stages. In the first, initial developmental phase, microforms grow in small colonies and, although they are most likely visible in the blood, are probably not detectable by physical sensations or symptoms. In the second, acute or chronic symptomatic phase, the complications and discomforts become obvious. Things are now bad enough that your body is complaining, throwing up warning signs, and pleading for help. A second-stage overgrowth may happen relatively quickly or take years to develop.

Even in this second, more serious stage, all you need to do to reverse it is to create an internal alkaline environment in your body that won't support the transformation and development of microforms. All that requires is alkalizing your blood and tissue pH with appropriate nutritional supplements and an alkaline lifestyle and diet like the one detailed in later chapters. Of course, it would be better still to stop them in their tracks they ever get that bad, which is why anyone will benefit from this program.

When your body goes from acid back to base, bacteria, yeast, fungus, and mold stop developing and can once again become benign. Their left-over toxins can then be bound up by certain fats and alkaline minerals and eliminated from the body.

WHEN THE FISH ARE SICK, CHANGE THE WATER

Think of your body as a fish tank. Imagine your cells and organ systems as the fish, bathed in fluids (including blood) that transport food and remove wastes. Then suppose I back up a car and put the tailpipe up against the air intake filter that supplies oxygen to the tank. The water becomes filled with carbon monoxide, making it acidic. Then I throw in too much food, or the wrong kind of food, and the fish are unable to consume or digest it all, so it starts to decompose. Toxic acid wastes and chemicals build up as the food breaks down, making the water still more acidic.

How long before the fish are goners?

You'd never do such things to the most ordinary of goldfish. Yet every day we humans do that very equivalent to our own bodies, our own blood and tissues, fouling them with pollution, excessive intake of food, acidic foods, and more. The fish are floating belly-up, but it is as if we can't see them, or don't know what it means.

Now, back to our polluted fish tank. If you've reached such a sorry state of affairs, what's the best thing you could do to fix it? Would you treat the fish for the illnesses they would no doubt develop? No—you'd change the water.

Do your body the same favor. Change the water. Clean up the internal environment. Then keep it clean. The diet and lifestyle program in this book shows you how.

HISTORY, LOST AND FOUND

Classical biology, based on the work of Louis Pasteur in the late 1800s, relies on the idea that disease comes from germs that invade the body from the outside. Yet in studying the dazzling but shamefully overlooked work of Pasteur's contemporary Antoine Béchamp and his followers, including Günther Enderlein, Claude Bernard, Virginia Livingston-Wheeler, and Gaston Naessens, I've learned that, in an acid environment, bacteria and other microforms can come from our own body cells.

Pasteur's "germs of the air" may contribute to illness, but they are not, contrary to popular belief, necessary for illness to occur. Their negative effects are simply *added* to the compromised environment already existing in the body.

Besides generating various microforms within our own bodies, we do also have them coming in through our respiratory system and intestinal tract (often via our food—but more about that later). Bacterial invaders appear to then grow in the body, wreaking their characteristic havoc. But what really happens is that their presence initiates a similar development in the bacteria already in the host—depending, again, on the internal environment.

An acid environment gives a big green light to this process. To contract an infection—or, as I think of it, produce an outfection—you have to be predisposed to it internally. You have to have some of the bug already in your system, and you have to have the acidity to allow it to take hold or to transform from body cells. This is why some exposed acidic people get sick, and some don't. Think for a minute of the flu epidemic of 1918. It ravaged the planet, killing about a hundred million people worldwide. But it would occur in one home but not the one next door, one family member but not the next. Why? If you throw seeds on concrete, they won't grow. They have to meet fertile soil. So it is with the germs of the air. Even if they do get into your body, unless it is nice and acidic, they can't grow and multiply and make you sick—or kill you.

MANY FORMS

The other key fact about microforms is that they can rapidly change their form and function. Bacteria can change into yeast, yeast into fungus, and fungus into mold. With this brilliant work and these critical observations and these crucial discoveries being overshadowed by Pasteur's influence, we have for more than a hundred years lost the critical knowledge that dis-ease and disease are conditions of our own inner environment, not something caused by attack from foreign entities.

This lost chapter of history reveals that there is something living independently in cells and body fluids that is capable of evolution into more complex forms. These elements are known as microzymas (*micro,* meaning "small," and *zyma,* meaning "being"), and all living things contain them. Degeneration and regeneration both originate with the microzymas. All cells evolve from them to begin with. In the right circumstances and environment, microzymas evolve into more complex life-forms, including bacteria and fungus. It is a two-way street: Bacteria can also de-evolve back to microzymas. Everything begins and ends with microzymas. What happens in between depends on the environment.

The ability of microforms to evolve, to change form and function depending on their environment, is known as pleomorphism (*pleo,* meaning "many," and *morph,* meaning "form"). My theory is that red blood cells do this, too: They can de-evolve and then re-evolve into any kind of cell the body needs—bone cells, muscle cells, skin cells, brain cells, liver cells, heart cells, and so on. In a kind of parallel process, bacteria, yeast, fungus, and mold are morbid evolutions of healthy cells (including red blood cells, brain cells, and liver cells).

You are already familiar with one chemical example of pleomorphism: the transition of plain water to steam—or snowflake. The chemical structure doesn't change—it is still just H_2O—but the form does, depending on the environment.

Now, I bet you can guess what kind of unhealthy environment spurs biological transformation of body cells into microforms in the human body. That's right: acidity. Microzymas don't always become bacteria, and bacteria don't always evolve into fungus, nor does fungus always become mold—it takes an acid environment. Harmful pleomorphic organisms do not, and cannot, evolve in healthy (alkaline) surroundings.

With a high-powered compound light microscope, a digital video camera, and a computer, I have been able to record the evolution of pleomorphic organisms from rod-shaped bacteria (bacilli) to spherical (cocci), and ultimately into yeast and fungus and mold—and back again. Pleomorphism has also been seen in recent electron microscope pictures of animal tissue. This transformation of matter across taxonomy lines is validated with CPR testing. But traditional Western medical research has not accepted or further seriously investigated these reports and findings.

Dramatic experiments have demonstrated the extent of the transformations possible. For example, one type of amoeba (a single-celled organism) feeds on bacteria and another, a dysentery amoeba, eats rice. The two have unique DNA specific to their form. But an amazing thing happens if you flip-flop their diets, gradually switching the one amoeba over to rice, and the dysentery amoeba to bacteria: Their genetic material actually changes! They literally switch into each other. That makes microform pleomorphism even more profound than the change of a caterpillar into a butterfly, and all the more fantastic because it can happen quite rapidly, sometimes in a matter of seconds.

Pasteur's friends in high places, his showmanship, and his ability to basically market himself and his work started the ball rolling in favor of "the germ theory" all those decades ago, and mainstream medicine adheres to this theory to this day. That tradition is so strong, and the alternatives so revolutionary, that even something that is plain to see, observable with your own eyes, nonetheless goes unseen. My fervent hope is that this ever-so-slowly evolving technology will soon gain momentum. The truth is, the future health of the world depends on it!

There is one more reason this lost history is so slow to be recovered. Just as microforms can evolve out of body cells, they can also revert to their original state. For example, in beer, only a trace amount of the yeast initially added to a batch is present after the fermentation of the grain, and it is no longer visible to the unaided eye. Only the alcohol—simply a mycotoxin—is left. Where did the organism go? It isn't really gone, of course, it has just returned to microzymas. Similarly, every cancerous tumor is surrounded by a pool of lactic acid—another mycotoxin—but the microform may or may not be there. So even those willing to look won't always find a bacteria or yeast, but they will find acid.

Those willing to look again and again, and with clear eyes, will be rewarded with the secrets to permanent health. We can heal ourselves by changing the internal environment of our bodies. Potentially harmful microforms of bacteria, yeast, fungus, and/or mold, then, will have nowhere to grow and will become harmless.

ACID IMBALANCE IS PERFECTLY NATURAL . . . WHEN WE'RE *DEAD*!

The chaos of acid imbalance and microform transformation and then overgrowth is an entirely natural and orderly process when life is ending. The body automatically becomes acidic upon death. Once a body stops breathing, oxygen levels of course rapidly decrease, creating the anaerobic ("without oxygen") environment in which microforms thrive (in addition to the acid they love). Then these little buggers get down to work. Their one big job—one reason they are a part of the normal human body—is that they are the principal "undertakers" when we die. Those mycotoxins are designed to decompose our dead bodies. The microforms and their toxins are here to reduce us into our simplest component parts—back to microzymas. Biologists call it the carbon cycle. It's the literal meaning behind "ashes to ashes, and dust to dust." In less technical or poetic language: Acid is what makes our corpses rot. (The really scary part is that it does the same thing to us when we are living!)

Thus, with dietary and metabolic acids that lead to microform transformation and overgrowth in overly acidic living bodies, that process is set in motion prematurely. Bacteria, yeast, and fungus start their takeover while we are still living. We are basically rotting inside. Fermenting. Molding. Take your pick!

Keep in mind, however, that there is nothing inherently bad about the microforms themselves. If anything, they are actually good. Cells all over the body must constantly break down and renew themselves to stay healthy and vigorous. Microforms are a stage of all transformed body cells and are there to handle the recycling, so the garbage doesn't pile up.

HOW ACIDIC ARE YOU?

You can check your pH levels at home with paper pH strips, available at many pharmacies, or with a battery-operated pH electron meter, available from health catalogs (see the resources section at the end of this book).

The strips, which are relatively inexpensive and should be easy to find, test the pH of your saliva or urine. The pH of saliva is much more variable, so you are better off testing your urine, which gives you a direct indicator of your tissue pH. Urine pH changes, too, in response to what you eat, so first thing in the morning, after you've fasted overnight, is the ideal time to test. This morning urine pH will reflect your lifestyle and dietary choices over the last twenty-four hours. Ideally, it will be mildly alkaline, pH at 7.2 or higher.

The strips change color to indicate acid or base, and are lighter or darker depending on the intensity of the reading. They come with a color chart to help you translate the color into a number.

If you also want to check your saliva, which ideally will also be above 7.2, test it before eating anything in the morning, and then a few times during the day. If you find that your results are below 7.0, you can correct it immediately by eating a bit of particularly alkaline food, like cucumber, broccoli, asparagus, or avocado, or taking three teaspoons of mineral salts in four to six ounces of water. Experiment a little and you will quickly get a feel for what successfully corrects your test results.

The meters can also be used to test saliva or urine, and the same recommendations apply: It is best to test your urine, and do it first thing in the morning. These meters are quite accurate and give you your pH with a number—no color charts to mess with. But they can be hard to find, and expensive, running into the hundreds of dollars.

So test yourself to see where you are right now, and then retest daily to keep tabs on your progress. You can also see for yourself the effect of meals on pH, by regularly testing with a meter throughout the day. Though the results are not definitive, you will at the very least be able to see trends. Test yourself after the basic meals like the ones described later in this book, and compare the result with those you got from your original diet. Anytime you have low pH readings, especially after eating, you know that you are deficient in alkaline reserves. Your body does not have enough of the minerals necessary to process food properly, and cannot adequately respond to the physiological crisis of acidic food or drink.

Your doctor can also do a blood pH test for you. As mentioned, the ideal blood pH is 7.365. The American medical establishment accepts 7.4, but that is too alkaline, and actually indicates tissue acidification: The body is collecting and storing alkaline minerals to tame excess acidity. If it isn't fending off acidity, the body has no need to become so overly alkaline.

Daily pH testing is a key health check. As long as you are keeping it at 7.2 or better, then you can rest assured your blood and tissues are also healthy. (People coping with serious health challenges may need to increase the pH of the urine or other bodily fluids in order to curb acidity.)

How to Test Your Own pH

Monitor your pH according to these guidelines every day for at least twelve weeks, or until you establish a pH balance at 7.2 (with the help of the program in this book). Once you are balanced at 7.2 or higher, you can reduce the number of tests to once a day or two to three times a week, just to keep an eye on things. Use a notebook to record all your pH results.

1. Upon waking, before you eat or drink or brush your teeth or smoke or put anything at all into your mouth, test your saliva with pH paper. Just wet the end of a test strip with your tongue. Note the color change and write down the corresponding pH number. The optimal result is 7.2.
2. Next, test your first urine of the morning. You just need a couple of drops on the end of a test paper. Note the color change and write down the corresponding pH number. The optimal result is 7.2 or more.

3. Test your second morning urine before eating any food. Your re-
    sult may differ from the first check, because with the first urine
    you cleared the acid load from the previous day. Again, you're
    looking for 7.2 or higher.
4. Eat breakfast—avocado soup, vegetable soup, Healing Soup (page
    274), or fresh almond milk or green drink. Wait five minutes and
    then check your urine and saliva again. After that good alkaline
    meal, your pH numbers should go up from the previous results.
    You're looking to be between 7.2 and 8.4.
5. Check your urine and saliva pH again between breakfast and
    lunch, and again between lunch and dinner. You're always look-
    ing to stay between 7.2 and 8.4 right after a meal, and at just
    about 7.2 a couple of hours after a meal.

You can run a simple pH test any time of the day after eating a few almonds. In a healthy person with adequate alkaline reserves, saliva pH will
go up almost immediately to 8.4.

Monitoring your pH puts the responsibility of caring for your health
back into your hands. It also lets you track your own results as you make
positive changes in your lifestyle and diet, giving you immediate feedback
that how you eat, drink, and live affects your body and your health—and
ultimately, the quality and quantity of your life.

LIVE BLOOD ANALYSIS

If your urine or saliva (or blood) are acidic, it's a safe bet that you have tissue acidosis and possible microform overgrowth. The simple fact is, most
people do.

Live blood analysis more directly detects overacidity and overgrowth. In
a standard lab evaluation performed by hospitals and clinics, drops of blood
are basically dried onto a slide to be examined under a familiar bright-field
microscope, where acidic patterns in the blood and many of these negative
microforms cannot be seen. Live blood analysis, by contrast, examines unal-
tered live blood, under special dark-field, phase-contrast compound micro-
scopes. The high-powered compound microscope can magnify objects up
to twenty-eight thousand times, so you can clearly view acid crystals, bacteria, yeast, and mold in exact detail in the blood. You can also see red and
white blood cells, crystallized microforms, mycotoxins, cholesterol, metals,

blood clots, undigested fats, and many other things—all in one drop of live blood! Bottom line: Though it can also provide a lot more information, live blood analysis gives you a plain view of how crowded your blood is with acid crystals and undesirable microforms.

When I look at live blood, I also look at the space between the cells, where the extracellular fluid, or plasma, is. I call this the negative space, or context. The blood cells, and the blood overall, are only as healthy as this plasma in which they are bathed.

The blood never lies. What you see when you look at it this way is a direct reflection of your health, and what you are eating, drinking, and thinking. In short, it shows how you are living. I have viewed the blood of thousands of people around the world—more than forty thousand blood samples in over seventy-two countries—and through my work I can tell you: There are only two types of blood: healthy and unhealthy! Whenever I analyze someone's blood, I always ask them the same questions. What are you eating? What are you drinking? What are you feeling? The people whose blood looks the best—the people who live the longest—are eating green foods, breathing clean air, drinking clean water, finding ways to manage stress, working outside, exercising daily, and getting lots of sunshine. And I can see the effects of all that in the blood, no question.

Live blood analysis requires some fairly expensive technical equipment, along with well-trained and experienced practitioners to interpret what is seen. We believe every hospital, clinic, doctor's office, medical lab, and nutritional center should have a properly trained live blood microscopist on staff. But that day is not yet here, so, although the test is quickly growing in popularity as its importance is better understood, it may not be easy to find a practitioner in your area. You can contact the pH Miracle Living Center via phone or Web site for a referral (see resources).

DRIED BLOOD ANALYSIS

After years of researching German techniques in dried blood analysis, I've developed a test called the Mycotoxic/Oxidative Stress Test (M/OST), which involves a small amount of blood allowed to dry and clot on a microscope slide. (Contact the pH Miracle Living Center for a referral; see resources.) Under the microscope, blood from healthy people forms a standard pattern—a dense mat of red areas interconnected by dark, irregular lines, called fibrin. The blood of people under mycotoxic/oxidative stress—meaning excess acidity and microform overload and the resulting harmful wastes—has a variety of characteristic patterns that deviate from that norm.

One common (and visually striking) abnormality is the presence of "clear" or white areas interrupting the standard pattern. The extent and shape of the clear areas reflect the symptoms that are likely to arise as a result of excess acidity, overgrowth, and cellular degeneration. That is, the pattern of the blood reveals not only the presence of microform overgrowth, excess acidity, and cellular degeneration but also the particular ways that overgrowth is affecting the individual. Certain patterns match certain symptoms, such as diabetes, arthritis, atherosclerosis, and even cancerous conditions.

In the end, however, getting all the details about your exact situation isn't absolutely necessary (though witnessing a live blood analysis may be motivating like nothing else!). Anyone on the standard American diet is, to a greater or lesser degree, imbalanced—acidic. If you have any symptoms, you can be sure you are imbalanced and overacid. On the other hand, if you follow the program outlined in this book, doing what you know is right for your body, you can rely on your body to handle the complex details of self-repair. Your results—how you look and feel—will speak for themselves. Freed from acid overload, you'll be symptom-free, full of energy, and mentally wide awake. You'll also reach your body's own best, healthy weight.

GET TESTED EVERY YEAR

You should have a live blood analysis done every year, and a dried blood analysis as well, assuming you are starting in a state of general good health. Annual testing will keep you conscious of what it takes to maintain a healthy and fit body, give you feedback on your success, and warn you of any looming problems.

If you are dealing with a symptom or condition, then live and dried blood cell microscopy should be done every seventy-two hours while you are symptomatic. As the symptoms improve, move to testing every twelve weeks. Once your condition has resolved, you can go back to getting tested once a year.

Testing the pH of your urine and saliva daily (as above) provides reassurance between blood tests.

WHAT CAUSES ACID IMBALANCE AND OVERGROWTH?

Overacidity and microform overgrowth are inextricably linked. Microforms are a major source of acid in the body. Acidification creates a comfy environment for microforms. We predispose ourselves to both conditions through various stresses. The main one is poor diet, although chronic toxicity from external sources and other physiological stresses (including poor digestion, more about which follows in chapter 4) play roles as well. Emotional upheaval, negative thinking patterns and other psychological stress, and lack of exercise, stretching, and deep breathing also contribute.

This is what I call the cycle of imbalance. And a vicious cycle it is, going round and round and round once it gets under way—unless you step in and take action.

First comes something that disturbs your body in some way, be it poor diet, polluted environment, negative thoughts, spiritual distress, under- or overexercising, or destructive emotions. Whatever it may be, that initial physical or emotional disturbance starts acidifying your body and disturbs your very cells. Cells work to adapt to the declining pH of their compromised acidic environment. They break down and evolve to bacteria, yeast, and mold. These in turn create their waste products—debilitating acids—which further pollute the environment. That in itself is a disturbance to the system, and in this way the whole cycle keeps rolling along.

THIS PROGRAM CHANGES ALL THAT

No matter how you got there, or how deep you're in it, a healthy, alkaline, electron-rich, plant-based diet and low-stress lifestyle with appropriate daily exercise will keep you in acid–base balance and housing only healthy happy blood and body cells. Eating the right kind of food is the single most important thing you can do for yourself and your health.

The pH Miracle diet and lifestyle program restores health, harmony, and balance to your body through a diet based on alkalizing vegetables, sprouted and soaked nuts and seeds, essential oils, unprocessed salts, low-sugar fruits, and alkaline water. You'll experience a new level of wellness, energy, and mental clarity. Normalizing blood-and-tissue pH will reduce the amount of symptom-causing acids and microforms in your body—and thus reduce symptoms. The closer your pH is to 7.365, the higher your level of health and well-being, and the stronger your resistance to disease. With this program, you can also have the lean, trim body you've always wanted. As you get back to basic, the body naturally begins to seek its own ideal weight.

The thousands of blood samples I've studied from all over the world reveal the amazing cellular changes that occur with diet changes. As a person eats more alkalizing foods, especially raw vegetables and greens, I see extreme improvement in red blood cell integrity, oxygenation of the blood, levels of acidity, and negative microforms. The same methods we covered for measuring acid imbalance and overgrowth will confirm for you that you are on the right path once you start eating according to this plan. Of course, you won't need the tests to tell you—the disappearance of your symptoms and your restored or renewed vitality will tell you all you really need to know.

Chapter 3

•

Confusing Symptoms and Disease

Unfortunately, Pasteur's confusion of disease with symptoms has come down through the generations as scientific law. To this day, conventional medicine operates under this central misconception, often identifying a pattern of symptoms and labeling them as a disease, without any consideration of the underlying cause of the symptoms. And if the underlying cause isn't considered, it can't be addressed. Symptoms may be masked with drugs, but that won't eradicate them. And it doesn't deal with the accompanying deterioration of the rest of the body, or, of course, do anything about the acids underlying it all.

The truth is, symptoms are just indications that you are overly acidic. Symptoms are caused by acidic food and lifestyle choices. The so-called disease is a general, underlying condition of acidity. If germs are involved, they are themselves just symptoms of that underlying acidic condition. Remember that germs come from within our cells, and that germs invading from outside the body can only contribute to a state of imbalance and stimulate secondary symptoms. What most people call disease is really just a collection of these secondary symptoms. Germs are really just the expression of the underlying so-called disease condition (overacidity and then evolutionary microform overgrowth). In the same way that a fired bullet does the damage, not the smoke from a fired gun, it is the acid that kills, not the associated germs.

Over the last century or so, mainstream science has told the public that it has identified the precise cause or causes of some so-called disease. An example would be the relationship of smoking and lung cancer or obesity and heart problems. And yet, for many other serious so-called diseases, scientists admit they are still baffled and need to do more research—and need more of our money for that research. It is important that if you want to be responsible for your own body and the future of your own health, you must start from the premise that acid is the immediate cause of all the symptoms that are bothering you.

You may know the joke about the inebriated fellow looking for his keys under the streetlamp: He dropped his keys up the block, but he was looking in this spot because that's where the light was. It's the same with medical research. They are doing almost no research where the problem is and where the solution lies . . . at the intersection of nutrition and blood. Instead, they are looking at symptoms because that's where the research money from the medical machine and the pharmaceutical companies is focused. The pharmaceutical companies support research that brings them more labels, products and profits . . . not research that's actually going to find the keys. Actually finding the keys would put them out of business!

So it is in this sense that I say, There is only one "disease." And that one disease is acidosis. Thus, the thousand-plus names for so-called diseases are simply a compendium of symptoms. These symptoms are the body's creative and intelligent ways of keeping acid focused on some less vital area of the body . . . and not the critically delicate balance of the blood. If all this acid were to get directly to the blood, you could be dead in days, or even hours.

COMMON PROBLEMS OF OVERACIDITY

Your body faces all kinds of breakdown if it is allowed to get too acidic or is forced to fight too hard for too long just to stay basic. As I said before and will no doubt say again, if you dig deep enough, these acidic-breakdown problems underlie just about anything that ails you. Sickness, dis-ease, and so-called disease of any kind is the result of acidity. This section examines some of the most common expressions of acidity.

Before we get to that, however, I want to point out that when you understand the wide variety of symptoms caused by acidity, you also realize that the treatment—even the cure—for virtually all chronic dis-ease and so-called diseases is as straightforward as making alkaline food and lifestyle choices.

WEIGHT

You can thank an overly acid internal environment for the excess pounds you are carrying around. In a defensive maneuver, the body creates fat cells to carry acids away from your vital organs to try to protect them. In one sense, your fat is saving your life! But that's why your body doesn't want to let it go. When you eat and drink to make your body more basic, your body won't need to keep that fat around anymore.

But excess weight also causes additional strain on the body, strain that can produce yet more acid. (And then more fat . . . it goes on and on.) Weight problems can also result from bacteria, yeast, mold, and fungus interfering with the alkalizing or digestion of food. The nutritional deficiencies created can actually trigger your body to pack on extra pounds, in part because you are always hungry. More commonly, blood poisoned by exotoxins and/or mycotoxins goes to the liver to be detoxified—and that added stress distracts the liver from efficiently metabolizing fat and sugar.

The chaos in an imbalanced body will exhaust the adrenal glands. The resulting low levels of energy contribute to weight gain. Another likely villain is fatigue of the thyroid gland—which controls the rate of metabolism. Cravings for acid food such as sugar, outsize appetites, and low blood sugar levels all follow dietary and metabolic acids and an overgrowth of harmful bacteria, yeast, fungus, and mold in the body, which then create even more acidic wastes. Taken together, these patterns all make it easier to gain fat and harder to lose it. To top it off, indigestion and possibly depression will develop or worsen, too. Those are only a couple of the myriad ways the chaos of imbalance can express itself, as it did for Tara (see the box). Ironically, though she had tried to control her weight for years, it was when Tara finally changed the way she ate—not to lose weight, but to address the symptoms plaguing her—that she finally did drop her excess pounds without even trying. Just as happened for Tara, when you alkalize, your fat will melt away, along with all of its acidic contents.

TARA'S STORY

I've been on weight loss diets for as long as I can remember—at least since I was eleven years old. I would starve my body into submission, but as soon as I returned to eating anything close to "normal," I would gain back all the weight I had lost—plus a few extra pounds.

Aside from my extra fat, I always considered myself healthy, strong, and energetic.

All that changed when, after a serious infection in my uterus, I had a hysterectomy for large fibroid tumors. I never felt as though I recovered from the surgery. I developed pain in my left breast. The doctors thought there was a lump, but after mammography and ultrasound decided it was just a cyst. Either way, it didn't explain (or relieve) my pain. I became fatigued to the point where, if I went to the grocery store one day, I had to spend the rest of that day, and all of the next day, in bed.

This went on for years. Doctors recommended antidepressants, but I refused them. What I was experiencing was certainly depressing, but I did not feel I was depressed. I have a wonderful husband, lots of interests, and many things I want to do with my life. We spent thousands of dollars pursuing many different avenues to restore my wellness, and eventually I was able to increase my energy from about 20 percent of normal to about 70 percent.

It was right around then that I ran across the Youngs' program. Within days, we had all the supplements we needed and began to change the way we ate. We had been off caffeine, alcohol, meat, and dairy for quite a while, so sugar was the only big challenge now. The first few days were rough. I was feeling sorry for myself and missing dessert. What I really wanted, however, was my health! It was the first time I went on a "diet" not to change my weight but for health alone.

After four weeks, we happened to be at a friend's house where I noticed a scale. We no longer owned one, as it had become an instrument of torture for me during my continuous dieting to lose weight. I stepped on and could barely believe what I saw: I had lost twenty-five pounds! I knew my clothes were getting looser, but I didn't feel as if I was really dieting because I wasn't going hungry. It turns out my husband, too, had lost twenty-five pounds. He's had to buy new pants with a four-inch-smaller waist.

Except for the extra weight, my husband thought he was pretty healthy—he went on the program to support me, and I will always be grateful for his loving help. But he got more out of it than he knew at the beginning. A blood test early on indicated a prostate imbalance, even though he had no other symptoms. Six weeks into the program, a repeat test showed that all signs of the imbalance were gone!

> We are both thrilled that our bodies are moving toward normal. Our energy levels are continually improving. Emotionally, we are more stable. Even under great stress, we don't overreact. I have no more pain in my breast, and the granulomas—little hard lumps on the skin—we both had are melting away. We are mentally more alert—and noticing how sleepy others seem. I think we spent most of our lives in a sugar fog.
>
> We have been checking our urine with pH paper. When we started, it was 6.0 or less. Now we run around 6.8 to 7.0. Best of all, our friends are overwhelmed at the changes they see in us. They all say, "You look great! What are you doing?" I tell them about our diet and supplements. But really I think about what we're doing as simply growing young together!

The yeast and fungus produced within an overly acidic body can feed on your protein and other nutrients, interfering with the absorption of everything you eat by as much as 50 percent. This can cause you to become excessively thin, which is no healthier than being overweight. As you restore a healthy balance in your body's environment on a basic (alkaline) diet, you will begin to gain weight, then stabilize at your ideal.

Healthy bodies are not overweight or underweight. A healthy body naturally maintains its own ideal weight.

ALLERGIES

The toxins produced by microforms within an overly acidic, oxygen-deprived body contribute significantly to what are commonly considered the symptoms of allergy. The exotoxins and/or mycotoxins severely stress the immune system, so it is constantly stimulated, overworked, and on edge. Imagine trying to clean your house while filth is constantly being tossed in through the windows! The irritation and inflammation caused by foods, airborne matter, or chemicals may get labeled hay fever, allergenic asthma (see Jennifer's story on page 37), environmental sensitivities, and food sensitivities or allergies. Soreness, swelling, watery eyes, runny nose, and eczema are all ways of eliminating acid toxins.

If you had no symptom-producing acid and/or bacteria, yeast, and fungus, it would be impossible for you to have allergies—another reason to keep your body in acid–base balance. Allergies are 100 percent reversible with an alkaline diet and lifestyle.

HECTOR'S STORY

When my wife undertook a radical change in her diet after a health crisis, I was not exactly on board. I still wanted my bacon and eggs for breakfast, and meat and potatoes for dinner, no matter what she was telling me about acidity and alkalinity.

All that changed after I attended a pH Miracle program myself. I agreed to go to better understand what my wife was doing, so I could better support her in her recovery, but I never really thought it would affect what *I* was doing. So I went, still basically a meat-and-potatoes guy, to see my own live blood for the first time. What a mess! My blood was full of yeast and bacteria from my acid diet. That's when I knew something had to give. I immediately switched over to an alkaline green diet and stuck with it during the entire weeklong workshop. That went well, so when I returned home, I just kind of kept it going.

Before long, I had dropped thirty unnecessary pounds. And two conditions that have plagued me for my entire life—allergies and acid reflux—have been totally eliminated.

In hindsight I can see how my initial refusal to make a change placed an additional burden on my wife while she was already under plenty of stress with her own serious health concerns, and I regret that. But I am so grateful for what we have now: a shared alkaline lifestyle, and mutual good health!

FOOD ALLERGIES AND INTOLERANCES

Food allergies or intolerances make millions of Americans miserable. They can even kill. As we commonly think about them, food allergies cause obvious symptoms as reactions to certain acidic foods, ranging from stomach pains to rashes to itching to swelling. There are many people who have these (or subtler) reactions and attribute their symptoms to other ailments. Either way, we're a little off base: All these symptoms are caused by acids from acidic foods and drinks. In fact, we *all* have food intolerances: Our bodies can't tolerate acidic foods.

True food allergies are usually immediate and occur within hours of ingesting the offending food or drink (which is always acidic!). Reactions appear suddenly, almost explosively. Some reactions can cause rapid collapse and even death, such as those to peanuts and shellfish. (Two of my top ten foods that should never be ingested by anyone, even setting aside allergies—see below.) Acidic reactions to food and drink can be delayed days, weeks, even months after exposure, because it can take time for acid residues to build up in the body to the point where it is overburdened and finally reacts. (The reactions are just the body trying to eliminate the acids any way it can.)

TOP TEN FOODS THAT CAUSE ALLERGIC AND ACIDIC REACTIONS

1. Dairy products.
2. Meat and shellfish.
3. All forms of sugar.
4. Vinegar.
5. Mushrooms and algae.
6. Peanuts and peanut oil.
7. Corn.
8. Fermented foods such as soy sauce and miso.
9. Eggs.
10. Alcohol.

Testing urine and saliva for pH can help determine if you are having allergic reactions causing common acidic complaints. So can live and dried blood microscopy (see chapter 2).

FATIGUE

Fatigue is probably the major symptom or complaint of an overly acidic body and/or a body overgrown with negative microforms (see the box on page 37, "Jennifer's Story"). It is the first stage of acidity. Microforms ferment the electron stores in our bodies that we would otherwise use for energy. Then, to add insult to injury, they spew out acid waste as a result. It's as if you were trying to fill your car's gas tank as someone else was siphoning off the gasoline. Without the energy it needs to keep going, your car won't get very far or perform very well. The toxins produced in an acidic body reduce the energy or electrons from carbohydrates, fats, protein, minerals, and other nutrients, which in turn weakens the body's ability to produce enzymes and hormones and the hundreds of other chemical components necessary for cell energy and organ activity. This also interferes with the reconstruction of cells and other necessary components of energy production. The result is fatigue, poor endurance, an inability to add muscle tone, and general weakness (as well as unwanted body weight changes and illness). The pancreas, liver, and adrenal glands, which play major roles in controlling energy levels, are all susceptible to the negative effects of exotoxins and/or mycotoxins.

Microforms—bacteria, yeast, fungus, and mold—also rapidly deplete your supplies of the B-complex vitamins, iron, and other minerals. That alone could cause fatigue. Another result of microforms draining off your body's nutrients is that you have rapid drops in blood sugar levels, which again create fatigue, poor endurance, and weakness. Dietary and metabolic acid and the increase of bacteria, yeast, and fungus unbalance the process that controls the water and mineral content of cells (electrolyte balance), which is necessary for cell activity, thus impeding the normal flow of energy.

Fatigue vicious circle number one: Low energy levels or electron levels encourage biological transformation of body cells and the overgrowth of harmful microforms.

With all this, you won't be surprised to learn that overacidity and microforms are the major players in chronic fatigue syndrome, which may involve bacterial, yeast, and fungus damage to nerve tissue and interference with nerve transmission thanks to the breakdown of neurotransmitters. In addition, acidic exotoxins and/or mycotoxins can strip away the myelin sheath that coats and protects nerves and enables transmission of impulses.

To give you just one example of the mechanisms behind the fatigue phenomenon, let's look at one mycotoxin, acetaldehyde, which is a by-product of the acid known as sugar (and by the end of this paragraph you'll have yet another good reason to stay away from sugar). Acetaldehyde can reduce strength and stamina, cause excessive fatigue, cloud thinking, and block ambition. One way that happens is that it reduces the absorption of protein and alkaline minerals, decreasing the normal healthy function of the organ systems, including the endocrine system that controls reproduction. Another way is that it destroys essential metabolic co-factors, reducing cell energy. Third, acetaldehyde directly destroys neurotransmitters, which are chemicals responsible for completing all nerve impulses. A fourth is that it binds to the walls of red blood cells, like molecular glue, making them less flexible and therefore less able to get into and through the capillaries of the circulatory system. That leads to starvation and oxygen deprivation in the tissues. Furthermore, the liver converts acetaldehyde into alcohol. That process depletes the body of magnesium, sulfur, hydrogen, and potassium, thus reducing cell energy. And of course the alcohol itself has negative effects. It can actually produce the same symptoms as being drunk, making you disoriented, dizzy, or mentally confused. Vicious circle number two: The less oxygen there is in the body, the more alcohol is produced.

JENNIFER'S STORY

Even when I first began playing volleyball on my high school team, asthma was a constant annoyance. The suffocating feeling of asthma always scared me, but I didn't let my breathing problems get in the way of the game I immediately loved so much.

But a year later, while I was playing for a nonschool team in the spring, my energy really began to flag. I thought my inhaler might be bothering me, so I went in for a checkup with my doctor. He gave me an extra inhaler to take in the morning along with the one I had been using before games.

So I wouldn't be dependent on inhalers, my family helped me change my diet to eliminate all sugar and dairy products. This helped a little with the asthma. But still, if I didn't use the inhaler before I exercised, I'd get an attack. I seemed to be tired all the time.

By the next spring, I was sleeping fourteen to fifteen hours a day. I could only handle one class at a time at school. I felt as though I was losing my bond with my friends, because on weekends I was too tired and depressed to get together with them. I had to use part of my summer to make up the classes I couldn't attend during the year.

It was another year before I found out about the pH Miracle, and how yeast in my system would cause extreme fatigue, sleepiness, and depression. I did a three-day fresh green vegetable juice fast, began taking supplements, and started eating whole green vegetables. Later I added turkey, grains, sprouts, and yellow vegetables.

I regained my strength and had more energy than before. I felt as though I could make something of life again. I lost five pounds the first week. I was able to complete a full volleyball session and join a volleyball club. I'm back to a full day of classes at school. I work out at the gym, work part-time, and have energy and vitality to be with many friends again. Best of all, my asthma is gone!

If it weren't for this program, I think the only way I could participate in volleyball would be to read about it on the sports page. Now when I read about my school's team in the newspaper, I often see my name as the high scorer!

MOOD DISORDERS AND NEUROLOGICAL IMBALANCE

As with Jennifer's experience, depression and other mood disorders are another result of acidic bodies. With body cell transformation followed by microform overgrowth, they have then reached epidemic proportions.

The usual pathway is exotoxin and/or mycotoxin interference with the production of coenzyme A, a pathway for the release of usable energy. Coenzymes combine with other compounds to make enzymes, which are necessary in almost every bodily process, including those of the brain and nervous system. When coenzyme A decreases, such conditions as depression, anxiety, panic attacks, irritability, mood swings, and PMS often appear or become worse. Other symptoms come simply from being poisoned: paranoia, not being in total control of one's actions, knowing the right thing to do but being unable to do it, mental incompetence, and a variety of other behavioral, emotional, and psychological disturbances. Another variation is hypochondriac-type reactions of neurotic behavior and emotional instability. People may be very aware of their behavior, and be miserable for it, yet still be unable to control themselves because the toxins stay in their bodies.

Excess dietary and metabolic acids lead to body cell transformation and microform overgrowth, causing an increase in acid. This leads to other neurological fallout, too, including headaches, migraines, inability to concentrate, memory problems, confusion, dizziness, that "fogged-in" feeling, and even MS-like symptoms such as slurred speech and lack of muscular coordination.

DIABETES

Low blood sugar (hypoglycemia) and high blood sugar (diabetes)—which are really just low energy and high acidity—are rampant today, and devastate a lot of lives. They both stem from—surprise!—dietary and metabolic acids and microform overgrowth.

Most people do not realize that sugar is *not* a source of energy but an acidic waste product from the breakdown of body cells. The more sugar or acid we eat, the more we risk an increase in bacteria, yeast, and molds. Their mycotoxins and exotoxins penetrate, overwork, and poison the pancreas, liver, and adrenal glands (among others).

For example, pancreatic cells are directly poisoned and destroyed by the mycotoxin alloxan. The pancreas produces not only alkalizing buffers—sodium bicarbonate—for alkalizing the food we eat, but also insulin, the alkalizing hormone that controls the blood acid sugar. A deficiency in alkaline compounds such as sodium and potassium bicarbonate and insulin leads to hyperglycemia or the high-acidity disease called diabetes.

Bacteria and yeast also feed on our electron energy resources and can cause energy deficiencies. Blood glucose is blood acid and is increased with an acidic lifestyle and diet, which can give rise to bacteria and yeast and more metabolic acids.

People with diabetes have low or normal blood sugar levels when their pH (as measured in urine) is up (alkaline, over 7.2)—and high blood sugar levels when their pH is down (acidic, below 7.2).

Type 2 diabetes is the natural physiological and metabolic result of consuming large quantities of sugars and refined carbohydrates and meat protein, especially without engaging in regular physical exercise (which could help compensate for such dietary practices).

Research has shown that in cases of diabetes, even one dose of sugar can create changes in the body, even at the genetic level, that increase the risk of complications of diabetes. Even short-term exposure to the sugar (acid) had long-term effects on the cells of the body. In a study on diabetic mice, cells showed the effects of a single dose of sugar up to two weeks later. Anatomical effects of sugar go beyond the response to one snack or meal itself, affecting the body's natural metabolic ability.

What that means, among other things, is that the solution is quite straightforward: Cut out all forms of sugar, eliminate animal proteins, and get regular exercise.

HIGH CHOLESTEROL

If your body is overacid—meaning there are too many acids for it to dispose of through urination, perspiration, defecation, and respiration—the body goes into preservation mode and releases cholesterol from the liver to buffer those acids in an attempt to protect itself from their toxic effects. Although we have been conditioned to think of it as harmful, the cholesterol is there to *help* us. It isn't cholesterol that causes heart attacks or strokes—dietary, environmental, and metabolic acids do. We have been trained to avoid high cholesterol at all costs, but lowering cholesterol with drugs, without also lowering our exposure to acids, is a recipe for disaster.

Your cholesterol level, and your risk for heart attack or stroke, rises as your acid level increases. Reduce your acid level by reducing acid foods in your diet, and exercising daily, and you'll reduce the cholesterol—your body won't need to protect itself against the acids by producing it—along with your risks. The pH Miracle diet and lifestyle program will naturally lower your cholesterol.

SALLY'S STORY

I am a nurse, but my medical training could not prepare me for the devastating diagnosis my youngest son, Gabriel, received after a routine doctor visit uncovered Type 1 diabetes. I was shocked. We had no family history of diabetes, and overall our family had been very healthy. Extensive testing showed that our beautiful, previously healthy six-year-old would probably be insulin-dependent within six months. The pediatric endocrinologist insisted there was nothing we could do to prevent this, and that no dietary changes were necessary or would help.

I did my own research, however, and discovered that Gabriel's diet, which I had thought was reasonably healthy, was actually far too acidic, with way too many carbohydrates. I changed him over to a totally alkaline way of eating, focusing on green veggies, healthy oils, good water, and mineral salts (Dr. Young's COWS plan). Gabriel's blood sugar levels almost immediately returned to normal ranges, and his weakened body returned to its previous vigor.

Our joy at this reversal was tempered four months later, when further blood tests revealed Gabriel had no measurable insulin left in his blood. Thankfully, he was still maintaining normal blood sugar levels (even this seemed impossible to our doctors), but we grieved at what appeared to be the loss of insulin production.

At just about this same time, our older son Nathan, who was ten at the time, was also diagnosed with Type 1 diabetes. At least this time, we knew what to do: He joined his brother in eating alkaline.

Two months later, the boys' doctor announced amazing lab results for both boys. Gabriel had once again begun to produce some insulin. And Nathan went from insufficient insulin to overproduction, compensating for the insulin antibodies present. Both were maintaining normal blood sugar levels. We felt overwhelmed with gratitude, and even more sure of our commitment to alkaline principles.

Two months later, we received still more great news. Our doctor sat us down to say Nathan no longer fit the diagnosis of Type 1 diabetes. In their labeling system, he was now considered Type 2. Gabriel, incredibly, no longer carried any diagnosis at all! All his insulin levels were considered completely normal.

A year since we first heard our son's name and *diabetes* in the same terrifying sentence, both boys continue to eat alkaline, though we are introducing some more carbohydrates, which they are tolerating well. It has taken some creativity to make this way of eating work in all ways for them (including radishes inside those little plastic Easter eggs—upon request), but we have adopted "an attitude of gratitude" as our motto, and both boys often hug me and thank me for their special foods and their renewed health. When people ask me how we can possibly live with this special diet, I answer the only way I can: With what we know now, how could we not?

OSTEOPOROSIS

Even conventional doctors recognize the fact that the body leaches calcium and sodium out of bones to handle the digestion of meat. Or, as I look at it, the body steals alkaline minerals that are *supposed* to be at work strengthening bone and uses them to protect itself from infusions of acidic animal protein by alkalizing it. The body strips away bone mass in a desperate attempt to neutralize excess acids in the blood and tissues. Osteoporosis is the direct result. Loss of bone density is an inevitable consequence of an acidic diet and lifestyle, especially the intake of animal protein.

Conversely, you can protect your bones (and muscles, and other organs) with an alkaline lifestyle and diet. Keeping the body alkaline (through diet and the right kind of exercise) is the best way to slow down aging in general, and avoid all disease processes, including bone loss and osteoporosis.

Conventional doctors paint bone loss as simply what happens with aging, and they'll explain it as changing hormones and so on. But the truth is that as adults on the standard American diet age, they are less able to excrete acid, so they experience more effects of the acid than they may have when they were younger, and *that's* why bone loss increases.

A study done by researchers at Tufts and Northwestern demonstrated the importance of alkalinity to bone health. Following groups of men and women for three months, they observed that the groups taking sodium or potassium bicarbonate along with calcium and vitamin D had lower levels of the marker for bone breakdown (resorption) and excreted less calcium when compared with those taking only calcium and vitamin D. The researchers noted in their write-up for publication that a high-acid diet accelerates calcium excretion (and therefore bone loss), adding that an alkaline diet can prevent bone loss because when vegetables are metabolized, they add bicarbonate to the body. They added that supplementing with bicarbonate was a good addition or alternative. (See chapter 12 for more on the benefits of sodium bicarbonate.)

If you follow the alkaline-by-design blueprint of your body, you won't have the body cannibalizing its bones and cartilage in order to buffer too many acids, and your bones will stay strong for life.

DARCY'S STORY

Everything was going well with my health until I hit my forties. First, I began gaining weight, slight but steady and totally unwanted. My doctor's response? Just: "Welcome to your forties." Then I, a person who had never been allergic to anything, became severely asthmatic, allergic to everything! My doctor informed me that as we age, we grow into allergies. I went into early menopause, and my thyroid began to fail. My doctor informed me that this was no problem, as we had medicines for these things. Then I had severe bone loss. Actually, the bones of a seventy-eight-year-old, though I was only forty-three! Once again, my doctor said no problem, handing me a prescription to stop bone loss. Then I started having skin outbreaks that turned out to be from an autoimmune deficiency. The doctor had a solution for that, too: monthly steroid shots to "mask" the outbreak. By this point, I was also very weak, having lost a lot of muscle mass, and chronically fatigued. But wait, there's more! Four years ago, a blood test showed my liver function was declining, and the results got worse each of the next two years. Then all the medications I was taking stopped controlling my asthma well, and a CT scan showed I had fungus in my lungs. Weeks later, I was diagnosed with cancer, an ocular melanoma.

For me, this was the breaking point. Within hours of returning home from my first oncology appointment I was reading about the pH Miracle program and preparing to begin it. For the first time in ten years of declining health, I understood the cause of every one of my health problems—the acid environment I was living in—and could see a true solution. I did a comprehensive urine and saliva pH test over two days, and discovered my body was at 5.0 pH. I had nowhere to go but up!

When I began an all-green raw diet with alkaline water, the changes were immediate. After just three days, the asthma was gone. Within two weeks, I had the energy level of my youth. After one month, I had lost forty pounds. The fifth week, a second CT scan showed no more fungus in my lungs. At my first checkup after my cancer surgery, my doctor said he had never seen cells regenerate the way mine had! Eight months after starting the pH Miracle program, I had a repeat blood test, which showed my liver function was back to normal after three years going downhill. As I continued to alkalize, I could see the direct correlation between the reversal of my health issues and increase in my urine pH, as it went from 5.0 to 5.9 to 6.4 to 7.0 to a steady 7.25–7.5. *The pH Miracle* saved my life!

KIDNEY CONDITIONS

The kidneys are responsible for eliminating acids out of the blood and recycling alkalinity back in. If acids are not eliminated from the blood, they move into the tissues. An acidic lifestyle and diet stresses the kidneys, sometimes to the point where they stop functioning well. Conventional doctors diagnose what they call kidney disease. Dialysis may be used to purify the blood, but the more obvious—and effective—solution is to alkalize the blood and tissues by leaving behind acidic choices and choosing more healthfully. You not only will have better electron fuel for the many internal and external operations of your body, but your kidney function will continue at normal healthy levels instead of deteriorating from too much acid.

INFANTS AND CHILDREN ARE PARTICULARLY SUSCEPTIBLE

Most childhood infections (or acidic outfections) and symptoms are caused by overacidity and body cell transformation leading to negative microform overgrowth, including diaper rash, thrush, ear infections, tonsillitis, colic, constipation, and diarrhea. Even the poorly understood sudden infant death syndrome (SIDS) is linked to dietary and metabolic acidity. As children become older, conditions such as attention deficit disorder (ADD), hyperactivity, aggressiveness, irrational behavior, poor self-esteem, learning disabilities, and short attention spans can develop when a child is overacid from an acidic lifestyle and diet.

A mother's acidity or overgrowth of negative microforms will certainly affect her newborn, and mother and child often have similar problems.

CANCEROUS CELLS

Cancer cells are once-healthy cells that have become cancerous. And they are a symptom of acidity. That is, when healthy cells are corrupted by dietary and metabolic acids, they can become cancerous. The more acid we have in our bodies, the greater the risk of developing cancerous tissue.

Healthy cells in the human body thrive in mild-, moderate-, and high-pH fluids (7.3 to 11 pH). They do not tolerate even a mild acid state. Cancerous cells, on the other hand, thrive in an acidic pH of 5.5. Cancerous cells become dormant at a pH slightly above 7.365, and transform back to the microzyma or die at a pH of 8.5 (while healthy cells live).

Prevention is the best cure, though the best ways to prevent cancerous conditions will also help reverse the symptom if you already have a cancerous condition. Better you should never get that far! Treatments such as surgery and chemotherapy do nothing to support the immune system or prevent buildup of acids in tissues. That's why cancerous conditions so often come back—nothing's been done to change the conditions that started them—acid!

But if you *do* change the conditions, you can prevent cancerous cells from ever cropping up in the first place. You need to eat, drink, and even move and think in ways that reestablish the body's alkaline design. Much research has shown that what we eat affects our susceptibility to cancer.

Some foods defend against cancerous cells, and some foods promote their development. Anticancer credit is often given to the antioxidants in beneficial foods, including vitamins C and E, beta-carotene, selenium, and the amino acid glutathione. And these do indeed protect healthy tissue from acidic damage that can cause a cancerous condition. But a larger point is often missed in that sort of discussion: The foods that support a healthy body are alkaline foods; the foods that are harmful are acidic. The diet for preventing all cancerous conditions is 100 percent alkaline. There is no room for any acidic foods when preventing and/or reversing a cancerous condition.

You can fight the development of a cancerous condition by increasing the alkalinity of your tissues, building in a diet based around green vegetables, fresh vegetable juice, unprocessed salts, good oils, and alkaline water together with nutritional supplements, exercise, and alkaline lifestyle choices (along the lines described in chapters 12, 13, and 14). You have to cut out acidic foods such as animal protein, alcohol, and sugar, and give up acidic habits as well. If a cancerous condition is your primary health concern, you'll particularly benefit from using alkaline mineral supplements (sodium, calcium, potassium, magnesium, cesium rubidium) and, even better, mineral salts like sodium, magnesium, potassium, and calcium bicarbonate, which are instantly alkalizing (see page 188).

KIM TINKHAM'S STORY

I was diagnosed with stage-three breast cancer just two days before my fiftieth birthday. I was stunned. I was not what I thought a cancer victim was. I mean, people who come down with cancer smoked cigarettes, drank hard liquor, ate lots of meat . . . none of which I did. I will admit there was a time much earlier in my life when I smoked and drank, and I once tried an all-protein diet for about two weeks, until my heart felt like it was going to explode out of my chest, but I had long since cleaned up my act. I was living what I thought was a fairly healthy life.

Sure, my hair was starting to thin a bit, but I *was* nearing fifty, after all. My skin was becoming drier, but that's what moisturizers are for! I didn't sleep much at night, but I was proud of my workaholic tendencies. My hot flashes were getting hotter and more frequent night and day, but that was normal, right?

A year prior to my diagnosis, I had felt a lump in my breast during my morning shower. But I'd read somewhere that too much caffeine can cause lumps, so I gave up coffee for two weeks and the lump went away. It came back a couple more times during the year, but always disappeared after I changed something I was drinking or eating.

Then, right around Thanksgiving, the lump came back and I didn't change anything about what I was doing during the holidays. I told myself that I would get on it after Christmas. The holidays came and went, but the lump stayed. In mid-January, I finally decided I needed to find out what was up and I went to the doctor. She examined me and scheduled a mammogram the following week. I was convinced the mammogram would show it was just a cyst, nothing to worry about.

Two weeks later, I was sitting down with a different doctor, who was telling me that all the tests they had run confirmed that I, in fact, had cancer. And it was already stage three. He recommended a mastectomy, followed by chemotherapy and radiation. He told me I had to begin immediately. He handed me the cards of a couple of surgeons, an oncologist and a cosmetic reconstructive surgeon. He told me to contact all of these people and keep in touch with him. I remember nodding my head okay, walking out of his office, and starting my drive home.

Somewhere inside me I knew that I had brought this cancer on myself. But I didn't want to make a decision based on fear. I had always believed that the human body was designed to heal itself if given the right tools, and I hadn't given mine the right tools. I realized now that I didn't even know for sure what the right tools were, but I didn't think they were the kind that would slice my breasts off my body and pour poisons into it. But I was determined to seek out another way to heal my body.

Needless to say, I faced plenty of resistance to my idea of finding another path. But I also discovered many people who supported my journey, as I went in search of answers from doctors and practitioners around the world. My path landed me on *The Oprah Winfrey Show* in March 2007, where I also encountered objections to ignoring the conventional treatments, but my appearance there also helped me reach doctors and researchers all over the world I may not have been able to access on my own.

I worked with massage therapists, reflexologists, nutritionists, and energy healers. I ordered crystals to take away negative energy and balance my chakras. I learned to reinvent myself. I got thermoscans that measured the heat in my body, having learned that cancer emits heat. (I was seeing a slight decrease in heat, but I still wasn't where I wanted to be.)

All the practitioners and researchers I talked with shared their findings with me and wished me luck. Occasionally I would talk to a doctor who expressed concern about my decision and my delay in getting Western medical treatment. I would always ask them one question, "What caused my cancer?" Not one could tell me. My logic told me that if they didn't know what caused it, they couldn't know the best way to treat it or how to make sure that it would never come back.

I had set myself a deadline of five months to learn all I could about how to rid my body of this cancer. Just as time was running out, I discovered Dr. Young's work. And here, at last, I found the answer I was looking for. What causes cancer? An acid lifestyle, diet, metabolism, and the environment.

I learned all I could about the pH Miracle program, and soon committed wholeheartedly to it. I was determined to rid my body of cancer/acids in the only way that made sense: cut out the acids, and maintain the alkaline design of the body. I cut out alcohol, coffee, tea, animal protein, and sugars of all kinds. I centered every meal around fresh green veggies, and liberally used sea salt and healthy oils from flax and hemp seed. I drank only alkaline water with alkalizing pH drops or baking soda, or green drink. I supplemented with magnesium oxide. I exercised every day, in ways that moved toxins out of my body and balanced my body and spirit. I got the sleep my body needed. I learned better ways to handle stress and express emotions.

Within four months (nine months after my initial diagnosis), I was cancer-free. Mainstream lab blood tests for cancer markers all came back clear, and live and dried blood cell analysis also showed no cancer.

I am healthy, happy, and have never felt better in my life.

I am still on this journey to continue my healing. I have permanently changed my understanding of food and nutrition and my lifestyle. In order to heal yourself from any disease, you must think differently and try to understand the true nature of your body and your responsibility to it. I believe that I am witness to the remarkable healing power of the human body and the ability of the body to heal itself if given the right tools. Dr. Young and his pH Miracle program were the tools I needed to bring my body back into its natural healthy state.

OTHER NAGGING SYMPTOMS

I hope by now I've made it clear that acidification and overgrowth of negative microforms in the body are root causes of every symptom, illness, and
so-called disease (all of which are really only symptoms themselves). Here I
just want to mention some of the common symptoms that are a direct result
of overacidification and bacteria and yeast overgrowth. That includes vaginal infections, menstrual difficulties, impotence, infertility, prostatitis, rec-
tal itch, urinary tract infections, and urgency and burning with urination.
Respiratory manifestations abound: In addition to allergies (see page 33),
congestion, excess mucus, postnasal drip, frequent clearing of the throat,
habitual coughing, sore throats, earaches, and even asthma and bronchitis
are often the result of overacid and yeast. So is the tendency to catch everything that's "going around"—coming down with every cold and flu, which
is the body removing excess dietary and metabolic acids. The skin also has
a variety of ways of manifesting excess acidity and microform overgrowth:
athlete's foot, jock itch, skin rash, hives, moles, birthmarks, dry browning
patches, ringworm, rough skin on the sides of the arms, fungal nails (nails
are modified skin), acne, and even skin tumors.

CARINA'S STORY

I was diagnosed with systemic lupus erythematosus when I was
only fifteen years old. The doctors put me on over twenty-five different prescription drugs (steroids, immune blockers, anti-malarial
drugs . . .), which were supposed to help with my symptoms, which
included arthritis, high blood pressure, face rash, and spleen/platelet
and kidney problems.

But I just got sicker and sicker. Sometimes the drugs gave me worse
side effects than the actual problem, which led me to take more drugs.
Ever-increasing weight gain was just one of those side effects. The
others included delusions, drug-induced hepatitis, depression, and
sleeping pill dependency. In my life, I've taken prescription medications for longer than I've done without them. I took prednisone for
almost fifteen years.

Until last summer, when I came across the pH Miracle program.
I started it right away. In the first week, I lost twenty pounds! And I
had more energy than I had in years. I hit plateaus where I didn't lose

weight, but I kept going back to eating alkaline foods because when I did I had less pain and felt much better. And my face rash disappeared. It's been seven months now, and I have lost eighty pounds. My goal is twenty more.

Even more important, however, is that I've been able to stop taking *all* prescriptions. I don't even need over-the-counter pain relief anymore—because as long as I am eating alkaline foods, I have no pain! (If I eat acidic foods, I start feeling it within an hour.) And when I went to see my rheumatologist last month—the one who told me I'd be on an anti-rheumatic drug for the rest of my life—she was astonished with my (drug-free) perfect blood work, organ tests, blood pressure, and overall health. She actually proclaimed me a walking miracle. I know it's a *pH* miracle.

Just as with all the other health conditions discussed in this chapter—and, in fact, any health issue, if you look to the root cause of it—restoring your body to alkalinity, as the program in this book is designed to help you do, will resolve your symptoms and restore you to good health.

Chapter 4

·

Digestion—and Disease

As I'll explain shortly, this chapter should really be called "Digestion and *So-Called* Disease." Good digestion is critical for good health. And a healthy digestive system is critical to good digestion. But the digestive system should really be called the alkalizing buffering system, because the key part of its work is not the breakdown of the food per se, but the alkalizing of that food. From the mouth to the stomach, to the duodenum to the intestines, the "digestive" organs are really all about trying to raise the pH of the food we eat to an alkaline state.

Still, we're all accustomed to talking of digestion and the digestive system, so we won't change those terms on you now. But we do want to impress upon you, once again, the importance of alkalinity throughout your system—and the central role the digestive tract plays in making and keeping you alkaline. Or not!

The human body requires efficient digestion and proper elimination in order to maintain well-being and optimal energy levels. The body needs access to the nutrients that carry the electron fuel, and it needs to be cleansed of acidic waste. The crucial function that allows for both is alkalization, which happens in several phases throughout the system (as we'll lay out for you in a moment). We all know the signs of a digestive system that isn't running at its peak. There is no more common physiological malfunction in humans than indigestion in all its many forms. Antacids, for taming just one of those forms of indigestion, are the number one over-the-counter remedy in the United States. (So we also already know the true cause of indigestion: acidity!)

When we tolerate or ignore indigestion, or mask symptoms with some drugstore chemical, we are missing the urgent messages our bodies are sending us. We must listen. Recurrent or chronic indigestion or nausea on its own can be deadly, gradually impeding intestinal function. These symptoms can go unnoticed until serious conditions exist, conditions such as Crohn's, irritable bowel syndrome, or even a cancerous colon. Digestive symptoms can herald or accompany just about any other health problem, anywhere in the body. The simple reason is that indigestion and all the diseases and dis-ease, ad nauseum, stem from the same root cause: over-acidity.

Digestive discomfort or difficulty is an early warning system. But only if we attend to it. The symptoms of digestive disturbance—and potential digestive disease—are a result of dietary and metabolic acids, including microform overgrowth and the resultant acid toxins. These symptoms pop up as a result of not chewing your food properly and, even more important, a lack of the alkaline buffer sodium bicarbonate in the system. We can't be properly nourished if we're not properly liquefying or digesting our food, and without proper electron nourishment, we can't be fully and permanently healthy.

A TOUR OF THE TRACT

Digestion happens in phases, and all of them must be in good working order to maintain good health.

The process begins as soon as you start chewing your food. You break the cell membranes within the food with your teeth, and once that happens, it will start to digest on its own. In addition, the tearing and grinding by your teeth releases enzymes or acids from the food. This triggers the salivary glands in the mouth to release sodium bicarbonate as saliva, to begin alkalizing the food as it is physically being broken down.

From there the chewed, partially liquefied food continues to the stomach, where the alkalizing continues. Cells in the stomach lining called cover cells secrete yet more sodium bicarbonate into ingested food to further alkalize it. The stomach manufactures sodium bicarbonate by pulling water, salt, and carbon dioxide from the blood. This can cause a drop in the pH of the blood. Conventional medical thinking is that the stomach should be acidic, with a pH of 1.5 to 3.0, but a healthy pH when food is present is at least 7.2, moving as high as 8.4 as the sodium bicarbonate is released from the stomach lining.

But for every molecule of that heavy-duty alkalizing sodium bicarbonate ($NaHCO_3$) substance produced, hydrochloric acid (HCl) is also produced, as a waste product. HCl destroys the electron potential of food. But the HCl never comes into contact—or *should* never come into contact—with the food or liquids you eat. The sodium bicarbonate rises to the surface of the stomach to meet incoming food and drink and alkalize it, but the HCl falls into the gastric pits of the stomach, away from the food. That is why you find residues of HCl in the stomach after the food has taken up all the alkaline sodium bicarbonate and moved on into the small intestines. The HCl in the stomach is evidence that the food has been partially or fully alkalized. Hydrochloric acid is not a cause of digestion, but a result.

By the time the food moves out of the stomach and enters the small intestine via the duodenum, hopefully it is both liquid and alkaline (ideally 8.2 to 8.4). And it has a new name: chyme. The pancreas squirts still *more* sodium bicarbonate into the duodenum as necessary, to raise the pH of the chyme as high as 8.2 to 8.4. Now it is ready to begin its long and winding journey through the small intestine (of which humans have up to twenty-seven to thirty feet). This is where the body absorbs all the good electron stuff it needs from the food we eat (and, if it's there, some of the bad stuff, too).

The next and final stop is the colon, or large intestine, where water and all alkaline minerals are absorbed back into the bloodstream. Sodium bicarbonate is taken up by the large intestine into the bloodsteam to be used again as an alkaline buffer. A large vein at the end of the colon takes up any leftover alkaline minerals and water. An alkaline environment (7.2 or greater) here supports appropriate travel time for the liquefied food passing through—enough time for it to be put to full use while still allowing for swift elimination.

Because after the colon, whatever is left, of course, you excrete. And that waste is acidic unless you are eating and drinking alkaline food, in which case it is alkaline and sweet smelling. There is no foul odor. (The exception is the newcomer to the alkaline diet in whom the hardened and encrusted feces of the large intestine are slowly softening and breaking down and are expelled over a period of time—often months. This matter does have a foul odor.) Bottom line, you don't want excretory waste hanging around any longer than necessary.

This is a neat and efficient system when it is working right. It is even pretty resilient. But we habitually overtax it with low-quality acidic food and drink that is pretty much devoid of alkalizing nutrients and electrical energy. Not to mention the acidic stress most of us live with. It's gotten to the point where, for the vast majority of Americans, digestion is simply not occurring as it should. But an alkaline digestive tract, from mouth to rectum, is essential for health—and for sustaining life itself.

THE SMALL INTESTINE

The twenty-seven to thirty feet of small intestine deserve a bit more attention than I gave them in that quick "Tour of the Tract." You also need to know that its inner walls are covered with little projections called villi, which serve to increase the surface area available. This means more places and more surface area for the liquefied food to contact on its way through, and thus more capacity to absorb the good stuff from that food. All told, you've got about seventy-two hundred square feet of surface area in your small intestine—about the same as a tennis court! And you need it. Your life literally depends on the transactions that happen here. I call the small intestine the root system of the body, just like the root system of a plant where nutrition begins and new cells are born.

Those villi grab the liquefied food passing through and transform it into stem cells and then red blood cells. These red blood cells circulate throughout the body and transform themselves into body cells of all different types, including heart, liver, and brain cells. I don't think you'll be surprised to learn that the pH of the small intestine must be alkaline in order for the food to be transformed into red blood cells. So the quality of the food you eat determines the quality of the red blood cells that determine the quality of your bones, muscles, organs, and so on. You are, quite literally, what you eat.

Furthermore, acid can damage and/or congest those villi. This can interfere with absorption, perhaps severely, to the point where you can be malnourished even if you take in decent levels of nutrients. But the creation of new stem cells (erythroblasts and erythrocytes) shuts down in an acidic environment, and over time, this can be disastrous.

If the intestinal wall is overgrown and coated with sticky acidic mucus (see page 57), these crucial stem cells and subsequent red blood cells cannot be properly formed. The ones that do get made are underweight, weak, and malformed, as can be seen under the microscope in live blood analysis. The body must then resort to making red blood cells from its own body tissue, stealing from bones and muscles, among other places. Why do body cells transform back into red blood cells? The number of red blood cells must stay above a certain level for the body to function—for us to live. We usually have about five million red blood cells per cubic milliliter, and the number rarely reaches less than three million. Below that, the supply of oxygen (which the red blood cells deliver) won't be enough to support the organs, and eventually they will stop working. Rather than let that happen, body cells begin to revert to red blood cells. This is an area only slowly becoming apparent to mainstream medical science.

That's why it is such a travesty to interfere the way most of us (unknowingly) do, creating acidic conditions that also allow explosive growth of bacteria, yeast, and fungus and the toxic effects that come in their wake. All microforms interfere with nutrient absorption and electron transport. They can cover large sections of the membrane lining the inside of the small intestine, preventing your body from getting the good stuff out of what you eat. This can leave you starving for alkaline minerals, chlorophyll, and oils regardless of what you actually put in your mouth. I estimate that more than half of adults in the United States are digesting, absorbing, and biologically transforming into stem cells less than half of what they eat or drink. This is directly related to the disastrous quality of food that our homes, schools, and agribusiness allow—even strongly encourage—our youth to consume. So by the time they are adults, the gut is already severely compromised, congested, and even damaged.

Overgrowth of microforms, which feed on the nutrients and electron energy we should be getting (and make their poisonous waste out of them), just make things worse. Without proper nutrition, the body can't heal or regenerate its tissues as necessary. If you cannot digest and assimilate food and transform chyme (or liquid food) into blood, you will begin breaking down body cells to make blood (body wasting) and eventually starve. That not only decimates your energy levels and makes you feel sick, but also accelerates the aging (or dying) process.

THE DANGERS OF SOME COMMON DIGESTIVE SUPPLEMENTS: ENZYMES AND PROBIOTICS (AND HCl)

You've probably run across recommendations for digestive enzymes and/or probiotics to improve the health of your digestive tract. In fact, I used to recommend them myself. But through live and dried blood cell analysis, my understanding has evolved, and now I want to emphasize the negative consequences of these supplements, and warn you to steer clear of them on your path to an alkaline lifestyle.

First, let me quickly address HCl. It hasn't been one of my recommendations, but still this is advice that often pops up on the Web, or in your health food store, or in health magazines or books. So let me just be clear: *Never* take supplements or drugs that contain HCl; it will compromise the alkaline pH of the digestive tract, leading to serious health challenges. Most pharmaceutical drugs contain HCl, and many nutritional supplements as well.

Enzymes and probiotics are a bit more complicated, because they may seemingly be beneficial in the short term. That's because they do help break down undigested matter from meat and dairy, and so can provide temporary relief from constipation. Think of it this way: Yes, they help to break down hard-to-digest animal protein and meat. But guess what. *You* are meat! It will break you down, too!

Enzymes and probiotics have many harmful effects over the long run. They are acidifying to the body, for one thing, and can damage healthy cells and tissues, including the delicate intestinal villi. They will eventually disrupt the alkaline process of creating stem cells and then red blood cells. This leads to blood disorders and then tissue disorders. When it becomes impossible to make healthy blood, it is impossible to make the healthy body cells that make up healthy body organs. This is one of the main reasons Type 1 diabetics are all underweight. They have done severe damage to their intestinal villi and can no longer create enough stem cells to make red blood cells; therefore body cells are broken down to make needed and lifesaving red blood cells. This process of transforming body cells into red blood cells increases the acids in the blood in the form of sugar or glucose. It's why a Type 1 diabetic goes to bed with normal blood sugar levels and then wakes up with high blood sugar levels. The symptoms of diabetes begin in the small intestine, not the pancreas.

Probiotics are transformations of what used to be healthy cells. There is no such thing as "friendly" or "healthy" bacteria. The presence of bacteria is evidence of an acidic environment. Ideally, the small and large intestines will be clean and free of all microforms. You don't want to be adding any in there!

The word *enzyme* means "ferment" when you trace it back to its Greek roots, broadcasting the fact that you should have nothing to do with adding more into your body. Enzymes are acids, the waste products of cellular breakdown. The enzymes in raw foods are released when you chew them—you are breaking their cellular membranes with your teeth—which is why alkalizing must start in the mouth. (Luckily, the enzymes in the food you eat actually turn on the alkalizing system, triggering the release of sodium bicarbonate.) The real benefit to you of raw foods is their electrical energy, not the enzymes.

Enzymes can help break down meat and dairy, which rarely completely break down on their own, but a far better choice is to eliminate all animal protein from the diet. In cases of extreme bowel constipation, enzymes may be used, but only for a very short period of time. You'd be a lot better off, though, using mineral salts such as magnesium carbonate or magnesium oxide to break up undigested proteins in the small intestine. You could also drink whole-leaf cold-pressed aloe vera juice to help break up undigested food in the bowel without any negative impact on healthy tissue and without damaging the delicate intestinal villi.

Best of all is to alkalize your body with electron-rich alkaline food and drink, thereby avoiding the problem altogether!

MEET YOUR COLON

The colon, or large intestine, is the sewer plant of the body. It moves out unusable waste while acting like a sponge, gathering and then squeezing alkaline water and mineral content out into the bloodstream. The large bowel should be alkaline, aiding prompt and thorough elimination of waste.

By the time your digested liquefied food hits the colon, most of the fluid material has been extracted. That's as it should be, but it does pose a potential problem: If the final phase of digestion doesn't go just right, the colon can get caked with old, toxic, acidic wastes.

The colon is very sensitive. Any injury, surgery, or other stress, including emotional upset and negative thinking, can change its alkaline state as well as its general ability to function smoothly and efficiently. Incomplete alkaline digestion here sets the stage for intestinal imbalance throughout the digestive tract, and for the colon to become a literal cesspool of acid waste.

Digestive difficulty throughout the intestines often prevents the proper breakdown of proteins. Partially digested proteins, not usable by the body, can still be absorbed into the blood. In this form, they serve no other purpose than to congest and feed the microforms, increasing the amount of waste they produce. These protein fragments also stimulate an immune system response to clean up the bloody mess.

Joy's Story

No one has time to be sick, especially when others depend on you. I'm a single parent also caring for a recently handicapped father, and I need all my strength to manage my home life. But I've been ill for more than two decades. It finally got to the point where I found it easier to stay home and basically remove myself from the human race.

One day at the library, trying to pull myself together after one of my excruciatingly painful attacks, I came upon a book with a chapter about irritable bowel syndrome—a condition I'd been diagnosed with, along with a score of other labels over the years. Its mention of aloe vera and acidophilus sent me immediately to a nearby health food store, where I started asking questions.

The clerk was quite helpful. She asked why I was seeking these products, and I told her about my IBS—and my thyroid and adrenal dysfunction, hiatal hernia, endometriosis, kidney infections, and numerous other infections. Antibiotics were a way of life for me. My doctors eventually just told me to learn to live with it, but the clerk assured me she knew of people with stories similar to mine who had reversed their conditions. She introduced me to one woman whose story was similar to mine. We clicked immediately, and she told me about how the Youngs' program had changed her life.

I knew beyond a shadow of a doubt what I had to do. I changed my diet immediately and started a regimen of antifungals as well as alkalizing minerals. Within two months I was no longer a prisoner to pain. I feel much better, on my way to 100 percent. An enormous weight has been lifted off my shoulders. My life has gone nowhere but up.

MORE ABOUT MUCUS THAN YOU EVER KNEW YOU WANTED TO KNOW

Although we tend to associate it with head colds and worse, mucus is, in fact, a normal secretion. It is a clear, slippery substance the body makes to protect the surfaces of membranes. One way it does that is by coating anything you ingest, even water. So it also engulfs any acidic toxin(s) you happen to take in, and in doing so it becomes thick, sticky, and cloudy (as we see when we suffer from colds) to "trap" the toxins and escort them out of the body.

The majority of foods Americans eat most often cause that thickened mucus. They either contain toxins or break down in a toxic way in the digestive tract—or both. The worst offenders are dairy products, followed by animal protein, white flour, processed foods, chocolate, coffee, and alcoholic beverages. (Vegetables do not cause the formation of this sticky mucus, which is just one more reason to feature them prominently in your diet.) Over time, these foods can encrust the intestines with thick mucus and the fecal material and other debris it traps. This slime is bad enough on its own before you consider that it creates an environment that also promotes the growth of negative microforms.

Emotional stress, environmental pollution, and lack of exercise all contribute to the buildup of that slime on the wall of the colon. With buildup, transit time for materials passing through the lower bowel increases. Low levels of fiber in your diet slow it still further. As the gooey mass begins to stick to the wall of the colon, a pocket is formed between the mass and the wall, which is an ideal home for microforms. Material gradually adds itself to the slime, until much of it stops moving altogether. The colon absorbs what fluids are left, the buildup begins to harden, and the home for unfriendly organisms becomes a fortress.

Heartburn, gas, bloating, ulcers, nausea, and gastritis (irritation of the walls of the intestines due to acidic gas and liquid) are all a result of a gastrointestinal tract overgrown with microforms. So, too, is constipation, which in addition to being an unpleasant symptom causes more problems and more symptoms. Constipation often shows up as, or comes along with, a coated tongue, diarrhea, cramps, gas, foul odor, intestinal pain, and various forms of inflammation, such as colitis and diverticulitis. (We've all heard the remark that a self-centered person thinks their "stuff" doesn't stink. The solemn truth is, it isn't supposed to! If it does, that's nature hammering a warning on the door that you are overacidic.)

Worse, the microforms and their acids can spoil healthy cells, giving birth to more microforms that can appear as if they are actually boring through the colon wall into the bloodstream. This means that the microforms not only have access to the entire body, but also bring their toxins and intestinal matter along with them into the blood. From there they can travel quickly and easily take hold anywhere in the body, invading cells, tissues, and organs with their acidic waste products. All this severely stresses the immune system (the janitorial system of the body) and the liver, as they desperately try to ward off what doesn't belong. Unchecked, microforms burrow deeper into the tissues and organs, the central nervous system, the skeletal structure, the lymphatic system, and the bone marrow, bringing their acidic-waste-making capabilities with them.

This is not simply a matter of clean pipes. This kind of impaction can affect all other parts of the body because it interferes with what should be automatic reflexes and sends inappropriate messages of its own. A reflex is a nerve pathway in which the impulse goes from the point of stimulation to the point of response without going through the brain—as when your doctor taps your knee with that little rubber hammer and your lower leg kicks out. Reflexes can also respond at places other than the one actually being stimulated. Your body is a mass of reflexes. Some key ones are in the lower bowel, connected via nerve pathways to every major organ system in the body. The impacted acidic materials are like a whole squadron of little rubber hammers banging away in there, sending disruptive impulses to other parts of the body. (This is, for example, a major reason for headaches.) That alone can disturb and weaken any and all body systems.

The body creates mucus as a natural defense against acids, as a way to bind them up and get them out of the body. So mucus is not, on its face, a bad thing. In fact, it is saving our lives! For example, when you eat dairy, the lactose sugar is fermented to lactic acid, which is then bound to mucus. If not for the mucus, the acid could burn a hole in your cells, tissues, or organs, causing cancerous cells. Lactic acid is one of the primary causes of all ulcerations and cancerous conditions. (If not for the dairy, there wouldn't be a call for that mucus.) It is just that if the diet continues to be excessively acidic, too much mucus is created and the mucus–acid mixture gets sticky and congestive, causing poor digestion, cold hands, cold feet, light-headedness, nasal congestion, lung congestion (as in asthma), and continual throat clearing. Even post-nasal drip is the body trying to eliminate dietary and/or metabolic acids and is always related to mucus.

RESTORING HEALTH

Eating animal products and processed foods, ingesting chemicals (including prescription and over-the-counter medicines), overeating, and excess stress of all types disrupt and weaken the alkaline state of the digestive tract. Acidity encourages the biological transformation of food and body cells to bacteria, yeast, fungus, and other microforms. This then invites parasites to the acidic party. Without the correct alkaline pH, the food you eat cannot be properly transformed into healthy blood cells. This will lead to unhealthy body cells.

Acidity in the stomach and colon varies depending on the food you eat.

High-water-content, low-sugar foods, like those recommended in the program, cause less acidity. High-sugar and high-protein foods increase acidity. As the food moves on into the small intestine, if necessary the pancreas adds additional alkaline substances including sodium bicarbonate to the mix to raise the pH (8.0 to 8.4). So the body has ways to moderate the acid or base to appropriate levels. But on our current highly acidic diets, we overtax those systems. Eating right to begin with keeps the stress off the body and lets the process proceed naturally and easily.

At baseline, we must replenish the alkaline design of the digestive tract with alkalizing compounds such as sodium bicarbonate. With a proper alkaline diet, bacteria and yeast will be eliminated. You can help move the process along with alkaline mineral salt supplements, such as sodium and potassium bicarbonate (see chapter 12).

Besides improving your overall health, following the pH Miracle diet and lifestyle program will clean your intestines and restore your alkaline state as well as balance your pH and control the growth of microforms. All of which, you can see by now, intertwine. As the alkaline pH of the bowel, blood, and tissue normalizes, and the intestines are cleansed, nutrient assimilation and waste elimination will normalize, too, and you'll be on your way to complete, radiant health.

KATE'S STORY

I went years with a collection of mysterious ailments before a doctor finally diagnosed me as having amoebas and parasites I had picked up in South America. My digestive system was so far gone that it remained out of whack even after I received treatment. Nothing I tried, mainstream or alternative, seemed to restore my normal good health. But with these straightforward dietary changes, and the addition of powdered concentrate of greens (including wheatgrass, barley grass, and kamut grass), I'm now able to digest my food, and I've seen tremendous improvement in my overall health and energy. I've got no more abdominal pain, gas, indigestion, or nausea. I am fifty-seven and feel twenty-seven.

I had been on a low-fat, low-sugar diet, and though I wanted to lose weight, I just couldn't cut back on the amount of food I was eating. Whenever I did, fatigue really hit. By just taking out the foods recommended here (for me, that meant mostly getting rid of meat, yeast products, dairy foods, refined white flour products, and most fruit)—yet still eating approximately the same number of calories and certainly never going hungry—I lost thirty-five pounds that wouldn't come off for the world before, through traditional diet and exercise schemes.

My husband is a medical doctor, and when he saw my results, he looked into the program for himself—and then changed his diet, too.

Part II

Eating (and Drinking) Alkaline

Chapter 5

•

Eat Vegetarian—Eat COWS

I realize all that information about dietary and metabolic acids, and micro-forms, mycotoxins, and mucus, can be a bit overwhelming—not to mention unappetizing! I do want you to get just a bit of the science behind our recommendations, so you really understand how you can best serve your own body. I also want you to understand the urgency of it. But don't worry—the solutions are a lot simpler than the problems. And they are well within your reach.

Parts 2 and 3 of this book lay out the specifics of exactly how to put this plan into practice in your everyday life. The recipes in part 4 will give you a great sendoff down this new path. But right here and now, I'm going to give you the most basic outlines of this diet: the foods to include, and the foods you must avoid.

The idea behind the whole thing is to keep your body basic, thereby eliminating dietary and metabolic acids, preventing the biological transformation of body cells into microforms, and ensuring radiant health. To that end, you're going to focus on foods that alkalize your body and avoid those that acidify it.

All food ingested releases electrons for energy, leaving an ash residue. This ash residue can be neutral, acidic, or alkaline, depending mostly on the mineral content of the original food. For example, potassium, calcium, magnesium, sodium, zinc, silver, copper, and iron form basic ash; sulfur, phosphorus, chlorine, and iodine leave acid ash. Most elements are alkaline.

Fortunately for us, it is easy to categorize which foods leave which kind of ash. In general, animal foods—meat, eggs, dairy—processed and refined foods, yeast products, fermented foods, grains, artificial sweeteners, sweet fruit, and natural and artificial sugars are acidifying, as are alcohol, coffee, chocolate, black tea, and sodas. Vegetables, on the other hand, are alkalizing. That includes a few that are technically fruits: avocado, tomato, cucumber, bell pepper. A few nonsweet citrus fruits, such as grapefruit, lemon, and lime, are also basic in the body, as are sprouted seeds, nuts, and grains. Grains are acidifying, though a few (millet, buckwheat, and spelt) are only very mildly so. Raw foods are more alkalizing, while cooked food is more acidifying.

We measure alkalinity and acidity along the pH scale. *pH* stands for "the potential of hydrogen"—its proton concentration. The pH scale also measures the potential of hydroxyl ions, or electron concentration. Foods saturated with hydroxyl ions, or electrons, are alkaline. Foods saturated with hydrogen ions, or protons, are acidic. In this way, the pH scale is also a measurement of the electrical energy in food or drink.

Alkaline foods are full of electrons or electrical energy. Electrons are, in fact, what make them alkaline. This is the energy the body runs on. You can measure it, as I do, with an alkaline electron meter. Alkaline foods provide electron energy to the body; acidic foods pull electron energy from the body. It's not much different, at heart, from batteries: New alkaline batteries are full of energy—they are saturated with electrons. Dead batteries have been drained of electrons, and they are acidic—saturated with protons.

Among many other things, electrons aid in digestion. Electrons or alkaline compounds are called upon to buffer the enzymes or acids of the food. Whatever the acids or enzymes within the food, the body will release alkaline compounds or electrons to buffer them. The lower the acidity of the food, the fewer alkaline buffers or electrons are required. The fewer that are required, the more the alkaline reserves and energy of the body are preserved. The conservation of all that potential, then, provides a boost in your overall energy. The body can make more alkaline buffers and provide more electrons or electrical energy, instead, for use by organs and tissues carrying on their metabolic functions, and to provide repairs associated with environmental, dietary, and/or metabolic acid or mycotoxic damage.

COWS

To make it easier to remember the key elements of this program, I call it the COWS plan—which stands for "chlorophyll, oil, water, and salt." For optimal health, alkalize the blood and tissues daily with all of these.

We'll start with how you get your chlorophyll—from plants.

C Is for Chlorophyll (Green Vegetables)

You get chlorophyll from plants. This is one of the main reasons green plants should be the focus of your diet, the majority of any meal you sit down to, the substance covering most of your plate—especially vegetables, and particularly green vegetables. Vegetables are your new best friends. They are some of the lowest-calorie, lowest-sugar, most nutrient-rich foods on the planet. They provide (as detailed below) vitamins and minerals, fiber, electrons, phytonutrients, and alkaline salts. And they are the way you get—the only way you can get—chlorophyll.

Chlorophyll is what produces a plant's—a vegetable's—green color. It is a key player in photosynthesis. In other words, plants need it to be able to get the energy they need from sunlight. I call chlorophyll the blood of plants because its molecular structure and chemical components are similar to those of human blood. Blood's hemoglobin is made up of carbon, hydrogen, oxygen, and nitrogen organized around a single atom of iron. Chlorophyll is the same with the exception of the central atom, which is magnesium rather than iron.

In the human body, chlorophyll helps the blood cells deliver oxygen throughout. (During World War I, when the troops ran out of blood plasma on the battlefield, doctors substituted transfusions of chlorophyll.) Chlorophyll also reduces the binding of carcinogens to DNA in the liver and other organs. If that is not enough of a benefit for you, keep in mind that it also breaks down calcium stones—stones that the body creates to neutralize and dispose of excess acid for elimination.

Green vegetables and particularly leafy greens have the highest amounts of chlorophyll. You want to focus your diet on a wide variety of vegetables, and, largely because of the chlorophyll, you should make the majority of those veggies green.

Vegetables are also an excellent source of the alkaline salts that protect against microform overgrowth and the associated mycotoxins, as well as helping to neutralize metabolic and dietary acids in the blood and tissues. (More about salts coming up.) So basically, the more, the merrier.

Vegetables, and particularly green vegetables, are incredibly nutrient-dense and provide just about all the vitamins, minerals, and micronutrients you could ever need. They are rich in antioxidants (as are all alkaline foods), which protect cells all over your body from oxidative damage by buffering dietary and metabolic acids and supporting the lymphocytes or white blood cells that release singlet oxygen, and hydroxyl radicals. This action serves to neutralize acids while protecting the delicate pH balance of the body. Antioxidants also buffer dietary and metabolic acidity.

Research has demonstrated the protective effects of a broad range of antioxidants in a wide array of symptoms and diseases—and the effects are mostly from diets rich in antioxidants, not supplements. The best way to get the full gamut of antioxidants is to eat a variety of green vegetables (and nonsweet fruits) every day.

Vegetables are also loaded with the fiber that is crucial to your diet. Besides the accepted benefits of fiber in reducing cancer and other serious health concerns, studies have shown that fiber markedly decreases mycotoxicity. Fiber acts like a sponge, soaking up acids from the body. It also works like a broom, cleaning out the intestines.

JULIA'S STORY

Doctor after doctor said I could never conceive without medical intervention because of an immunological disorder. After ten years of fertility treatments, my body was full of fertility drugs and needle scars. Now that the treatments were over with, I was a great candidate for cancer. There was a solution for that problem, too: birth control pills and further hormonal roller-coaster rides. Worst of all: still no baby.

Then we learned about the pH Miracle program. I felt I was blessed with a second chance, and started "cleaning house"—in my own body, using sound nutrition to undo all the mistakes I had made in my twenties and early thirties. The knowledge of how my body truly works gave me the power to control the way I looked and felt, which brought with it inner peace and confidence. More than the physical effect, I felt a spiritual change come over me. It seemed as though my once depressed, tired, and preoccupied self became one hopeful, energetic, and peaceful entity. Internal dueling was replaced by a sense of clear purpose.

Several months after I started on this program, I became slightly ill and discovered, to my complete surprise and joy, that I was pregnant! It came as an enormous shock to me, considering all the difficulty I had in the past, to become pregnant without even trying. Our bouncing "Green" baby was born last year, our own miracle child. She is happy, healthy, and smart and beautiful! After six months of breast-feeding, she started on solid foods, which I prepare myself using almond milk, organic grains, and veggies (broccoli, cabbage, carrots, celery, green beans, spinach, parsley, cilantro, dill), avocado, new potatoes, and yams. She loves munching on cucumbers and peppers. She loves pureed salads with lemon juice and olive oil. I know our happy ending would never have been possible without our new way of life.

The very best dietary source of chlorophyll is grasses. What I said about the benefits of green fruit and vegetables goes double for grasses.

Right off the bat, you may have experienced a bit of cognitive dissonance here, because despite your need for green grasses, and despite your very real need for a COWS program, you are not, in fact, a cow. Cows don't read books. And I am not suggesting that you save the lawn clippings when you mow the grass, even if they do have lots of chlorophyll.

Not to worry. While you can get wheatgrass in most health food stores, and dishes flavored with lemongrass at Thai restaurants, that's pretty much the limit for the grasses sold for human consumption. I predict that this will soon change, but for now you need more. So what I recommend is using a supplement to get your grasses—either taking capsules of powder or, preferably, mixing the powder into water for a green drink. I'll get more into the details in later chapters, as all "greens" supplements are not created equal. Basically, you want to look for a wide variety of grasses (such as wheatgrass, barley grass, oat grass, dog grass, kamut grass, lemongrass, and shave grass) while avoiding all algaes, mushrooms, and such (see "What to Avoid" on page 101 for details).

Grasses are incredibly nutrient-dense, even more so than vegetables as a general rule. (After all, how do you think a cow gets by?) Wheatgrass and barley grass are particularly good sources of chlorophyll, for example, and it is the chlorophyll that gives grasses the power to regenerate our bodies at the molecular, cellular, and emotional level. To give you just two examples:

- Wheatgrass contains more than one hundred food elements, including every identified mineral and trace mineral and every vitamin in the B-complex family. It has one of the highest pro–vitamin A contents of any food, and is rich in vitamins C, E, and K. Wheatgrass juice is 25 percent protein, a higher percentage than in meat, fish, eggs, dairy products, or beans. In addition, it has high amounts of an antifungal, antimycotoxic substance called laetrile.

- Barley grass boasts four times as much thiamine (vitamin B$_1$) as whole wheat flour, and thirty times as much as milk. It has even more vitamin C than oranges (actually, seven times as much!).

O IS FOR OILS (ESSENTIAL FATS)

One of the most dangerous fad diets is the no-fat obsession. Fats play a crucial role in our bodies, and getting none at all opens our bodies up to nutritional deficiency and the degeneration that comes with it. The key thing is to get healthy fats, not the artery-clogging, zero-nutrient varieties most Americans eat (primarily saturated fats and partially hydrogenated oils—liquid oils chemically altered into solids). Approximately 20 percent of your calories should come from these healthy fats. On the pH Miracle COWS plan, most of those healthy fats will come from delicious natural oils.

The long-chain polyunsaturated fats from fish, seeds, fruits, and vegetables are alkaline, and buffer acids created through diet and metabolism. On the other hand, saturated fat—found mainly in animal proteins—is acidic. And we don't need any of that.

What your body does need from good oils are the essential fatty acids (EFAs). EFAs are, well, essential—vital to good health. They are the building blocks of the fats that strengthen cell walls, including blood cell walls. Polyunsaturated fats such as flax, borage, evening primrose, grape seed, and hemp oils help construct cell membranes, produce hormones, and bind and eliminate acids. Most oils contain both monounsaturated and polyunsaturated fats, and those that are predominantly monounsaturated, such as olive oil (as well as raw nuts and avocados), are also beneficial. They are used for cellular energy—meaning our body runs on those instead of sugars when we finally get in balance.

EFAs strengthen immune cells; lubricate joints; insulate the body against heat loss; provide energy; are used to make the hormone-like prostaglandins that protect against heart disease, stroke, high blood pressure, arteriosclerosis, and blood clots; and are necessary for energy metabolism and immune system health. EFAs can also help relieve arthritis, asthma, PMS, allergies, skin conditions, and some behavioral disorders, as well as improve brain function.

Nuts, seeds, olives, avocados, and their oils are all good sources of healthy fats, including the omega-3s and omega-6s you may have heard about (sometimes called fish oils because fish is another good source if you are not vegetarian). EFAs are found in the highest concentration in flax seed oil, borage seed oil, and hemp seed oil. We like the brands Essential Balance from Arrowhead

Mills, sometimes sold as Omega Nutrition, and Udo's Choice. You might try those or similar combination oils found at your health food store. Pomegranate seed oil is the best source of omega-5 CLA oils. And since you eat the whole seed, including its oils, when you eat a pomegranate, eating the whole (low-sugar) fruit is as good for you as using the oil. Look for cold-pressed oils, extracted and packaged without being heated. And don't heat the oils yourself! Add them to vegetables after warming or steaming, or make a flavorful salad dressing simply by combining with lemon juice and seasoning. Beware of rancid oils. Buy only what you'll use up pretty quickly, store it in dark containers in a dark place, and use only what smells fresh.

W Is for Water (Alkaline Water)

Chapter 7 looks at water in depth, but the main message bears repeating: Plenty of water—correction: clean, pure alkaline water—is absolutely crucial to creating a healthy pH and a healthy body. The body is 70 percent alkaline water overall. Your eyes are 98 percent alkaline water! Your blood, 94 percent. So we should provide all the parts of the body with a lot of this basic component. That includes foods that are actually high in alkaline water. That means—you guessed it—green electron-rich vegetables and low-sugar fruits! And of course you should also drink up. As you'll see in chapter 7, the human body thrives with plenty of electron-rich alkaline water with a pH of 9.5.

Getting the right water in the right amount is the single most important part of the pH Miracle plan for health. Fully hydrating the body with good water is the quickest and easiest way to reach and maintain good health.

The Dangers of Dehydration

Chances are that you're among the 75 percent of Americans who are chronically dehydrated, meaning they don't get the eight 8-ounce servings of water each day—about two liters—recommended by mainstream health experts. The average person gets only about *one* liter of fluid a day—much of it from acidic coffee, tea, and soft drinks, many of which actually *rob* the body of water. And to get even to that minimal level requires estimating the amount they get from food. Oh, and sometimes they get it from drinking actual water, though it is likely to be inadequate in quality as well as quantity. Fully 10 percent of respondents to a survey done for the Nutrition Information Center at Cornell Medical Center reported drinking no water at all!

For ideal health and weight, you need much more water—good water—as I'll detail later. The average adult loses about two and a half to three liters of fluid a day through sweating, breathing, urinating, moving, even sleeping, and the body becomes dehydrated if it isn't replaced.

If you don't get enough water, you'll get fat. Simple as that. For one thing, even mild dehydration slows metabolism by as much as 3 percent. For another, we are so poorly attuned to our bodies' thirst signals that we interpret them as hunger pangs. That is: If we don't drink enough, we eat too much. Third, if we don't get enough water, our bodies will actually retain water, and we'll feel bloated and uncomfortable—and look even fatter than strictly necessary! An acidic body pulls water into the tissues to try to neutralize the acids there.

Most important, the body uses water to neutralize acids, to dilute excess acid, and to literally wash them (and all toxins) out of the body via urine and sweat and through the bowels. Without enough water, your body becomes too acidic and goes into preservation—fat-storing—mode. A drop of just over 2 percent in body water content is enough to make that happen. In case you think that sounds like such a big change that it's unlikely to ever happen to you, take note: It's not unusual to lose 2 percent of your body water during an average hour of exercise.

If that's not enough to get you to drink up, let me add that in addition to fat, not getting enough water will also make you sick and tired. In fact, lack of water is the number one cause of daytime fatigue. Without enough water, you won't have enough energy. You'll feel tired and weak.

That 2 percent drop in body water can result in a measurable decrease in physical performance. The acid that builds up in your tissues when you don't get enough water acts like a meat tenderizer, making your muscles flabby—and weak. Studies show that a 3 percent drop in water causes a 10 percent drop in muscle strength and an 8 percent drop in speed, as well as lower muscular endurance.

By the time you get to a 4 percent drop in water, you'll experience dizziness—and a fall of as much as 30 percent in your capacity for physical labor. Drop another percentage point and you'll have problems with concentration, drowsiness, impatience, and headaches (one of the most common signs of dehydration, along with dry skin). Losing another percent can cause your heart to race and your body's temperature regulation to go out of whack. Hit 7 percent, and you could collapse.

Even in the earliest stages, dehydration can also lead to muddled thinking, short-term memory problems, trouble with basic math and expressing yourself verbally, and difficulty focusing on a computer screen or printed page. Light-headedness and cold hands and feet can also result. The list goes on: anxiety, irritability, depression, sugar cravings, and cramps.

As for making you sick: When the dehydration gets a little more severe, symptoms include acid reflux (heartburn), joint and back pain, migraines, fibromyalgia, constipation, colitis, and angina. Serious dehydration is linked with asthma, allergies, diabetes, hypertension, and skin problems like eczema, rashes, spots, blemishes, and acne. Degenerative conditions including morbid obesity, heart disease, and cancer are all linked with serious long-term dehydration. If you lose 15 to 20 percent of your body's water, it can be immediately life threatening.

In short: Lack of water can kill you.

In fact, although you could go about thirty days without eating, you can't live seventy-two hours without water. Your body uses as much water in cold weather as it does in warm, and as much when you are sleeping as when you are awake. In an average day, even with no physical activity or environmental extremes (a hot and/or dry climate, say), and no particular drains on your body's water supply (like air travel, or time in a high-rise building), you can lose 1 percent of the water in your body. Although the most serious symptoms we're listing here don't come from spending an hour or a day with low levels of water in your tank, most people exist in a chronic state of low-level dehydration for most of their lives. No wonder so very many of us are fat and sick and tired!

Hydrate for Health

Fortunately, this is a relatively easy problem to solve. Finding the right water may take some doing, as you'll see, but essentially you just need to drink up! Those who do provide their bodies with a crucial element for normal performance, in everything from temperature regulation and toxin excretion to joint lubrication and fat metabolism. Water helps process just about every biological, mechanical, and chemical action that takes place in your body. It cushions and protects vital organs, transports nutrients within each cell, and dispels acidic wastes. Your lungs need water to humidify the air they move. The digestive system uses several gallons of water daily to process food. Your brain needs water to perform the chemical reactions required to run your body. Your pancreas uses water to alkalize food coming out of the stomach and into the intestines. Water keeps your skin soft and supple, increases oxygen in the blood, and maintains normal electrical properties of the cells, improving cell-to-cell communication.

One study published in the *Journal of the American Dietetic Association* showed that women who drank more than five glasses of water a day had 45 percent less risk of colon cancer. Another from the same journal showed a 50 percent decrease in the risk of bladder cancer in people who drank two and a half quarts of water daily, and a 79 percent drop in the risk of breast cancer. A survey of more than three thousand American adults conducted at the New York Hospital–Cornell Medical Center indicates that eight to ten glasses of water a day could significantly reduce back and joint pain for up to 80 percent of sufferers. Drinking plenty of water also helps prevent kidney stones.

A University of Washington study showed that one glass of water shut down hunger pangs for nearly all dieters in the study. And German researchers found that drinking water increases the rate at which you burn calories. Just two cups of water increased metabolic rate by almost a third— and it stayed up for about half an hour. When they reported their findings in the *Journal of Clinical Endocrinology and Metabolism,* they calculated that getting an additional one and a half liters of water a day for a year would mean burning off an extra 17,400 calories—or about five pounds.

S Is for Salt

We cannot live without healthy alkalizing salt. Salt is essential to human nutrition and physiological processes. It is as important to our bodies and our health as water or air. We need all three to survive. Our bodies contain about a *pound* of salt. Our blood, sweat, and tears all contain salt. So does your saliva. In fact, *all* body fluids are salty.

Pure salt consists of the elements sodium and chloride (hence the chemical name, sodium chloride, and symbol NaCl). In addition to their individual roles in the body, sodium and chloride are used to build magnesium, potassium, and calcium. All five of these elements are mineral salts, and the primary forms of electrolytes—substances that conduct electricity— in the human body. These electrolytes perform an elaborate balancing act in the body to maintain hydration, blood pH, and nerve and muscle function at optimal levels.

Salts also help normalize the volume of blood in the body, and regulate fluid pressure, including blood pressure, within cells. Salts play an important role in making the heart beat correctly, and in the regulation of metabolism. The body uses salt to make the iron from which it builds the hemoglobin of the red blood cells. Calcium salts help build strong bones. Magnesium salts help balance body temperature. Sodium and potassium salts keep the correct balance of water in and around the cells, regulate the acid–alkaline balance in our blood, and are required for proper muscle functioning. Salt is important in the digestion of food. The body uses salt to make sodium bicarbonate (see chapter 4).

And, of course, salt is famously involved with blood pressure. But it does not *cause* high blood pressure. Dietary and metabolic acids do, when they are not properly eliminated through urination, defecation, perspiration, and respiration. Blood pressure also naturally increases with age.

The truth is, salt is the key to reducing and normalizing blood pressure (and to maintaining a healthy pulse rate below seventy beats per minute). But it has to be the right kind and the right amount of salt, which we'll get into shortly. The wrong salt can cause blood pressure problems, especially if you are living and eating acidic.

Without enough salt, we get muscle cramps or weakness, dizziness, and exhaustion—and those are just the initial outward signs that something is awry inside our bodies. In extreme cases, this can ultimately lead to convulsions and even death.

Salt concentration in the blood must be kept constant, and the body has various ways to maintain this tight control. If you don't get enough salt, the body drastically reduces its excretion of salt (via urine and sweat), but has to try to maintain blood salt concentration nonetheless so it increases secretion of water. You get dehydrated, perhaps severely, and that can become a medical emergency. (Getting too much water can be similarly dire if the water is acidic and is taken in such a way that it throws off the salt balance; see chapter 7.)

We all have a role to play, too, in keeping the salt concentration correct. We need to replenish the salt our body uses up in maintaining our normal health, vigor, and alkalinity, so it should be a regular part of our daily diet. But *not* the processed salts most of us sprinkle on indiscriminately, and certainly not the sodium loaded into processed foods of all kinds. You need alkalizing salts like sea salts, cell salts, and mineral salts.

Processed Salt

The salt you're most likely getting (if you are like most Americans—in fact, like most people in the world) is highly processed salt that has been bleached white and contains additives, preservatives, anti-caking agents, moisture absorbents, fluoride, and dextrose (sugar!). But it has been stripped of its natural mineral content. It often contains dangerous preservatives not required to be listed on the label, such as aluminum hydroxide, which improves the salt's pour-ability. Aluminum is a light alloy that forms deposits in your brain—a contributor to Alzheimer's disease. Iodine is commonly added (this time, promoted on the label), but it is potentially toxic and there are no health advantages to using salt with this additive. The essence and purpose of this foundational element has been destroyed, making an acidifying mess out of what should be full of good alkaline properties.

Table salt has been dried in huge kilns where temperatures reach twelve hundred degrees F, and "chemically cleaned." The heating process is powerful enough to alter the natural chemical structure of the salt, as some of the elements are blasted into the air as a gas. This form of sodium can't satisfy the body's needs for sodium chloride. And it is an irritant—the body treats it as something completely foreign. It requires a tremendous amount of energy for the body to try to metabolize and eliminate. And this is what most of us have been eating all of our lives! Processed salt is bound to upset your fluid–salt balance, and overburden your elimination systems. For every gram of unnatural salt that your body cannot get rid of, *twenty-three grams* of water has to be drawn from inside the cells to neutralize it. This causes excess fluid in your body tissues (which contributes to cellulite, rheumatism, arthritis, gout, and kidney and bladder stones) on top of cell dehydration and their resultant premature breakdown.

So, in a way we are right when we think that salt is bad for us. Standard overprocessed, demineralized salt *is* bad for us—and at our current rate of intake (the average person consumes between four and six thousand milligrams of salt each day, with heavy users getting up to ten thousand), it's literally killing us. Table salt is absolutely useless, and potentially destructive. Yet it is in almost everything we eat—certainly in every preserved product.

THE SALT TEST

Try this experiment: Mix a spoonful of the salt you usually use into a glass of water and let it stand overnight. In the morning, if you can see salt down in the bottom of the glass, you can be sure it is processed salt. If it's natural salt, there'll be nothing to see but clear water: Natural salt dissolves—naturally!

Salt that does not dissolve in water cannot dissolve in your body. Like any foreign substance that collects in the body organs and tissues, it will eventually cause the malfunctioning of essential body processes and you'll end up with heart disease, arthritis, hardening of the arteries, calcium deposits in the joints, or something similar. Natural organic salts, on the other hand, will not cause calcification in the body—and in fact can help dissolve damaging calcium deposits.

Good Salt

Despite the bad news about common American salt, you cannot consume too much *natural, unrefined* salt. Salt that hasn't been processed or denatured, salt that is still whole, full of minerals, and contains all of its natural elements, is healthy and alkaline. This salt will provide potassium, calcium, and magnesium, and in fact every known mineral in at least trace amounts. Even more crucially, it will energize the body. It acts as a catalyst in the transport of electrical energy from cell to cell. If that transfer of energy stops—you die. Processed salts cannot conduct electricity.

Sea Salt and Rock Salt

A healthy ocean is maintained by the same alkaline mineral salts as the healthy human body, namely, sodium, chloride, magnesium, potassium, and calcium. So the ideal salt for our bodies would be sun-dried from the waters of a healthy sea. (Really, all salts come from a sea—the oceans that once covered the earth left a generous supply of salt beds and underground deposits.)

Unfortunately, most of today's sea salt is not nearly as healthy as it used to be—because the oceans are not as healthy as they once were, thanks to chemical dumping, toxic oil spills, and all sorts of pollution. Furthermore, 89 percent of all sea salt producers now refine their salt.

Unprocessed, crushed, natural rock salt is whole and intact and contains all its original minerals, so it should be alkalizing. But the body often cannot metabolize and absorb the valuable elements found in rock salt. Mixing it into alkaline water to create a salt solution will help.

Look for Celtic salt, Himalayan salt, and Real Salt from Redmond, Utah. (See resources.)

Mineral Salts

Your best bet is mineral salts. Look for an equal combination of the four most important salts for the body: sodium, potassium bicarbonate, and magnesium and calcium carbonate mineral salts. This is a powerful alkalizing compound. The combination of salts helps ensure adequate levels of the four main electrolytes in your body. These salts are naturally occurring in all the fluids of the body, and help in the reduction of acidity in the lymphatic, circulatory, and digestive systems. The salts themselves have a pH around 8.4.

Our brand is called Young pHorever pHour Salts, but you may find something similar at your health food store. Innerlight's 4 Salts powder and capsules are available via the Internet. Tri-Salts is another example. It contains magnesium, potassium, and calcium carbonates, but no sodium. You may find something similar, and that'll do if you can't find all four together. You can take sodium bicarbonate in addition (see below), or add in whichever of the minerals is missing. Look for mineral salts from the Great Salt Lake, Dead Sea, Celtic Sea, or Himalayas.

As a backup plan, get some good sea salt and eat as much of the darkest green foods as you can.

To maintain health, energy, vitality, and the alkaline design of the body, use salts liberally in your water or on your food. You'll need more than what you get that way, though, so stir up a salt solution: Take one teaspoon in three to four ounces of alkaline water, three times a day. This will keep the pH of your urine and saliva at 7.2 or above.

Liquid Colloidal Mineral Salts

Another excellent choice is liquid colloidal mineral salts. This is salt suspended (dispersed evenly through, but not dissolved within) water. Colloidal salts are ideal because the vital minerals (including calcium, potassium, and magnesium) and trace elements in the salts are in particles so small that the cells can easily absorb them. There is no need for them to be broken down. They are already in their bioavailable state, which is the big difference between colloidal salt and salt crystals or rock salts.

Our product is called Young pHorever pH Miracle pHlavor Mineral Salts, which is salt from the entrance or North Shore of the Great Salt Lake. Or look for a liquid mineral salt in your health food store. Make sure you get one containing sodium and potassium bicarbonate in a liquid form. The mineral contents will be on the label. Choose a product uncontaminated with any toxins or environmental pollutants.

Colloidal salts are ideal. If you can't find that, you can get almost as good results by stirring salt into water yourself. Once the salts are dissolved, they are colloidal. The resources section at the end of the book provides other sources for good salt.

Whatever you go with, use it liberally on your food and in your cooking. (See chapter 13 for more on using liquid colloidal mineral salts as salt therapy.)

Sodium Bicarbonate

Sodium bicarbonate—which you probably already know as baking soda—can be used on its own or in conjunction with mineral salts for best results. It has a pH in the 8s, and when you use it, you'll see the results almost immediately if you are testing the pH of your urine. It'll turn that paper purple, meaning a pH above 8, up to as high as 10.

I recommend our own liquid bicarbonate product—it's the only liquid form on the market—but you can also make your own solution of baking soda in water. Make sure you get aluminum-free baking soda (check the label). Be sure to use a baking soda with no aluminum in it. Bob's Red Mill brand is a good option.

If you cannot find or afford the liquid bicarbonate product, just mix one teaspoon of baking soda into anywhere from four to sixteen ounces of water. One teaspoon is fine in up to a liter of water, so you can use more water to dilute it if you're not wild about the taste. Take this two or three times a day. Use more baking soda, up to a tablespoon at a time, if you are struggling with a serious health challenge. The goal is to keep the pH of your urine at 7.2 if you are healthy and 8.4 if you are experiencing a serious health challenge.

Using Salts

It is difficult to get enough of the proper relative quantities of the interrelated salts (sodium, chloride, potassium, magnesium, and calcium) without supplementing a proper alkaline diet. I recommend ten to twelve grams (three to four teaspoons) unprocessed mineral salts daily, and drinking one liter of salt water every day. You can take it first thing in the morning to flush the alimentary canal of all impurities. See chapters 7 ("You Are What You Drink") and 10 ("Putting It Together") for more information.

You can sprinkle sea salt (or spray liquid sea salt) on your food or in your water. Add it to soups or shakes. You can even just take a bit straight. That's especially useful if you feel light-headed, dizzy, weak, tired, fatigued, or are having a sugar craving.

You see the alkalizing effect in the blood and tissues right away if you test your urine: The pH will be over 8 almost immediately. You should also experience an immediate increase in energy level, along with a disappearance of sugar cravings (which are often really a signal of a need for salt).

I do want to caution you that *alkalizing mineral salts at these levels are only for people committed to an alkaline lifestyle and diet.* They could cause blood pressure problems and rapid pulse or heart rate if your diet and lifestyle remain acidic. Using salts properly gets even more important as you get older, as blood pressure naturally increases with age.

GREEN ATHLETES

We exercise a lot—running, lifting weights, and walking and hiking every day—and we rely on this program to sustain us. Alkalizing increases athletic performance, building stamina and muscle as well as providing pure energy. So while the pH Miracle program can be a literal lifesaver for sick people, it is also a boon to even the fittest and healthiest among us. It will make anyone well, but it will also keep you from getting sick in the first place and keep you functioning at peak levels, physically.

We've seen the results in ourselves, of course, but on a more objective level we've seen the results in all kinds of stellar athletes. We advised two biathletes in training for the 2002 Olympics, one of whom attributed his third-place finish in a European competition (the Europeans dominate the sport) to the concentrated greens he takes. When he sought us out, he was having trouble even completing some events! We also work with the top soccer team in Trinidad, which uses concentrated green powder to fuel them through all their top-flight international matches. We've also started the West Point gymnastics team on the program (more about that in a moment).

The one that really blows our minds is Stu Mittleman. In the summer of 2000, Stu ran from San Diego to New York City in fifty-six days (running approximately two marathons every day). And he did it all powered by alkaline foods, appropriate supplements, and daily green drink (actually, several daily green drinks). He also holds the world's record for long-distance running: If you want to challenge him, you'll have to do better than one thousand miles in thirteen days, or approximately three marathons every day.

He does eat fish almost every other day, and he also has a steak now and again. But for the most part Stu is a living, breathing pH Miracle. Vegetables are by far the largest portion of his diet.

You don't have to be at that kind of extreme to experience how the pH Miracle program can enhance your athletic abilities, though we find it inspiring to know what it can do even at the extremes. It is important to note that it is a two-sided coin. Exercise itself accelerates the lymphatic process (that is, sweating), getting rid of excess acids and wastes through that all-important "third kidney"—the skin. So the program is good for exercising; exercising is good for the program.

Now, about those gymnasts. Here we've got something more than just anecdotal evidence. No matter how impressive Stu is, he's still just one guy, doing his thing. But at West Point, I (Rob) was able to do a controlled study. I divided the eleven army college gymnasts into two groups (A and B) and gave one of them (A) concentrated green powder and pH drops to add to their water every day. (I also had them each wear a special pendant designed to mitigate the negative effects of electromagnetic frequencies, or EMFs.) Group B had just plain water (and a placebo pendant). Their diets stayed the same, and they made no other changes to their lifestyle.

Over the course of the season, their coach kept statistical results on each gymnast for every meet, on all six events (floor exercise, vault, high bars, parallel bars, pommel horse, and rings), including the number of routines attempted and the number of routines "hit" (successfully completed). The five competitive gymnasts taking the supplements, group A, hit 66 percent of all their routines. The other six, group B, hit 38 percent. Group A outperformed group B by almost 100 percent! And this was just with the addition of green drink, pH drops, and the pendant—not even the full pH Miracle program.

In addition, although this is more subjective, I think it is still worth noting that group A gymnasts reported increases in strength and endurance, longer practice time, improved attitudes toward workouts, and, most important of all, less time in recovery after workouts and meets compared with their group B teammates and to themselves at the start of the season.

I also took before-and-after blood samples of all the gymnasts and found that the blood of group A participants was significantly healthier and stronger than that of men in group B.

None of this surprised me. Think about it: Many of the strongest animals in the world are herbivores (vegetarians) subsisting almost exclusively on greens—raw ones, of course!

80–20

For sustainable energy, health, and vitality, the body needs to be maintained in an alkaline state; everything you drink, everything you eat, every activity you engage in should be alkaline. Yet the standard American diet is almost 100 percent acid. As such, it is at the heart of the American health crisis. It is the reason so many are sick, tired, and dying. It is the reason diabetes, cancer, and heart disease are on the rise.

To maintain a balanced pH in your blood and tissues, your diet should consist of at least 80 percent basic foods—that is, no more than 20 percent acidifying foods. And at least half of that 80 percent should be raw. These are visual measurements, not by weight or calories. The more alkaline your diet, the more rapid your improvement will be. Unlike the familiar food pyramid, which has an overall acidic effect, this program will bring you back to basic.

The initial phases of the program (as described in part 3) are the most restrictive. The guidelines here are essentially for maintenance, once you've gotten your body on track. These general principles I have divided into two sections: what you should eat, and what you should avoid, with all the whys and wherefores. First, we'll look at what you must include in your diet: the good alkalizing foods, including electron-rich, high-chlorophyll vegetables and fruit, mono- and polyunsaturated oil, raw foods, pure alkaline water, and unprocessed sea salt. Then we'll dive into the acidifying foods you must avoid, such as meat, sugar, and yeast.

Eat Like Royalty

But only at breakfast. To keep your body more alkaline during the times of the day when you are most active, you want to eat your biggest, richest meal for breakfast ("Eat like a king"), scale back bit for lunch ("Eat like a prince"), and dine lightly at dinner ("Eat like a pauper"). That way you're fueled when you need it, and you have less acid to buffer and eliminate while your body rests at night.

Raw Foods

Raw foods contain electrical energy or life force (technically, they are what's known as biogenic), which they can transfer to you, while cooked foods are dead or depleted of electrical potential or electrons. That's because heat (over 118 degrees F) destroys the electrical potential of food. Cooked food requires the body to produce all the necessary electrons (energy), creating an unnecessary stress and diverting resources from other jobs.

Sometimes, however, a little bit of cooking or other processing can actually be helpful. Cooked carrots provide more vitamin A than raw ones do, for example, though raw carrots provide more fiber. So—eat them both raw and cooked! Cooking improves some characteristics of tomatoes, too (see page 89).

In general, though, the more of your vegetables you eat raw, the better. Aim to have at least 40 percent (visually) of your food uncooked—working up to 75 to 80 percent as you get used to this program. Think salads. Great big salads. In infinite variety. And when you do cook your food, do so for as short a time as possible.

Fresh, Organic Foods

Fresh food is essential, and organically grown is preferable. Organic foods let you avoid exposure to pesticides and all the other chemicals routinely dumped on most produce. They are usually more nutritious, as well, since the soil (where plants draw their nutrients from) is less depleted than it has become with the harsh treatment on standard farms. Organic produce is as much as 300 percent higher in nutrients than non-organic.

Eating your food as fresh as possible is also key. The minute something is picked, the nutrients begin to break down. Ideally, we'd still be living in the kind of world where we all could walk out into our gardens, pluck our dinner, prepare it immediately, and sit down to enjoy it within the hour. I realize that's not feasible for most of us, most of the time, but to get the most out of what you eat, look to get as close to that experience as you can. Currently 90 percent of the money Americans spend on food is spent on processed food. No wonder we are sick and tired. We *must* do much better!

And we are beginning to. Organic food has become mainstream, and you can find it in most grocery stores today, not just health food stores. And home vegetable gardening is starting to take off in a similar upsurge. We urge you to consider trying it for yourself. Grow a garden, plant in a kitchen atrium, or build a greenhouse. Pretty much anyone can grow a lot, if not all, of the produce for their own families. People who live in apartments can garden on rooftops or in neighborhood co-op gardens. Greenhouses make gardening possible in any climate. You can organize a garden group among parents at your local school or church or other community organization. Now, *that's* organic!

When organic is not a choice, get the freshest produce you can and clean thoroughly with the vegetable washes available at the health food store, or soak for ten to fifteen minutes in electron-rich alkaline water with pH drops of sodium chlorite or sodium and/or potassium bicarbonate added. The alkaline compounds will break up any acidic residues or toxic chemicals on your vegetables. Rinse lightly in plain alkaline water.

CHEW THIS OVER

Besides not using up alkaline reserves and electron energy, the best thing you can do to help conserve energy is to chew your food extremely well. Chewing your food is the first and only time when the literal digestion of that food takes place. Chewing breaks the cellular membranes of the food, which starts its transformation and the release of electrical potential or energy needed by the body. The idea is to drink your solids and chew your liquids. That means chewing solid food long enough to convert it to a liquid consistency in the mouth—and not gulping liquids without mixing them a little with your oral secretions. Although the latter process may not be featured in the etiquette books, it gives the digestive process the boost it needs to extract all the value from food it can.

You should also be sure to take small bites. When solid food is properly chewed, it expands considerably. Large initial mouthfuls then provoke premature swallowing of food, which cannot be adequately liquefied in the stomach or the intestines. The food needs to be liquefied in the mouth or it puts undue stress on the root system or intestinal villi of the small intestine. Remember, the body cannot convert chunks of food into stem cells and then blood cells. Food must be in the liquefied state called chyme to be able to fall into the crypts of the intestinal villi and then be transformed into stem cells, erythroblasts and then erythrocytes. Finally, stop eating before you think you are full, and give your stomach a chance to register it has had enough.

Phytonutrients, or phytochemicals as they are also known, are highly biologically and electrically active and extremely beneficial. They exist in astounding number and variety. Some phytochemicals give plants their color, such as the yellow, orange, and red in summer squash, carrots, and peppers (though it is chlorophyll that takes care of the green, of course). One large group of phytonutrients are the bioflavonoids, water-soluble companions of vitamin C that abound in the plant kingdom.

Phytonutrients help prevent cancer, lower cholesterol, relieve arthritis and osteoporosis, stop hormones from being turned into acids, and more. Some argue that this is because they counter free radicals, but in truth, although the effects have been observed, the pathway is rarely understood. I believe their secret is, rather, their ability to eliminate harmful microforms and their acidic toxins. Phytonutrients generally bind to (thereby neutralizing or eliminating) acids.

Chapter 6

•

What to Eat, What to Avoid

You already know the main principles of what to eat to experience the pH Miracle in your own life: COWS. If you are like most Americans, putting all this into practice is going to involve a major transition. As mentioned, part 3 of this book helps you with the practical details of how to do that. Here, we're more focused on the *why* to do that. Now that you have the general outlines, I want to fill in a few more details about specific foods you will be building your diet on.

We'll begin with vegetables, those plentiful sources of the electron energy that is needed for just about every chemical activity in the human body. There are thousands of alkaline vegetables, and we need them all for our overall energy reserves and good health. Plant-based diets provide micronutrients that improve overall health and prevent chronic disease. Government guidelines recommend five to six servings of fruits and vegetables a day. That would be a good start, but we really should be eating three to four times that!

GET YOUR FRESH VEGGIES HERE!

Here is a partial list, in alphabetical order, of excellent dark green and yellow vegetables and fruit. For as long as you are having symptoms, go easy on the high-sugar vegetables such as carrots, beets, and winter squash. But in general, you can eat these freely:

Asparagus
Beet greens
Broccoli
Brussels sprouts
Burdock
Cabbage
Carrots
Cauliflower
Celery
Cucumbers
Eggplant
Garlic
Green and yellow squash (zucchini and summer squash)
Green beans
Greens of all kinds (including spinach, mustard greens, collards, kale, lettuce, watercress, and Swiss chard)
Okra
Onions
Parsley
Parsnips
Peas (fresh)
Radishes
Red and yellow and green peppers
Rutabagas
Salsify
Scallions
Sea vegetables such as nori, wakame, and hijiki
Sprouted grains or beans or seeds
Turnips
Water chestnuts

WHAT TO EAT

Avocados

Avocados (technically a fruit) are just about as close to a perfect food as you can get—an alkalizing, energizing, hydrating fuel for your body! Avocados are a great source of protein, monounsaturated fats, essential fatty acids, beneficial plant sterols, chlorophyll, and a broad range of micronutrients, all while having no starch and very little sugar, and being high in fat content and protein.

Avocados rank as the most easily digested rich source of fats and proteins in a whole food. In fact, they are about 80 percent healthy fat and 15 percent protein. They provide more protein than cow's milk. They contain all of the essential amino acids (the building blocks of protein)—eighteen in all. And avocados are rich in healthy monounsaturated and essential fatty acids (seven varieties, including omega-3 and -6). Their good fats are useful in cellular construction, and help lower cholesterol. And they serve as an energy source for the body to burn for fuel. That's a better alternative than burning glucose (sugar) or even protein, because those leave acidic ash waste in the blood. This also makes them especially useful to people with diabetes, Type 1 or 2, who should eat two or three a day.

As with nuts and olive oil, the healthy fats in avocados signal your brain when you are full, helping to ward off overeating. Researchers at the University of California–Irvine found that foods that contain the unsaturated fatty acid oleic acid (such as avocados) stimulate production of a compound called OEA (oleoylethanolamide)—which suppresses appetite. OEA is released in the small intestine, connecting with nerve endings there to tell the brain that the body doesn't require any more food. Other studies confirm that increased OEA levels help with weight loss—and lower blood cholesterol and triglyceride levels to boot.

Avocados also have high levels of helpful phytosterols, or plant sterols. Certain sterols can help lower blood cholesterol levels, and some have been shown, in animal studies, to inhibit the growth of tumors.

In addition, avocados contain a wide range of antioxidants and other nutrients, including vitamins A, B-complex, folic acid, C, E, H, K, along with glutathione, a key nutrient you'll learn more about in chapter 12. They've recently been discovered to contain nearly twice as much vitamin E as previously thought, making them the highest fruit source of that nutrient. Vitamin E helps slow the aging process and protect against heart disease, and is a powerful buffer of metabolic and digestive acids. Avocados have also been recently found to be a source of lutein, a carotenoid that helps prevent some types of cancerous conditions, particularly in the prostate and cervix, and plays a major role in eye health. Glutathione helps prevent various cancerous conditions and heart disease by buffering dietary and metabolic acids—and avocados are an excellent source of glutathione.

Avocados are also full of the alkaline buffering minerals so critical in neutralizing excess acidity, including magnesium, copper, iron, calcium, and potassium (more than bananas!) as well as other trace elements. Avocados contain fourteen minerals all of which regulate body function and stimulate growth. Iron and copper, in particular, aid in red blood cell regeneration and prevention of nutritional anemia. They contain ionic sodium, which gives them high alkaline reaction without all the acidic sugar.

We rely so much on avocados to keep us healthy and happy that it seems only natural to us that we now operate an organic avocado ranch (where we grow grapefruits and pomegranates as well). In our research there, we've found many ways to extend the benefits of avocados, from avocado oil to avocado-based super-antioxidant supplements, a liquid avocado extract of glutathione, and shampoo, conditioner, moisturizer, and cleanser all made with an avocado base. The dense nutrients of this incredible food are good for you inside and out!

We recommend eating at least one avocado every day. If you have a serious health condition, make it two to three. Of course you can just enjoy slices as they are, or with a squirt of lemon or salt, or atop pretty much any salad. They pair especially well with tomatoes. Or try an AvoRado Kid Greens Shake or Pop—or any of the many recipes in part 4 of this book that feature avocado. Use avocado oil on your salads, in your green shakes, and on your foods. Or you can just drink one ounce of avocado oil each day. (You can get some of the benefits of avocado from glutathione supplements, available in the health food stores, but they are from animal sources and so are not right for everybody. Some veggie powders include avocado, so that's another option for adding the benefits to your diet.)

Freshly picked avocados ripen in two to three weeks at room temperature. They last longer when refrigerated.

Tomatoes

Tomatoes are another great vegetable—though also technically fruits. They are low in sugar and chock-full of antioxidants. They also have a high water content. And tomatoes are a great source of a very valuable nutrient: lycopene. Lycopene is a carotenoid found in many fruits and vegetables, but most abundant in tomatoes. (Carotenoids are what give red, orange, and yellow fruits and vegetables their color.) Lycopene helps maintain the alkaline design of the body so strongly that there's evidence it plays a major role in preventing cancerous conditions, particularly in the prostate, breast, and cervix.

Tomatoes are at their most alkalizing when eaten raw. When cooked, they become mildly acid forming. Cooking also destroys much of their vitamin C. But cooking also breaks down cell walls in the tomatoes, releasing lycopene and dramatically increasing the amount available to the body. Olive oil helps the body absorb lycopene more easily. So tomatoes dressed with olive oil is a great combination. And if you are cooking tomatoes, try doing so in olive oil. Drying tomatoes (low-heat dehydration) boosts their nutrients, including lycopene. Dehydrating retains all the electrical potential that is destroyed by cooking. Rehydrating them from powder into tomato paste maximizes the beneficial properties.

We recommend combining tomatoes and avocados for an ideal pairing that is not only unfailingly delicious, but also allows lycopene and lutein to work together. When they do, they produce even better results than either on their own. I have a bowl of avocado and tomato for breakfast almost every morning, topped with lemon juice, sea salt, and olive, hemp, or flax oil.

Sprouts

Full of vitamins, minerals, and complete proteins, sprouts are just about the best food you can eat. They are living plant foods that are biogenic— meaning they can transfer their life energy to you! Seeds become more alkaline as they sprout.

In the sprouting process, plant hormones are activated, proteins are predigested into easily assimilated amino acids that work better in the human body, fats are broken down into more easily assimilated fatty acids, and starches are broken down into easily assimilated vegetable sugars. The body needs *no* sugar—sugar is an acidic waste product of food breaking down or energy being consumed. All the hard sugars compromise the pancreas as an alkalizing gland and sap energy supplies!

Sprouts—and soaked nuts and seeds—are alkalizing, life-generating, revitalizing, high-energy foods. They are high in electrical energy or electrons, predigested complete proteins, chelated minerals, nucleic acids, vitamins, RNA, DNA, and vitamin B_{12}. Their plant phytochemicals are activated, their starches broken down into easily assimilated vegetable sugars, their proteins predigested into easily assimilated free amino acids, and their fats broken down into soluble fatty acids. And their nutrient content skyrockets: Biotin content increases by 50 percent at sprouting, vitamin B_5 by 200 percent, B_6 by 500 percent, folic acid by 600 percent, and riboflavin (B_2) by 1,300 percent!

You may think of sprouts only as the familiar bean sprout and alfalfa sprout. But sprouts from just about any beans, grains, or seeds are healthful and delicious. To give you some examples, we enjoy mung bean sprouts, chickpea sprouts, green lentil sprouts, sesame sprouts, sunflower sprouts, buckwheat sprouts, hemp sprouts, and wheat sprouts. As mentioned, sprouted is the best way to eat soy. In fact, it is the ideal way to eat all legumes: When sprouted, they are much easier to alkalize and will not produce intestinal acidic gas as they do when full-grown and cooked.

While sprouts are available in health food stores and supermarkets, growing your own ensures absolute freshness and maximum living energy. Sprouts are easy to grow in your own kitchen, in any season, providing you with fresh organic produce year-round. (More about how to do this in chapter 10.)

Lemons, Limes, and Grapefruit

Although you must avoid almost all fruits (see details later in the chapter), lemons, limes, and (nonsweet) grapefruit are actually beneficial. (Usually, white grapefruit is less sweet than pink, though taste is your best indicator on how sweet it is.) Fruit itself is not unhealthy per se—in fact, most fruit is rich in nutrients—but the sugar it contains ferments like any other acid sugar, wreaking the familiar havoc in your system. It is crucial to strictly avoid high-acid-sugar fruit when you are embarking on this program, though once you are thoroughly back in balance, your body will be able to tolerate a piece of fresh fruit, in season, once in a while for a treat.

Though lemons, limes, and grapefruits are chemically acid, my tests show that when they are metabolized in the body they actually have an alkalizing effect because of their high concentration of sodium and potassium bicarbonate salts. They have very little acid sugar (lemon and lime 3 percent, nonsweet grapefruit 5 percent). And they contain an abundance of oxygen. Remember, microforms do not live well in the presence of oxygen, so these foods prevent microform overgrowth and an increase in mycotoxins.

Squeeze fresh lemon or lime into your purified water throughout the day—and especially before going to sleep for the night. Don't take lemon or lime within half an hour before a meal, or for ten minutes after you finish eating. It is best to drink an hour before eating, then wait until digestion has taken place to drink more.

Pomegranates

Pomegranates are alkalizing low-sugar fruits, rich in vitamins C, E, and B_6, and containing significant amounts of folic acid, B_1, B_2, and niacin as well. On the mineral front, pomegranates are a good source of potassium, copper, and iron. They contain other antioxidants as well, along with lots of flavonoids. Pomegranate seeds are loaded with omega-5 CLA oils, which neutralize acids among other benefits (see chapter 12 for more on the omega oils).

The juicy jewel-like seed sacs inside the pomegranate are the part of the fruit that is most commonly eaten. And they give you the most nutritional benefits, because you get the juice and the oils all at once. But you can also use pomegranate juice or pomegranate seed oil for even more concentrated nutrition.

Pomegranates support optimal health because they are alkalizing, antioxidant, and anti-inflammatory. The juice and oils help to build healthy red blood cells. These characteristics and their particular nutrient content also make them particularly beneficial for people with certain health challenges, especially high blood pressure, heart disease, gout, obesity, and digestive problems including diarrhea, cramps, and flatulence. Recent studies published in medical journals show a positive relationship between pomegranate consumption and lowered rates of cancerous prostates and hypertension. (Pomegranate is also helpful in getting rid of intestinal parasites, but the active ingredient for that, an alkaloid called pelletierine, is only in the rind and membranes of the fruit. Those are edible, or you can look for supplements made from those parts of the pomegranate.) The juice is also antiseptic, and so is useful to apply to cuts.

For all these reasons and more, we are proud to grow pomegranates alongside the avocados and grapefruits at our California ranch. Even those of you who can't walk out your back door and pick a fresh one off a tree should be sure to make pomegranates, pomegranate juice, and pomegranate seed oil a regular part of the diet.

Herbs and Spices

Herbs and spices provide both flavor and nutrition. Herbal teas can also be very beneficial. Freshness is again key: Herbs and spices can get moldy during processing (drying) and storage.

Juices

Although you lose the benefits of fiber, juicing enhances all the other benefits of vegetables and grasses. (Fruit juice, however, you should avoid. Details follow later in this chapter.) When you "drink your vegetables," your body is receiving a greater concentration of rapidly usable alkaline salts, vitamins, minerals, chlorophyll, and electrons, and can assimilate them more easily and rapidly.

Juice from green vegetables is highly alkalizing. If you are having any symptoms, you should limit the amount of beet and carrot juice you use, as they are sweet because they are relatively high in the acid sugar (11 percent and 13 percent sugar, respectively). Carrots are generally alkalizing, but concentrated the way they are in juice, they can quickly add up to too much acid sugar.

Though not technically juices, I also want to mention vegetable broths here, since they, too, are so alkalizing—particularly cucumber, onion, and garlic. You can make your own or buy premade (just check to make sure it is preservative-free and contains no yeast).

Low-Carbohydrate Vegetables

Complex carbohydrates make a lot of acid when they break down, and so should not exceed 20 percent of your diet. So the vegetables you choose should be mainly those that are low in carbohydrates (like the fresh veggies listed in the box on pages 86–7), and you should enjoy legumes and grains in limited quantities because they are high in complex carbohydrates.

Diets with 50 percent or more complex carbohydrates—which would encompass a lot of seemingly "perfect" low-fat, vegetarian diets as well as the official food pyramid—provide a favorable environment for microform overgrowth even in healthy digestive tracts. Simple carbohydrates—fruits, sugars, white flour—are even more conducive to overgrowth, and the typical American diet is full of them.

High-carbohydrate vegetables, including potatoes, winter squash (acorn, butternut, pumpkin), yams, and sweet potatoes can be eaten in moderation. When you do eat them, make sure they are fresh, not stored for a long period of time, and check them carefully for fungal spots (especially potatoes). Red new potatoes are the best choice in the potato family because they are this year's potatoes. Idaho potatoes and others could be years old by the time you get them, having been stored in silos. Red potatoes are fresher than other potatoes (except those you pick from your own garden), but still should be used sparingly.

If we lived in an ideal world, you'd be able to choose fresh legumes (beans and peas) as well. But almost all legumes sold in the stores are dried or canned—though I do get frozen edamame (soybeans) in my local health food store. Avoid the canned beans, by all means, but if you pick over, soak, and rinse the dried beans thoroughly before cooking, you can use them in that 20 percent of your diet. Beans are actually quite antifungal—even if you find a few bad beans, you never see the whole bag get moldy, so in moderation they are a good choice. Their starchiness is the main reason to limit quantities. The best choice of all is to eat sprouted beans (see page 163).

Most legumes are primarily starch: kidney beans, pinto beans, adzuki beans, black beans, white beans (navy beans), chickpeas (garbanzo beans), split peas, black-eyed peas (cowpeas), and lima beans. Two are primarily protein and so are okay to include more often: soybeans (especially edamame, the fresh, whole bean) and lentils.

The grains you eat must also be fresh, not stored. Stored grains are any grains stored into the next season. Look for a supplier that can assure you you're getting this season's grains—grains not more than three months away from having been harvested. Ask at your store to ask their supplier. Stored Grains are full of fungus and their mycotoxins (see "Stored Grains" on page 110 for details). Grains form acids when they are broken down, so limit how much you eat of them, and use only fresh, organic grains. Sprouted (see page 90) are best.

The most common complex-carbohydrate grains are the most acid forming: wheat and rice. (They make mucus, too.) They have to stay in that 20 percent of your diet. You should eliminate all wheat and rice, however, if you are sick or tired; a balanced, healthy body will be able to handle them in small amounts. Corn you should avoid altogether (more about that coming up). On the other hand, amaranth, quinoa, and spelt are only slightly acidic, and millet and buckwheat hover between neutral, slightly acid, and slightly alkaline, so they don't contribute to the formation of sticky acidic mucus.

There are other benefits to these grains as well. Buckwheat groats (really a seed, strictly speaking, but used like a grain) and millet are high in protein and digest slowly, keeping blood sugar balanced. Spelt contains more protein, healthy fats, and fiber than wheat. Spelt is also plentiful in mucopolysaccharides—vital complex sugars that literally glue the body together, lubricate joints, and support immune function. It is also high in B_{17}, which is an anticancer vitamin.

Non-Animal Protein

Here's a question we get a lot: "Where do you get your protein?" The inquiry presupposes, first, that protein comes only from meat, dairy, and eggs, and second, that getting enough protein is somehow difficult.

Expert research suggests we need only 25 grams—just one ounce—a day of protein. The average American who eats meat, eggs, and dairy probably gets 75 to 125 grams a day—three to five times more than we actually need. I believe protein should comprise roughly 5 to 7 percent of our total healthy diet.

Our bodies are just 7 percent protein (and 70 percent water, 20 percent fat, 1 to 2 percent vitamins and minerals, and 0.5 to 1 percent sugar). Most meats are 20 to 25 percent protein—therefore providing more than the human body requires. If you don't eat meat, never fear: Spinach and other greens are higher in amino acids (the building blocks of protein) than steak!

Cow's milk, too, is protein-rich. In contrast, a protein source specifically designed for human consumption—breast milk—is only 5 percent protein (and some sources put it as low as 1.4 to 2.2 percent). And that's meant to be the sole source of nutrition for a human who is growing and developing faster than at any other time of life—doubling or tripling body mass and size within the first year of life. If we really needed super-concentrated proteins for good growth and health, surely mother's milk would contain a much higher percentage. As it is, I believe the innate intelligence of Mother Nature reflects the body's actual requirements.

Some of the strongest animals in the world—take, for example, the gorilla, the horse, and the elephant—eat no meat. They are obviously not hurting for protein. What do they subsist on? Grass and leaves.

The truth is, there is plenty of protein in green plants. And if you are getting enough calories to be healthy, and you are eating a reasonable variety of foods, you're getting enough protein. Don't just take my word for it: A clinical study published in the very mainstream *Journal of the American Dietetic Association* analyzed the diets of meat eaters, vegetarians who eat dairy and eggs, and pure vegan vegetarians, using strict requirements about how much protein would easily cover the requirements of growing children and pregnant women. Not only did all three diets provide enough, they all actually doubled requirements. The take-home message is: No one has to worry about getting enough protein. If you eat a reasonable amount of alkaline foods, you will.

Most people seem to think protein needs to come from meat and dairy products. Even those more "in the know" about alternative health subscribed for a long time to the theory that vegetable proteins were somehow second-class and required proper "combining" to be complete. But vegetables carry all the amino acids (the building blocks of protein) the body needs. Not every vegetable has every one, of course, but if you are eating a wide variety of vegetables, especially dark green and dark green leafy vegetables, and supplementing with grasses, you are getting plenty of all the essential amino acids.

The body has a free amino acid pool, which contributes about seventy grams of protein daily. We all have these protein reserves, so unless you have specific symptoms of protein deficiency (muscle tissue loss, hair falling out, brittle nails), you can be sure you are getting enough protein.

We eat fish maybe once every other month. Other than that, we eat tofu a couple times a month. We often eat sprouted legumes, and get plenty of raw nuts, sprouted seeds and grains, like flax seed and hemp seed, and lots of avocados, all of which have high-quality protein that is better assimilated than animal proteins. All the rest of the protein we need we get from greens. The key to providing your body with protein is quality, not quantity. In fact, eating more protein than you need can make you tired, weak, and sick, especially the animal proteins that contribute sulfuric, nitric, phosphoric, and uric acid to the body.

PERCENTAGE OF CALORIES FROM PROTEIN IN ALKALIZING FOODS

Food	Protein Calories	Food	Protein Calories
Vegetables		Dandelion greens	27%
Alfalfa sprouts	40%	Eggplant	12%
Artichoke	29%	Fennel	28%
Asparagus	25%	Garlic	20%
Bamboo shoots	26%	Kale (leaves)	60%
Beet greens	22%	Leek	22%
Broccoli	49%	Lettuce, Boston	12%
Brussels sprouts	49%	Lettuce, green-leaf	42%
Cabbage, Chinese	12%	Lettuce, iceberg	27%
Cabbage, red	20%	Lettuce, loose-leaf	13%
Cauliflower	27%	Mustard greens	22%
Celery	10%	Okra	24%
Chard, Swiss	24%	Onion (green)	15%
Chives	18%	Parsley	36%
Collards (leaves)	48%	Pepper, green	12%
Collards (stems)	36%	Pepper, red	14%
Cress	26%	Pepper, red hot	13%
Cucumber	10%	Radish	10%

Food	Protein Calories	Food	Protein Calories
Rhubarb	11%	Pea, green fresh	6%
Seaweed, dulse	25%	Red bean, dried	23%
Spinach	49%	Soybean, dried	34%
Turnip greens	30%	Soybean, fresh	11%
Watercress	22%	Soybean sprouts	6%
Wheatgrass	25%	Tofu	43%
Zucchini	26%		
		Nuts and Seeds	
Fruits		Almond	19%
Avocado (California)	22%	Brazil nut	14%
Avocado (Florida)	15%	Filbert	13%
Grapefruit, sour	5%	Pumpkin seed	29%
Lemon	13%	Sesame seed	19%
Lemon juice	5%	Sunflower seed	24%
Tomato, green	12%	Sunflower seed, sprouted	33%
Tomato, red	18%		
		Grains	
Legumes		Barley	10%
Chickpea	25%	Millet	10%
Lentil	30%	Rice, brown	8%
Lima bean, fresh	9%	Wheat	17%
Mung sprouts	38%	Wheat bran	16%
Navy bean	26%		

SOY

Soy is a smart addition to your diet, as a source of protein and a wide variety of nutrients. Soybeans contain a host of beneficial chemicals:

- Isoflavones, a type of phytoestrogen ("plant estrogen"), help prevent the growth of hormone-dependent cancers, such as many breast cancers.
- Daidzein, a particular isoflavone, inhibits the growth of cancer. It also promotes cell differentiation in animals—cancerous cells being undifferentiated.
- Genistein is a phytochemical that can inhibit tumor growth and promote cell differentiation. Studies have shown that it helps block the growth of prostate cancer cells and breast cancer.

- Protease inhibitors (more phytochemicals) block the action of enzymes or acids that may promote tumor growth and work against a wide range of cancers, including some of the most common—colon, breast, and liver cancers.
- Physic acid chelates mycotoxins that promote tumor growth, binding to them and taking them out of the body. Studies have shown that it can help reduce the size and number of tumors in laboratory animals fed mycotoxins.
- Saponins, studies have shown, lower the risk of certain cancers, including those of the breast, prostate, stomach, and lung. (Saponins are also found in chickpeas and ginseng.)
- Soy works to help prevent some cancers, protect the heart, and balance the endocrine glands.

Your best bet is fresh soy sprouts (see "Sprouts" on page 90) or a soy sprout supplement (see chapter 12). Other choices are soybeans, edamame, tofu, soybean oil, and non-GMO lecithin (a soy by-product that comes as liquid or granules to be used in recipes or sprinkled on salads and soups, or taken as a supplement). Soy milk, however, is usually not a good option, as almost all kinds contain added rice syrup to sweeten them—and the syrup ferments and creates more acidity. Nonsweet soy milk is okay. Organic is best, as always, and fresh is crucial.

I recommend sprouts without reservation, but whole beans are slightly acidic, and processed soybeans require some cautions. In processing soybeans, the intact bean is altered—cells broken, protective coating removed—which activates the inherent microzymas to start decomposing their surroundings. And of course, many soy products (such as soy hot dogs) are just as refined and processed as any junk food. I wish we all had access to fresh tofu whenever we wanted it, so we could eat it on the same day it was produced. But in this reality, your best bet is simply to use a packaged brand that is dated, rinse it thoroughly, and use it as soon as possible. Don't let it sit in the refrigerator for long.

With that in mind, tofu is a very good source of protein, it's certainly far better for you than animal and dairy foods, and it's alkaline when combined with calcium carbonate. (One study pinpointed eating tofu as the single factor associated with a lower risk of developing prostate cancer among Japanese men living in Hawaii. Another found a strong correlation between consumption of soy foods and a decreased risk of developing breast cancer in Chinese women.) Tofu is a good food for making the transition to a vegetarian diet, and occasionally as part of a balanced, wholesome diet.

On the other hand, you must avoid fermented soy products such as miso, tempeh, and soy sauce (see page 113).

Fresh Fish (Occasionally, or as a Transition Food)

Fish is rich in healthy omega-3 oils (essential fatty acids), protein, and several nutrients. Still, it shares the properties of all animal foods: It has no fiber and forms acid and sticky mucus. And it's hard to know if it has come from clean water, whether river, lake, or ocean. On balance, fish is still a good choice for making the transition to a vegetarian diet, or used on occasion in the context of a healthy (basic) diet.

If you do choose to eat fish, it must be absolutely fresh. If it isn't newly caught, or you can smell that fishy smell, it is already spoiling—so you must avoid it. You want to make sure it comes from unpolluted water. Choose sea bass, salmon, trout, red snapper, swordfish, and tuna, for their high levels of omega-3 oils, but be sure to avoid shellfish altogether. Shellfish are scavengers—they eat anything and everything, including the feces of other fish. As a result, they are full of toxins. Skip dried fish, which is used in many Asian dishes, especially soups, as it has fungus and mycotoxins on it. (Although the FDA has declared that swordfish and tuna have potentially high mercury levels and so should be restricted or avoided, at least by women of childbearing age, I believe the good oils you get from these fish far offset any risk for mercury poisoning when following the program in this book, which limits the amount of fish you eat.)

THE pH OF FOOD

The following is a list of common foods with an approximate, relative potential of acidity (−) or alkalinity (+), as present in one ounce of food.

Vegetables and Low-Sugar Fruits

Peas, ripe	+0.5
Asparagus	+1.1
Artichokes	+1.3
Comfrey	+1.5
Green cabbage (March harvest)	+2.0
Lettuce	+2.2
Onion	+3.0
Cauliflower	+3.1
White radish (spring)	+3.1
Rutabaga	+3.1
White cabbage	+3.3
Green cabbage (December harvest)	+4.0
Savoy cabbage	+4.5
Lamb's lettuce	+4.8
Peas, fresh	+5.1
Kohlrabi	+5.1
Zucchini	+5.7
Red cabbage	+6.3
Rhubarb stalks	+6.3
Horseradish	+6.8
Leeks (bulbs)	+7.2
Watercress	+7.7
Spinach (March harvest)	+8.0
Turnip	+8.0
Lime	+8.2
Chives	+8.3
Carrot	+9.5
Lemon	+9.9
French-cut beans (green beans)	+11.2
Fresh red beet	+11.3
Sorrel	+11.5

Spinach (harvested other than March)	+13.1
Garlic	+13.2
Celery	+13.3
Tomato	+13.6
Cabbage lettuce, fresh	+14.1
Endive, fresh	+14.5
Avocado	+15.6
Broccoli	+16.2
Red radish	+16.7
Cayenne pepper	+18.8
Straw grass	+21.4
Shave grass	+21.7
Dog grass	+22.6
Dandelion	+22.7
Kamut grass	+27.6
Barley grass	+28.7
Soy sprouts	+29.5
Sprouted radish seeds	+28.4
Sprouted chia seeds	+28.5
Alfalfa grass	+29.3
Cucumber, fresh	+31.5
Wheatgrass	+33.8
Summer black radish	+39.4

Nonstored Organic Grains and Legumes

White rice	−18.5
Brown rice	−12.5
Wheat	−10.1
Buckwheat groats	−0.5
Millet	−0.5
Spelt	−0.5
Lentils	+0.6
Soy flour	+2.5

Tofu	+3.2	Almonds	+3.6
Lima beans	+12.0	Hemp seeds	+7.6
Soybeans, fresh	+12.0		
White beans (navy beans)	+12.1	**Fats (Fresh,**	
Granulated soy (cooked,		**Cold-Pressed Oils)**	
ground soybeans)	+12.8	Sunflower oil	−6.7
Soy nuts (soaked		Ghee	−1.6
soybeans, then air-dried)	+26.5	Coconut milk	−1.5
Soy lecithin, pure	+38.0	Olive oil	+1.0
		Pomegranate oil	+ 3.1
Nuts and Seeds		Borage oil	+3.2
Wheat kernel	−11.4	Flax seed oil	+3.5
Walnuts	−8.0	Evening primrose oil	+4.1
Pumpkin seeds	−5.6	Hemp oil	+4.7
Sunflower seeds	−5.4	Marine lipids	+4.7
Macadamia nuts	−3.2		
Hazelnuts	−2.0	**Water**	
Flax seeds	−1.3	Distilled water (neutral)	
Brazil nuts	−0.5	Fresh coconut water	+9.04
Sesame seeds	+0.5		
Cumin seeds	+1.1	**Fish**	
Fennel seeds	+1.3	Freshwater fish	−11.8
Caraway seeds	+2.3		

WHAT TO AVOID

Sugar

Sugar is an acid waste product created in the body as a result of metabolism. And it causes healthy body cells to biologically transform into bacteria and yeast. Sugar feeds biological transformation like gasoline feeds a fire. All forms of sugar (white sugar, brown sugar, processed beet, cane, and corn sugars and syrups, maple syrup, honey, molasses, sucrose, fructose, maltose, lactose, glucose, mannitol, sorbitol, galactose, monosaccharides, date sugar, turbinado sugar, candy, soft drinks, pastries, ice cream, chocolate, carob, and, yes, even "natural" sugars from fruit)—especially those that cause a rapid rise of blood sugar (cane sugars and corn sugars)—create an environment for the birth of bacteria, yeast, and mold from within the body. That's because all sugars are acid and can produce acetaldehyde (a toxin and carcinogen) and alcohol in the body. The more sugar the body gets, the more harmful microforms evolve internally, and the faster they will reproduce. And the faster they reproduce, the more they are decomposing and fermenting your body from the inside. Cut them off by alkalizing.

Contrary to popular belief, the body does not need sugar. It needs energy or electrons, and energy or electrons come from alkaline food and drink. You will find some sugar in the vegetables we recommend, but our organs are much more able to handle these gentle vegetable sugars, and can eliminate them efficiently.

Be sure not to replace sugar with artificial sweeteners, which are just as bad or worse (see page 115). If you really need to sweeten something, consider the green herb stevia, or chicory, which you can find at health food stores. Even though they are better choices, they are acidic, too, and should never be used when dealing with a serious illness.

Australian researchers have found that over the long term, acidic eating habits, and especially a diet with a lot of sugar, can actually damage our genetic material, DNA. Even a single dose of sugar can affect cells for up to two weeks, changing the body's metabolic response to food, switching off genetic controls designed to protect the body against dietary and metabolic acids, leaving the door open to symptoms of diabetes, heart disease, and cancer. With that kind of input regularly, over time, the effects are amplified, and genetic damage can result. It can last months or years, or even be permanent—and heritable. An alkaline diet without sugar keeps your genes protected, so they can protect you.

Simple Carbohydrates Are Simply Acid

Simple carbohydrates are sugars and cause the same acidic problems. This category includes white flour (and anything made from it, such as bread and pasta), white rice, corn (which you should be avoiding because of its fungal content, anyway), and potato.

Even complex carbohydrates may have to be restricted (or temporarily eliminated; see chapter 11), especially if you have more serious symptoms, since complex carbohydrates break down into simple ones—or complex sugars—and from there into straight glucose: sugar or straight acid.

Refined and Processed Foods

You've got to skip the "junk food" (I hate to even dignify it by calling it food!). Yes, that means chips and cookies and doughnuts and just about anything you can get at fast-food restaurants, and so on (and on, and on, and on). But it also includes many foods you may not have been concerned about before, such as the low-calorie frozen dinner you had last night, or the frozen burrito, or the canned soup. All these things are refined and processed to within an inch of their lives, and whatever nutrients they may have had to begin with are trashed in the process, even in the so-called enriched products. On top of that, they are loaded with sugar, processed or refined salt, artificial colorings and flavorings, additives, preservatives, and butter, margarine, or hydrogenated or partially hydrogenated (hardened) vegetable oil—and deficient in fiber. They are, of course, all acidifying.

Fruit

Though fruit has many good vitamins and minerals, and is rich in fiber, it is also filled with the acid sugar. (Pineapples are 28 percent sugar, bananas 25 percent, honeydew melons 21 percent, mangoes 18 percent, apples 15 percent, oranges and cherries 12 percent, strawberries 11 percent, and watermelon 9 percent, just to name a few.) Despite what some nutritionists claim, there is no difference in your body between natural sugars and any other kind. Sugar is sugar—and acid is acid—it doesn't matter if it is honey, agave, jelly beans, maple syrup, or a berry or a piece of melon. In any form, microforms love it and will ferment it into alcohol and other mycotoxins and create an acidic environment in your body. So with the exception of lemons, limes, and occasionally nonsweet grapefruit, which actually turn out to be basic, fruit must be avoided to gain a healthfully balanced body. You can get all the same nutritional benefits from vegetables and low-sugar fruit without the negative side effects. Once you are in balance, a small portion of fresh seasonal fruit, eaten by itself, can make a nice treat.

By the way, here's a little insight into why fruit gets sweeter as it ripens: The complex carbohydrates are fermenting into simpler and sweeter ones (acidic sugars), which are then fermented further as yeast evolves out of the fruit cells. The fruit is actually turning into alcohol and mold—rotting, basically. Appetizing, huh?

Fruit juice is even worse, as the acid sugars are more concentrated and the fiber has been lost. Most of it is also processed and pasteurized, and it is almost always made from second-quality fruits—those that were too damaged or dirty or diseased to sell whole—and already contaminated with harmful microforms and mycotoxins.

THE pH OF FRUIT

The following is a list of common foods with an approximate, relative potential of acidity (−) or alkalinity (+), as present in one ounce of food.

Rose hips	−15.5	Black currant	−6.1
Pineapple	−12.6	Strawberry	−5.4
Mandarin orange	−11.5	Blueberry	−5.3
Banana, ripe	−10.1	Raspberry	−5.1
Pear	−9.9	Yellow plum	−4.9
Peach	−9.7	Italian plum	−4.9
Apricot	−9.5	Date	−4.7
Papaya	−9.4	Cherry, sweet	−3.6
Orange	−9.2	Cantaloupe	−2.5
Mango	−8.7	Fig juice powder	−2.4
Tangerine	−8.5	Grapefruit	−1.7
Currant	−8.2	Watermelon	−1.0
Gooseberry, ripe	−7.7	Coconut, fresh	+0.5
Grape, ripe	−7.6	Cherry, sour	+3.5
Cranberry	−7.0	Banana, unripe	+4.8
Pomegranate	−7.0		

Dairy Products

Like most animal foods, dairy products contain acidic hormones and pesticide residues, microforms, mycotoxins, and saturated acid fats. Layered on top of all those goodies, milk sugar (lactose) breaks down like any acid sugar and causes the biological transformation of healthy body cells into bacteria, yeast, and mold. All dairy products produce lactic acid. Furthermore, dairy cows feed on stored grains laced with acidic hormones and antibiotics made from sugar and fungi, which are then concentrated in milk. Then, too, cheese and yogurt are made by fermentation. And dairy is the leader of all foods in forming sticky mucus. It is highly acid forming. It can increase risk of cancers, including ovarian and endometrial. Furthermore, pasteurization destroys the beneficial electrons milk starts out with. And pasteurization doesn't even really work! Pasteurized milk left out will rot and stink, whereas raw milk curdles naturally and is still edible.

With all that to recommend them, you can see why all dairy products should be eliminated from your diet. Try soy, almond, or hemp milk as alternatives (though look carefully to avoid the vast majority of them that are filled with added sugar). If you must have milk, use unprocessed goat's milk from organically grown and grazing goats. It contains the antifungal caprylic acid.

No matter how many times you were told by teachers and parents to drink your milk, and no matter how cute the milk mustache ads starring highly paid athletes and movie stars are, the idea that dairy products are healthy is pure hype—a cultural myth. Even if cows lived in some kind of bovine utopia and produced the perfect milk, let's face it: It simply isn't a human food. It is designed for baby cows, whose requirements are far different from those of humans. Milk is full of components of no use to us, and they must either be converted to use (wasting our body's resources in the process) or eliminated as toxins. No other animal species drinks milk beyond infancy—and certainly not from a species outside their own!

Milk is only the beginning of the problem. Consider that it takes ten pounds of milk to make one pound of hard cheese, twelve pounds to make one pound of ice cream, and more than twenty-one pounds to make one pound of butter. Remembering that it takes twenty parts alkalinity to neutralize one part acidity, just imagine what it takes to counter the effects of so concentrated a source of acid! If it would take 20 cups of something alkaline to neutralize 1 cup of milk (already bad enough, don't you think?), you'd need twelve times as much—240 cups, or fifteen gallons!—to neutralize a cup of ice cream.

No wonder so many people do so poorly on dairy foods. No wonder so many suffer with osteoporosis while still ingesting so much dairy. No wonder so many people have allergic reactions to dairy foods, or are lactose-intolerant. No wonder people can gain weight quickly on dairy foods and lose it so quickly when they go off these very concentrated foods. They are just too concentrated, and are ultra-acidic in the bloodstream.

WHAT ABOUT CALCIUM?

We get asked this question a lot. It is true that calcium is vital for many functions in the body, but the current rage for getting huge doses of the mineral—through large quantities of dairy products daily as well as supplements—is based in faulty understandings of how the body uses it. Many people worry—totally unnecessarily—that if milk products are eliminated, their diet will leave them deficient in calcium.

The fact is that all leafy, green vegetables and grasses are inherently high in calcium (as well as iron, magnesium, vitamin C, and many of the B vitamins, but that's another story), as are celery, cauliflower, okra, onions, green beans, avocado, black beans, garbanzo beans (chickpeas), tofu, almonds, hazelnuts, and sesame seeds. In short, you get plenty of calcium with a diet that looks like the one described in this book. When we're asked about where we get our calcium, we often answer with a question of our own: Where does a cow get hers?

It is also important to evaluate how much calcium you really need to keep your bones and body healthy. To do so, you must understand that one of the things calcium does in the body is neutralize the acid created by eating animal protein. When you eat these acidic foods, the body tries to return to its alkaline state the only way it can—by withdrawing calcium from your bones if there isn't enough on hand in the food itself to do the job. Your kidneys also rob your bones in order to eliminate the excess nitrogen found in animal protein.

The current recommendations for a thousand milligrams or more a day of calcium assume an average American diet—which consists of one and a half to four times as much protein as necessary, creating an unnatural and unhealthy demand for calcium. Many experts blame the seeming epidemic of the bone-weakening disease osteoporosis on this protein overdose. It isn't really a lack of calcium at all! Rather, it is a calcium-robbing problem, not a calcium-deficiency problem. We need to stop worrying about not getting enough calcium and pay attention instead to not getting too much protein. In the meantime, we're living the irony that getting plenty of calcium-rich dairy products can actually leave us with a negative calcium balance by the time all that protein is buffered.

Just to confirm, in a way that even mainstream science could understand, that we're getting enough calcium in our own bodies, we both recently had bone density tests. We have been essentially vegan for approximately twenty years now, and both of our tests came out with densities well above average. Shelley's rating was similar to a twenty-year-old's (when bone density usually peaks)—though she was forty-six at the time. Rob was also in the very highest percentile at age forty-eight.

CALCIUM CONTENT OF ALKALIZING FOODS

Food	Calcium	Food	Calcium
	(per 100 grams/4 ounces of food)		
Vegetables		Spinach	93 mg
Artichoke	51 mg	Turnip greens	246 mg
Asparagus	23 mg	Watercress	151 mg
Bamboo shoots	13 mg		
Beet greens	119 mg	**Fruits**	
Broccoli	103 mg	Avocado (California)	10 mg
Brussels sprouts	36 mg	Avocado (Florida)	10 mg
Cabbage, Chinese	43 mg	Grapefruit, sour	16 mg
Cabbage, red	42 mg	Lemon juice	7 mg
Cauliflower	25 mg	Tomato, green	13 mg
Celery	39 mg	Tomato, red	13 mg
Chard, Swiss	88 mg		
Chives	69 mg	**Legumes**	
Collards (leaves)	250 mg	Chickpea	150 mg
Collards (stems)	203 mg	Lentil, dried	79 mg
Cress	81 mg	Lima bean, fresh	52 mg
Cucumber	25 mg	Mung sprouts	118 mg
Dandelion greens	187 mg	Pea, green fresh	26 mg
Eggplant	12 mg	Red bean, dried	110 mg
Fennel	100 mg	Soybean, dried	226 mg
Garlic	29 mg	Soybean, fresh	67 mg
Kale (leaves)	249 mg	Soybean sprouts	48 mg
Kale (stem)	179 mg		
Leek	52 mg	**Nuts and Seeds**	
Lettuce, Boston	35 mg	Almond	234 mg
Lettuce, iceberg	20 mg	Brazil nut	186 mg
Lettuce, loose-leaf	68 mg	Filbert	209 mg
Mustard greens	183 mg	Pumpkin seeds	51 mg
Okra	92 mg	Sesame seeds	1,160 mg
Onion, green	51 mg	Sunflower seeds	120 mg
Parsley	203 mg		
Pepper, green	9 mg	**Grains**	
Pepper, red	13 mg	Barley	34 mg
Pepper, red hot	130 mg	Millet	20 mg
Radish	30 mg	Rice, brown	32 mg
Rhubarb	96 mg	Wheat	46 mg
Seaweed, agar	567 mg	Wheat bran	119 mg
Seaweed, dulse	296 mg		

Processed Salt

The negative effects of processed salt are well known, and yet the typical American diet is crammed with it, starting with a saltshaker on just about every dining table in the country. Even if you never use a saltshaker, you can easily overdose on processed salt with processed foods—boxed, bottled, bagged, frozen, or canned—restaurant food, and junk food, all of which are, unless specifically labeled otherwise, generally loaded with salt.

Aim to eliminate all added processed salt from your diet.

Saturated and Other Unhealthy Fats

As healthful as the essential fatty acids are, the wrong fats are devastating. You know the litany of bad effects: clogged arteries, heart disease, cancer, and so on. The villains are hydrogenated or partially hydrogenated (saturated, solidified) vegetable oil, margarine, butter, saturated fats, and almost all animal fats (from meat, poultry, eggs, and dairy—fish alone escapes).

Your aim here, too, is to eliminate all these dangerous fats from your diet. Don't cook your food in fat or oil (steam it), and don't smother it with them afterward.

I want to be clear, here, however: I am not advocating a nonfat diet. Your body needs good fats to survive, and to be fully healthy. Use good oils like olive, flax seed, and grape seed (and our favorites: Udo's and Essential Balance, which are blends!).

Meat and Eggs

Like dairy foods—like all animal products—meat (pork, beef, lamb, chicken, turkey, and so on) and eggs are filled with acidic hormones, pesticides, steroids, antibiotics, microforms, mycotoxins, and the saturated fats that contribute to heart disease, strokes, and cancer, among many other things. (While I agree that the fat itself is part of the problem, consider also that fat is where animals' bodies store the toxins they've been fed and exposed to.) And they are highly acidic. Eating animal protein results in uric, nitric, sulfuric, and phosphoric acids in the body. (If you test the pH of your urine first thing in the morning after eating animal protein the previous day, you'll see a dramatically lowered acidic pH.)

The animals feed on stored grain and pass along all the associated problems in their meat (see "Stored Grains" on page 110). What I'm trying to say is: Don't have anything to do with them.

There is a strong correlation between animal protein and several kinds of cancer, particularly breast, thyroid, prostate, pancreatic, endometrial, ovarian, stomach, and colon cancers. Studies show that people who get 70 percent of their protein from animal products have major health difficulties compared with those who get just 5 percent of their protein that way: seventeen times the death rate from heart disease, for example, and five times the likelihood of dying of breast cancer (for women).

The consumption of eggs, alone, is associated with increased risk of colon cancer. I'm not surprised, as eggs from grain-fed chickens have been documented to contain mycotoxins. (My own observations have revealed that fifteen minutes after eating an egg, people will show bacteria, or an increase in bacteria, in their blood.) Dairy products were also incriminated in the same study, with the highest association being with cheese. Interestingly, increased consumption of red meat did not increase risk. I attribute this fact to the study being done in Argentina, where the beef cattle are usually pasture-grazed rather than grain-fed. This is not to say that red meat from grazing animals is good food—just that it may be the lesser of two evils.

An Australian study also turned up a positive association between egg consumption and colon cancer, as well as links with intake of red meat, liver, dairy foods, and poultry.

Researchers studying the effects of a Western-style diet in Japanese women found that it was linked to a higher risk of breast cancer because of the much larger amounts of meat included. Scientists started down this track after noting that breast cancer was rare in Japanese women before World War II.

Another study linked poultry, ham, salami, bacon, and sausage to increased risk of thyroid cancer, as well as cheese, butter, and oils other than olive oil. (Olive oil is generally free of mycotoxins.)

Yet another study supported the fact that the type of dietary fat consumed influences the occurrence of endometrial, ovarian, and stomach cancers—with animal-derived fats contributing to an increased risk. People in the study who developed cancer ate more bacon and ham, used more butter in cooking, and drank more whole milk.

A Swedish study found a number of dietary factors to be associated with pancreatic cancer, including higher consumption of fried and grilled meat (as well as margarine on white bread—just to remind us that simply being vegetarian isn't enough to solve the whole problem).

Processed meats and cheeses are even worse, thanks to their nitrosamines, and are a risk factor for brain and spinal cord tumors.

Besides, animal foods are simply dead or absent of electrical potential or electrons. Vegetable foods, alive with electron energy, and phytonutrients, are far superior in every way.

All meats properly aged for human consumption are, by definition, partially fermented, and thus permeated with microforms and their toxins. It is yeast, after all, that causes the aging, and the final taste and texture is determined by the nature of the microbial aging process. (That's on top of the mycotoxins in the animals' feed, which then show up in their muscles—the meat.) One of the specific mycotoxins involved has been linked to diabetes. In case you were wondering, most mycotoxins are heat-tolerant, so cooking doesn't get rid of them, even if it kills off some of their creators.

Whatever nutrients may be in animal foods, they simply are not worth the risks—not to mention the stress they put on the body during digestion and through the energy required to extract what nutrients they contain.

Anatomically and physiologically, humans are just not meant to be carnivores or omnivores. The long, complicated human digestive tract is designed for the slow absorption of complex and stable plant food. Carnivores have short, simple bowels to allow for minimum transit time of unstable, dead animal food. Their intestinal microorganisms are different from humans', too.

On the other side of the coin, starch digestion in humans is quite elaborate, whereas carnivores eat little or no starch. If humans were carnivores, we'd be sweating through our tongues instead of our skin. Flesh eaters have teeth and jaws designed for tearing apart freshly killed animals. Only our hand tools allow us to override this obvious natural limitation, not to mention the fact that we get none of the nutrition contained in fur, feathers, organs, and bones, the way true carnivores do. Finally, we seldom eat raw flesh. We almost always need to cook it to kill parasites and other harmful microforms, and to disguise the corpse that it is, none of which is necessary for real meat eaters. Humans are designed to be vegetarian, and our bodies will never work their best if we keep forcing them to do something they are not equipped to handle.

Stored Grains

Stored grains means last year's crop. Grains that are stored will usually begin to ferment within ninety days, and in short order are full of mycotoxins. They also harbor harmful microforms. So you want to get this year's crop, preferably within three months of being harvested. The only way I know of to get fresh grains is to ask the store manager to check the dating on the packing (if you buy in bulk), or to check with the supplier. It is always important to read the labels.

Unstored grains are a healthy part of your diet, generally, though you should cut them out for the initial eight to twelve weeks at the beginning of our program—after a cleansing, or for as long as you have symptoms.

Eating stored grains is, not surprisingly, damaging to the body. For example, a 1991 study found positive correlations between eating stored grains and esophageal cancer. That same year, researchers identified cooked cereal (a form of stored grain) as a risk factor in stomach cancer.

Stored potatoes are similarly risky. To take just one example: In pregnant women who consume large amounts of potatoes, two mycotoxins produced by fungi commonly found in potatoes have been incriminated as a cause of spina bifida in their offspring.

Yeast

You must scratch all yeast—brewer's and baker's and "nutritional"—and yeast-containing foods from your diet. Obviously, you don't want to be taking in pure microforms. Besides, the most common ways to get yeasts are bad for you for other reasons, too: beer and wine (double whammies, as alcohol is a danger) and breads and baked goods (a triple whammy because of the stored grains the flour is made from and the sugar and other simple carbs they contain).

Eating yeast and anything made with yeast can spur microform overgrowth and increase mycotoxins (increasing the amount created in your own body, in addition to whatever's in the product itself). If you need anything else to discourage your use, you should know that yeast food products can cause kidney stones (and stones in the liver, gallbladder, and even brain), bone deposits, osteoarthritis, rheumatoid arthritis, kidney disease, heart disease, diabetes (in a 1990 study, all mice fed a diet containing 10 percent brewer's yeast developed diabetes), sarcoidosis (an autoimmune disease affecting the lungs, eyes, and skin), cirrhosis, and many cancers, particularly breast, prostate, and liver. Other resulting symptoms include Crohn's disease and colitis.

Read labels carefully to make sure all your foods, condiments, and seasonings are yeast-free.

"Edible" Fungus

Mushrooms of all kinds and in all forms—besides the obvious problem that they are themselves the fruiting bodies of yeast or fungus—form acids as they are digested. They also contain mycotoxins that poison human cells and lead to degenerative diseases. In my opinion, there is no such thing as a good mushroom. The "edible" ones are just less poisonous than the ones that kill you immediately! Don't eat them, don't drink them, don't even sniff them. Mushrooms all contain various amounts of the mycotoxin amanitin, which, in large amounts, will kill you almost instantly. With smaller amounts the result is the same—it just takes a little longer.

In a 1979 study, a leading cancer researcher administered mushroom mycotoxins to mice in their drinking water. She noted twenty-one different types of cancer as a result. Now we know that all mushrooms contain at least five active ingredients that exhibit carcinogenic properties in animals.

Many impressive health claims have been made for some mushrooms, but they do have occasional toxic side effects—and all the same problems as any other mushroom. I believe all of their alleged benefits can easily be obtained in other—safer—ways.

Spirulina and Algae Supplements

We wish we could go along with the glowing recommendations for spirulina and algae supplements. After all, they are green plants rich in chlorophyll, protein, minerals, and other nutrients. But they thrive in acid conditions. And just think of what they really are: the scum you see growing on the surface of stagnant ponds and lakes. Toxins in algae have been shown to harm the liver and nervous system, and one seems to spur tumor growth in animals.

Algae supplements do contain vitamin B_{12}, which is not found in veggies—including this one in its pure state. Rather, it is made by bacteria that get into the algae via bird feathers and droppings. Call me crazy, but since we have our own intestinal bacteria that can make B_{12}, I'd rather not get my B_{12} from bird droppings!

Fortunately, any benefits from a day's dose of algae differ little from those in a serving of organic broccoli, so you can reap the benefits without facing the risks.

Fermented and Malted Products

This includes condiments such as vinegar, mustard, ketchup, steak sauce, soy sauce, tamari, mayonnaise, salad dressings, chili sauce, horseradish, miso, monosodium glutamate (MSG), and any kind of alcohol, as well as pickled vegetables such as relish, green olives, sauerkraut, and, of course, pickles. And tempeh. All are acid forming and create sticky mucus and, with the exception of MSG, are fermented by fungus.

Malt products such as malted milk and certain cereals and candy are also fermented by fungus and, besides containing high levels of sugar, are acid-forming and create sticky mucus.

Alcohol

Alcohol is an acid. And think about it this way: Alcohol is a mycotoxin made by yeast. That includes wine, beer, whiskey, brandy, gin, rum, and vodka, to name just the most popular. You already know that abuse of alcohol causes disease, including cirrhosis of the liver, brain damage, cancers, fetal injury, and death. That's before you even factor in the damage any mycotoxin can do—and it doesn't take what mainstream medicine considers abusive quantities for serious harm to be done. On top of that, the liver can convert alcohol into yet another mycotoxin (acetaldehyde), with its own harmful ways.

Caffeine

The main sources of caffeine are chocolate, cocoa, tea, sodas, and all forms of coffee—even decaffeinated contains enough to have a negative effect on you. All are acid and produce a lot of acid and a lot of mucus. I have seen it under the microscope. Tissues are compromised as well, which can be seen in a decline in urine pH in people eating caffeine.

Now think about the foods commonly eaten along with a cup of coffee or tea (often traditional breakfast foods and desserts), all of which are also acid producers, and you'll see it is a recipe for disaster.

Furthermore, caffeine is addicting. You could take the word of researchers at Johns Hopkins School of Medicine for it—or simply observe your own headaches when you've been deprived of your morning jolt. Eighty-two percent of volunteers for that Johns Hopkins study showed withdrawal symptoms when they were given a placebo instead of their usual dose of caffeine. Official estimates are that more than 80 percent of adults in the

United States regularly consume enough caffeine to produce addiction. Do your part to bring down that grim statistic!

Corn, Corn Products, Peanuts, and Peanut Products

Corn contains twenty-five different mycotoxin-producing fungi, including recognized carcinogens! Peanuts contain twenty-six. On top of that, broken and ground nuts (of any kind) are ready targets for airborne mold spores and quickly become rancid. You can see it on the nuts as a dark or black discoloring. Contamination occurs during the growing process because the plants themselves are not resistant. Humans who eventually ingest them are also eating the fungi and their toxic waste, inoculating their digestive tracts with negative microforms.

Research has linked corn consumption with cancers of the esophagus and stomach, and peanuts with pancreatic and liver cancer.

Cashew nuts and dried coconut are similarly contaminated, and should also be avoided.

Heated Oils

Any oils that have been cooked, or heated in processing, have been nutritionally destroyed, including the biggest brands of corn, canola, and other vegetable oils. Look for cold-pressed virgin oils instead, such as many olive oils, choosing from the healthy varieties, of course.

Microwaved Food

First of all, microwaving your food depletes the electron life energy, just because it is cooking it. But it gets much worse. The Russians, who have done the most diligent research on microwave ovens and their biological effects on food and humans, outlawed their use. In their research, foods that were exposed to microwave energy increased in cancer-causing effects and decreased in nutritional value. Vitamins and minerals were made useless in every food tested, and the bioavailability of nutrients, including the B vitamins, vitamins C and E, and essential minerals, decreased. Meat proteins were rendered worthless (not that we're recommending nonmicrowaved meat, but just to show you how powerful these machines are—in generally unacknowledged ways). Microwaving also interfered with the digestibility of fruits and vegetables. To top it all off, microwaving makes all foods acid forming. In my own work, I see a higher-than-normal percentage of abnormal blood cells in the blood of people who eat microwaved foods.

Artificial Sweeteners

Artificial sweeteners are acidifying. The bad guys include aspartame (NutraSweet), saccharine (Sweet'N Low), neotame, sucralose (Splenda), acesulfame (Sunett, Sweet & Safe, Sweet One), and cyclamates. They all break down into deadly acids in the body. For example, when you ingest aspartame, one of the ingredients, methyl alcohol, converts into formaldehyde, a deadly neurotoxin and known carcinogen! But that's not all. From there, it turns into formic acid (which is, by the way, the poison fire ants use in their attacks). And that's just one ingredient in one of the many artificial sweeteners.

A wide variety of symptoms can be caused by artificial sweeteners, including headaches, migraines, dizziness, vertigo, seizures, depression, fatigue, irritability, increased heart rate, heart palpitations, insomnia, vision problems, hearing loss, ringing in the ears, weight gain, numbness, muscle spasms, joint pain, breathing difficulties, anxiety attacks, slurred speech, and a loss of taste. Artificial sweeteners can also trigger or worsen arthritis, chronic fatigue, diabetes, fibromyalgia, brain tumors, MS, Parkinson's, Alzheimer's, systemic lupus, mental retardation, birth defects, thyroid disorders, lymphoma, and epilepsy. Don't let them into your body to do their worst.

Safer sweeteners to use would be natural plant sources such as the herb stevia or chicory, which you can find in your natural food store. Even these natural sweeteners are acid, though. So use them if you must, but ideally you'll skip all forms of sugar.

The pH of Food

The following is a list of common foods with an approximate, relative potential of acidity (–) or alkalinity (+), as present in one ounce of food.

Root Vegetables

Corn	–9.6
Stored potatoes	+2.0

Meat, Poultry, and Fish

Pork	–38.0
Veal	–35.0
Beef	–34.5
Ocean fish	–20.0
Chicken	–18.0 to –22.0
Eggs	–18.0 to –22.0
Oysters	–5.0
Liver	–3.0
Organ meats	–3.0

Milk and Milk Products

Hard cheese	–18.1
Quark	–17.3
Cream	–3.9
Homogenized milk	–1.0
Buttermilk	+1.3

Bread, Biscuits (Stored Grains/ Risen Dough)

White bread	–10.0
White biscuit	–6.5
Whole-meal bread	–6.5
Whole-grain bread	–4.5
Rye bread	–2.5

Nuts

Pistachios	–16.6
Peanuts	–12.8
Macadamia	–11.7
Cashews	–9.3

Fats

Margarine	–7.6
Corn oil	–6.5
Butter	–3.9

Sweets

Artificial sweeteners	–26.5
White sugar (refined cane sugar)	–17.6
Beet sugar	–15.1
Molasses	–14.6
Dr. Bronner's Barley Malt Sweetener	–9.8
Dried sugar cane juice (Sucanat)	–9.6
Fructose	–9.5
Turbinado sugar	–9.5
Milk sugar	–9.4
Barley malt syrup	–9.3
Brown rice syrup	–8.7
Honey	–7.6

Condiments

Vinegar	–39.4
Soy sauce	–36.2
Mustard	–19.2
Mayonnaise	–12.5
Ketchup	–12.4

Beverages

Liquor	–28.6 to –38.7
Fruit juice sweetened with white sugar	–33.4
Tea (black)	–27.1
Beer	–26.8
Coffee	–25.1
Wine	–16.4
Fruit juice, packaged, natural	–8.7

Rick Laurenzi's Story[*]

I'd been a student of holistic health for all of my adult life, but that didn't stop me from eating my way up to being over 360 pounds a few years ago. I started to eat all acidic all the time after a near-fatal motorcycle accident and a six-week hospital stay left me wheelchair-bound for months. I was so happy just to be alive, I didn't care *what* I ate. Good thing, too, because I couldn't really shop or cook (still can't cook!), so for months on end I lived on delivery (pizza or Chinese) and fast food. And ice cream. Lots of ice cream. I was also lonely and isolated, essentially stuck in my house, and eating to try to stuff my emotions. And the anticlotting drugs I was taking (side effect: rapid weight gain) meant I *really* packed on the pounds.

Things got worse before they got better. My mother's health declined to the point I had to go live with her to take care of her. She died a year later, followed just weeks later by my brother. Across the country from most of my friends, I was still lonely and isolated even once I was no longer homebound, and more and more sought emotional comfort in food. And continued to do so for a total of five years.

I will never forget the day I stepped on a scale—though it took all my courage to do so—and watched the needle rocket up to the highest available number: 350. Yet that needle was nowhere near settling when it got there. I was now BS—Beyond Scale. I could only guess my real weight. Maybe 370 pounds, maybe more. My T-shirts were size 5X—I had to special-order them on the Internet—and I could barely fit my entire silhouette in my hallway mirror.

I could barely fit behind the wheel of my car. I couldn't fit in just one airplane seat. Putting on socks was beyond me. I took only showers, afraid that if I got into a tub there may be no way out. I plodded along with great effort, slow as a turtle. Walking through my house took so much energy, I'd have to stop for rest breaks. Me, a guy who used to bike a hundred miles at a clip, who used to run up Pikes Peak. Now I could barely stand, certainly not for any period of time. I developed sleep apnea, which can be fatal, and I thought the resulting sleep deprivation might kill me if the oxygen deprivation did not. Mentally, I was always in a fog.

Then one day I uncovered a box of documents and the paper on top of it caught my attention: my brother's death certificate. Dead at fifty-two. And all I could think was that I didn't want to join him. I really didn't. Something deep inside me roared, *I want to live!* Really live, a full life, not the scaled-back, constrained life my weight had forced me into. I knew I had to change. Change or die. Half measures weren't going to do it.

I decided to dig back into all I had learned in what seemed like a previous life, when I was an athlete and student of alternative health. From somewhere in my memory banks this insight floated up: *I ate my way into this problem . . . I gotta eat my way out.* I had read long ago about the value of going raw; I even had a water alkalizer and a case of pH paper. I'd checked myself a lot, but got discouraged because I was never alkaline. With my new mission, however, I finally found the way, thanks to the pH Miracle program.

I made a commitment to eating only the most alkalizing, energizing food. I was going to put my health back together one meal at a time. Meals with energy, with tons of electrons, blood-building meals. But hearty meals, fill-my-tummy meals, meals that worked on my seemingly insatiable hunger. *Delicious* meals. Eating alkaline, I never counted calories and never felt hungry. And right from the start, I was losing one to two pounds a week. With no exercise! At my size, I found meaningful exercise all but impossible.

Before I knew it I was down sixty . . . eighty . . . a hundred pounds. My energy level was back up. My mind was clear and quick again. By losing weight, I was getting healthier. By getting healthier, I was losing weight.

Along the way I kept tweaking lots of little things, constantly improving my results. For all my adult life I had prided myself on never using salt, but I learned the error of my ways, and added alkaline sea salts to my program. I also made sure to get healthy oils—a quart a week. I started drinking green drinks. I noticed a difference with even very small changes, like when I stopped using soy sauce, gave up cashews, and cut out stevia. With all this I brought my total number of pounds lost to *150!*

That's when I started to exercise. For one thing, now I physically *could* exercise without a problem. And I had the energy to do so. More that that, I wanted optimal health and wouldn't settle for less. I knew by now that the weight would come off without it. But I also knew that for the best good health, I'd need exercise and all the health benefits it brings, starting with pumping the lymph system to flush stationary acids.

I'm now down 180 pounds. In the last two years I've lost almost as much as I weighed before I started my five-year slide into obesity! I've shed the body weight of a whole other adult male. I was once literally twice my size now. I've gained a significant amount of muscle mass. I think I look pretty darn good. And I know I feel great!

* Rick Laurenzi has produced a documentary about his pH Miracle experience titled *Losing a Ton and Having Fun*.

Chapter 7

•

You Are What You Drink:
Water, Juice, and Green Drink

At least as important as how you eat is how you drink, beginning with the fact that most of us simply don't drink enough. Then, when we do drink, most often we don't drink what is good for us. If you don't get proper hydration—or "hydrate" with the wrong things—you compromise your health. At the very core of this program are three simple ways to change all that: drinking alkaline water, juice, and green drink. This chapter looks at each in turn, explaining its benefits, pointing out the pitfalls you must avoid, and describing what you need to know to make sure you get the best for your body.

THE RIGHT WATER

The single most important thing you can do to be healthy is to drink good water—and plenty of it. Water is of the utmost importance to becoming and remaining healthy. But water quality (tap and bottled) around the country is already atrocious, and going downhill fast. And, as they say in the Catskills, *we get so little of it!* Centuries ago, the drinking water around the planet was alkaline. But because of industrialization and pollution in general, this is no longer true, not only in America, but in many parts of the world.

Bad water can actually make you sick—and tired. Getting alkaline, electron-rich water is just as important as eating alkaline, electron-rich food.

Like the earth on which we live, our bodies are 70 percent water—10 to 13 gallons of the stuff. All living organisms are composed largely of water.

Your muscles and heart are 75 percent water, your brain and kidneys 83 percent, your lungs 86 percent, your blood 94 percent, and your eyes 95 percent. You need to keep every cell in your body properly hydrated if you want to experience optimum good health.

You are, literally, what you drink. If you drink acidic water, you're going to be acidic. If you drink alkaline water, your body will be alkaline. Proper hydration keeps all your cells healthy and pH-balanced, so your body can be healthy and pH-balanced. If your cells don't get the buffering they need from what you provide them, they are going to pull alkalizing mineral salts from the bones and muscles and elsewhere in the body, leaving those areas undefended. For optimal health, you need water that's pure, alkaline, charged with electrons, and has ideal molecular structure.

Pure Water

Body cells are only as healthy as the fluids they are bathed in. If you subsist on polluted water, imagine the devastation to our bodies. Come to think of it, you don't have to "imagine"—chances are you are experiencing it right now. Almost all easily accessible water is acidic, and will make your body acidic. When your water is acidic, it can't act as a buffer, or help flush acid out of your system. Alkaline water, on the other hand, neutralizes stored acid wastes from diet and metabolism and, if consumed every day in conjunction with a good diet, gently removes the acids from the body.

Unfortunately, the water you need is *not* flowing from your tap. And it's not in your bottled water, either, no matter how pricey or how many "natural" claims are on the label. Even if it looks clear and tastes good (and let's face it, the taste isn't always so great, especially straight from the tap), it's probably not something you should really drink. Even if you filter it (with the popular but not sufficiently effective Brita systems, or the like)—it is not healthy.

Most municipal water supplies are a disgrace, especially those poisoned with chlorine and fluoride, which means most of them. According to the Natural Resources Defense Council (NRDC), more than 240 million Americans use water from contaminated public water systems every day. Bottled water, though usually better tasting, may also contain many impurities, or simply be dead from processing and storage.

Commercial drinking water standards ignore thousands of potential pollutants. The EPA lists around two hundred primary, major water pollutants for which municipal and commercial drinking water must be tested. There are thousands more unidentified, and thousands more that are variants or combinations (but not listed). Physicians for Social Responsibility reports more than seventy-five thousand toxic synthetic and chemical compounds identified in our nation's water supply. No one can screen for all possible poisons in all water supplies as it is. And that's before you consider the fact that some well-known contaminants don't even have standards set for them—no one is officially counting (or maybe no one knows) if your water has safe levels or not. When someone is keeping track, testing procedures are often inadequate, or very expensive. Tests for some of the worst contaminants run up to twelve hundred dollars—for each separate chemical! And do not be fooled by taste. Some of the deadliest pollutants are tasteless (one reason official standards can ignore them). I've tested waters from around the globe myself, bottled and from the tap, and I've found precious few that I'd put to my own lips. Pretty much all readily available drinking water, including most bottled, reverse-osmosis, and distilled waters, may reasonably be expected to contain some contaminants.

I could write a whole chapter on the specifics of the pollutants in our water in this country—in fact I have, elsewhere—including their impressively long scientific names and very scary lists of their proven health effects. I could point out which ones are common fuel additives or poisonous heavy metals, which ones are used to kill termites, which ones are an effect of aggressive mining operations, which ones are pharmaceuticals, or mold, and which ones are found primarily in household cleaners. But the heart of the matter is, whatever they're called, whatever they are meant to do, wherever they come from, *they don't belong in your water.* Or in your body.

We have to face facts: We have to take responsibility for our own water. Pretty much nothing out there is good for us simply as is. Once upon a time glacial melt must have been about perfect, or springwater, or rain water, or high mountain streams. But air pollution and acid rain and contaminated groundwater and ocean dumping have changed all that. And we've established that we can't count on processing by today's standards to result in a product that's up to *our* standards.

Fortunately, there are ways to purify your water that anyone can do at home, and we'll explore them later in the chapter.

Alkaline Water

In addition to being free of pollutants, your water also needs to be alkaline—that is, above 7 on the pH scale. Any alkaline pH will be better than any acidic water, but ideally I recommend water that's at least 9.5 (and, for people dealing with serious health conditions, as high as 11.5 to 12.5).

Most tap and bottled water, however, doesn't even make it up to a neutral 7. (Distilled water is a 7, but there are problems with distilled water; see "Don't Drink Distilled Water" on page 127) The contaminants we discussed above can, among other problems, make the water they are in acidic.

When you drink acidic water, your body has to draw on stores of alkaline substances in the body just to buffer the water. So those substances aren't available for any other alkalizing work—a problem when the substance is, say, calcium that's supposed to be strengthening bone. When you drink alkaline water, however, your body can use it to wash acids out of your tissues. And negative microforms can't survive in an environment flooded with alkaline water. Furthermore, alkaline water may contain alkaline minerals your body needs, including calcium, magnesium, and potassium. That's actually the ideal delivery system for these minerals—suspended in water, the best way for your body to absorb them.

I know from the testing I've done around the world that you're extremely unlikely to be drinking alkaline water already, no matter what water you are drinking. But there are simple ways to alkalize your water, which I'll get to as soon as I finish describing all the properties of healthy water.

Water Charged with Electrons

For optimal health, your water must be energized—saturated with electrons. Water like that is highly charged and full of potential energy. It's also alkaline. In fact, water is alkaline because of the negative charge from all its electrons, while acids are dominated by positive charged protons. It is the attraction of electrons to protons that allows alkaline substances to neutralize acidic substances.

In chemistry, the addition of an electron is called reduction, and the removal of an electron is called oxidation. The value known as ORP ("oxidative reduction potential") lets you quantify the electron activity, or energy potential, of water (or anything else) by numbering its electrons. Reduction stores energy in a substance. A negative ORP, expressed in millivolts (mV), lets you know the water is alkalizing.

Water with a negative ORP provides a safe source of free electrons to block the oxidation of normal tissue by free oxygen radicals. In other words, it's an antioxidant—and a more powerful one than any food or supplement, thanks to the large mass of electrons, all ready to be donated, that it contains. It is fast acting and able to reach all tissues of the body in a very short time. The effects of drinking reduced water are immediate.

You want water with an ORP of at least –250 mV and greater than –1,250 mV. But most tap water registers between about +400mV and +1,250 mV—it's proton-saturated, and apt to acquire electrons and oxidize other molecules. It is water with no energy. In fact, it will actually steal energy away from your body. So you have your work cut out for you in finding healthy water. We do have a solution, however, coming up in the section on how to create the water you need for optimal health.

RESEARCH REPORT

Researchers at Texas University demonstrated the life-giving properties of alkaline water charged with electrons. They raised three groups of mice on three kinds of water—tap water (pH 7.5, ORP +600), reduced (pH 9, ORP −400) and hyper-reduced (pH 10, ORP −600). The mice in the middle group, given alkaline water but not the *most* alkaline water, lived longer than the mice drinking tap water. And the mice sipping hyper-reduced water lived longer than either of the other two groups (346 days, on average, as against 235 days for those on tap water, and 287 days for the other group). Mice getting alkaline water had stronger immune systems (as measured by four different markers). They had higher levels of antioxidants in their systems as well. No wonder they lived so much longer!

Molecularly Structured Water

Electron activity takes place on the surface of a molecule. More surface area means more electron activity. The H_2O molecules that make up any water tend to cluster in groups of ten to twenty, which decreases surface area. When you break up or shrink those clusters in the water (which you can, at home, even without a PhD in chemistry!), you increase the surface area and, therefore, the energy in the water. Breaking down the molecular clustering increases the electrical potential of the water—it increases the negative charge.

Smaller clusters also allow the water to permeate cell membranes more readily, so cells can be fully hydrated from the inside out. I think of it as "wetter" water. Water with larger clusters has a hard time getting into the cells of the body, so if you're drinking the wrong kind of water, you could be dehydrated no matter how much you consume. When you do get good water, it inhibits excessive fermentation in the digestive tract and abnormal fermentation of intestinal microbes.

Your water should have no more than five to six molecules clustered together. (This is sometimes referred to as small-diameter water because of the size of the molecules.) Ideally, in fact, you'd get monomolecular water—water with each molecule standing alone. Tap water is typically composed of clusters of between ten and forty molecules. The average bottled water is arranged is clusters of about twenty molecules.

Water molecules cluster together when they lose their electrical charge, or the charge is compromised by acid. All acidic water has larger molecular clusters.

MAKING GOOD WATER

The best way to get the best water is with an ionizing water processing machine. This is sometimes also called electrolysis. Ionizing or electrolysis reverses the charge of water from positive to negative by breaking up clusters (generally getting them down to between four and six molecules each). This increases not only the ORP (creating electrically charged water), but also the pH of the water (making it more alkaline).

I know this is tooting my own horn, but I know of only one home appliance that creates ideal water, alkalizing, purifying, structuring, and charging it: the Young pHorever Ionizer. It's an electrical appliance about the size and shape of a large dictionary, standing on its end, which connects to your kitchen water supply and sits on your countertop or under your sink. Another good machine is the Jupiter Orion ionizer, though it does not have quite as high a range in pH or ORP (see the resources section).

Your tap water runs through a plastic hose into the unit, where it passes through multiple types of filters (micromesh, carbon, tourmaline, and coral calcium mineral filters) to remove any chemicals (including chlorine), pollutants, bacteria, yeast, mold, parasites, drugs, and heavy metals (including mercury). (Other machines may actually transfer some contaminants into water, or concentrate them.) Then the water passes into an ionization chamber where it runs across seven self-cleaning titanium/platinum ionization plates, which use magnetism to attract more electrons to one side of the chamber and more protons to the other. (These titanium plates are what give the highest and lowest pH and ORP of any machine on the market.) Here the water is divided into two different streams as two types of water are created: 70 percent is electron-rich alkaline water, and 30 percent is proton-rich acidic water. The good stuff—with a pH between 9.5 and 11, small clusters of molecules, and an ORP between −150 and −450 mV— proceeds to your faucet, ready for you to drink.

Actually, the other water is "good," too, for certain purposes. The positively charged acidic water (a pH of about 4) is a great disinfectant. It can withdraw electrons from bacteria, killing them. Use the oxidized water from your ionizing unit to clean hands, kitchen utensils, fresh vegetables and fruit, cutting boards, and minor wounds. In addition, tests have shown it to be effective in treating athlete's foot, minor burns, and insect bites.)

The equipment to create healthy water at home this way will run you about two to three thousand dollars. But the cost to operate it, including electricity, is generally low—about two to three cents per liter of water processed.

Reverse Osmosis

Another useful technology is a reverse-osmosis system. This is a multifilter process that purifies water of toxic chemicals and large mineral deposits. These units do <u>not</u> alkalize or energize water. But they may be more affordable and more readily available than ionization machines (see resources). If you use a reverse-osmosis system, I recommend adding pH drops (see below) to the filtered water, which will increase the electrical potential of the water and decrease its proton or hydrogen concentration.

pH Drops

If you can't afford a machine to structure and correct the ORP level of your filtered water, or temporarily don't have access to such a machine, *do not* let that keep you from doing the things you *can* do to optimize your water. Filter your water with high-quality water filters. And use alkaline pH drops to correct the water pH to 9 or 10.

However you process your water, you can make it more alkaline as necessary with the addition of pH drops such as sodium/potassium bicarbonate ($NaHCO_3$ or $KHCO_3$) or chlorine dioxide (ClO_2). When using a 5 percent solution of sodium chlorite, I recommend fifteen drops in each quart or liter of water; with an 8 percent solution of sodium/potassium bicarbonate solution, I recommend five drops. Look for sodium chlorite ($NaClO_2$) at the health food store, or regular or liquid sodium and/or potassium bicarbonate at the health food or grocery store (see resources).

The pH drops help reduce the size of the molecular clusters in the water and increase electron activity. These substances react with and release oxygen in the water, increasing its energy potential. When added to pure water, and thus added to your bloodstream, pH drops act as an oxygen catalyst, alkalizing, neutralizing, oxygenating, and pH-balancing the body. You can drink alkaline water before, during, and after meals to help the stomach alkalize the food ingested.

Don't Drink Distilled Water

Distillation is the evaporation and condensation of water, mimicking the natural rain cycle. Many health experts (including us) have recommended distilled water for its neutral pH. But distilled water is electrically neutral; it has no energy and can give no energy. (When you think about it, the water in the body isn't distilled. And it *is* alkaline.) And because it lacks bicarbonates and minerals, it is slightly acid forming in the body. So we no longer promote distilled water among the best answers to the question of what to drink.

Distilled water is an excellent aid in detoxification and chelation because its purity pulls on toxicities in the body, but day in and day out it will not work as effectively as using alkaline electron-rich water.

Adding pH drops of sodium chlorite or sodium and/or potassium bicarbonate to distilled water increases the electron concentration, making it a suitable alternative when you can't get ionized water.

If you take just one thing away from this book, let it be to get your body plenty of water. And not just any water. You need water that's pure, alkaline, charged with electrons, and has ideal molecular structure. In liberal amounts.

Drink Up!

Ideally, you'll get at least four liters of good water (about one gallon) every day. This may seem like a lot at first, so you can build up to that gradually. And your body will quickly become accustomed to the proper hydration.

On this program you may not feel a need to drink with meals, because so many of the vegetables you'll be getting contain so much water (many are 70 to 90 percent water). So following a schedule of drinking *between* meals is especially important.

We like to squeeze fresh lemon or lime juice into our drinking water to boost its alkalizing effects. And it is, of course, also very tasty!

But good water isn't just going to come out of your tap. Not unless you improve the municipal supply in the above ways. And you can't just buy a bottle of good water. (The only reasonable bottled waters are ionized and bottled in glass, like pH Miracle Water, Essentia, Evermore, and Trinity— see resources.) But investing in the right equipment for your home, and adding pH drops as needed, you can provide your body with what it is truly thirsty for: good water that can hydrate the cells, buffer dietary and metabolic acids, water that's alkalizing and energizing. Water that supports a stronger, healthier, and more vibrant you.

JUICE

Eight ounces of fresh vegetable juice is an ideal beginning to any meal or an excellent snack. All the benefits of vegetables (and grasses) can be enhanced simply by juicing them. The nutrients are more concentrated and more quickly and easily available to the body. You do lose the fiber with juicing, but that is what frees the nutrients or electrons. (Chewing does the same thing, just not as completely as juicing does.)

You do need fiber, so you wouldn't want to get all your vegetables this way. But when you "drink your vegetables," your body is getting a greater concentration of rapidly usable alkaline mineral salts, vitamins, minerals, chlorophyll, and electrons, so vegetable juices are very alkalizing. They also have an important cleansing effect in the intestines. Juicing vegetables you might otherwise cook also provides alkalizing relief to the digestive organs.

The best, most alkalizing juice is made up mostly of green vegetables and grasses. (Fruit juices must be avoided, especially early in this program, because of their large amounts of sugar acids.) At first, when your taste buds may not yet be accustomed to the more subtle sweetness found in greens, you may want to add some carrot, beet, or red, yellow, or orange bell peppers. You can even use butternut squash and sweet potato sparingly. These vegetables are sweet because they have higher levels of sugar acid, so use them moderately, keeping them to 20 percent or less of your juice—meaning 80 percent green. (Beet can also be a vigorous lower bowel cleanser, another reason to go easy on it, especially at first.) As your body gets more basic, green juices will taste better and better to you, and then you may want to lower the proportion of carrot or beet juice to 10 percent or less to get even more greens. (Peppers are not high in sugars, so you can use them freely.)

The recipe section provides many ideas for juice combinations, and the resources section includes some good juicing books if you want to explore more. In addition, all juicers come with some recipes. Experiment a bit to find the combinations you enjoy most. All green vegetables are terrific for juicing (we use a lot of celery, cucumber, broccoli, green bell pepper, zucchini, green beans, lettuce, cabbage, beet greens, and leafy greens of all kinds). Tomatoes are also great for juicing—as you probably already know. But don't rely on processed and canned stuff—make your own! (And consider starting your own garden.) Juicing grasses is a good way to reap their benefits without feeling as if you are chewing your cud. You can juice sprouts for a kind of double bonus, concentrating still further the nutrients that are already so dense and making them even more alkalizing than they are whole. Also think about spicing up your juice with jicama (very mild), parsley, radish, ginger, and garlic.

Because of the way juice concentrates everything, using quality produce is particularly important here. Use organic whenever you possibly can, and, as always, get it and use it as fresh as you possibly can. Wash it well, particularly anything that's not organic, and perhaps soak it in pure alkaline water (twenty drops to the gallon of ClO_2 or liquid sodium and/or potassium bicarbonate).

Peel heavily waxed vegetables. But there are plentiful nutrients in the skin, so leave it on whenever you can. Don't forget to use green vegetable tops, too, such as beet and carrot greens. When you can't get organic or newly picked vegetables, you can bolster your juice by adding some dried, powdered "greens" (like the ones described in chapter 12). You can use wheatgrass juice powder as an alternative to juicing wheatgrass itself (if it is difficult for you to buy fresh, or if your juicer isn't up to the task).

When you spin, whip, shake, and press vegetables into juice, the microzymas excrete acid waste, making the juice mildly acidic despite coming from alkaline vegetables. So make your fresh juices highly alkaline by diluting them with distilled water (just one part juice to ten to twenty parts water), then adding pH drops (ten to twenty drops for ten to twenty ounces).

Making your own juice is the best option, for freshness. And drink it up as soon as you make it. Don't let it sit for more than a few minutes. (If it is going to sit more than ten or fifteen minutes, maintain its goodness by adding three to five drops of colloidal vitamin C to the juice container as it begins to fill, or dissolve 250 to 500 milligrams of crystalline vitamin C in a few ounces of pure water and add that to the juice container before beginning.)

Your own juice will always be better than packaged, preserved products. Pasteurizing juice—and almost all of it, even in health food stores, is pasteurized—destroys the electrical life force therein.

Take the time and trouble to choose a quality juicer—it's worth it. You'll find a wide range of prices, though more expensive does not necessarily mean better. If possible, talk to owners of different machines and see what they think—and see if they'll let you test-drive theirs. Look for an efficient one that has the ability to juice continuously—stay away from hand-press juicers and hand wheatgrass juicers—and is easy to clean (has few moving parts and disassembles and reassembles easily). To juice grasses or parsley, you'll need a high-powered juicer (check the packaging for voltage and wattage). There's even one juicer available (the Green Power Juice Extractor) that ionizes the juice, which is a bonus in my opinion. It also does a beautiful job with grasses, which not every juicer can claim (see resources). That machine does not heat the juice, as some do. Make sure you get a machine that does not heat the juice! A juicer that whips or spins the juice will cause it to heat up as the molecules bounce off one another. As with pasteurization, heat causes the electrons to evaporate and reduces or destroys the life force. My juicer is rotary-geared and has a gravity fall for the juice (versus a centrifugal spinning juicer that needs the filter changed).

Juan's Story

Two years ago, I came down with what I thought was the flu—until I noticed blood in my urine. I got myself checked out by my doctor, who told me my kidneys were failing and admitted me to the hospital. I went home a week later with the diagnosis of kidney disease, though I was told I would pretty much be able to go back to my regular life. But as the months went by, I just got sicker and sicker. Going to work and doing my normal daily activities felt almost impossible. I was in and out of the hospital four times, and more than once I didn't think

I'd make it out alive. Even on my good days, I felt like I was slowly dying.

Two days after I first heard about the pH Miracle program (and before I'd done anything about what I'd heard), I collapsed in church with a fever of 104 degrees and was rushed to the hospital. My wife ordered concentrated green powder and pH drops—although my doctors dismissed them out of hand—which I started on as soon as I got home. After about a week, I started to have a little more strength, and I made a commitment to changing my life and undertook the whole program. With a radically new diet, I saw incredible results within a month. I had no more blood in my urine; I wasn't tired all the time; I felt up to playing with my children. It's been almost a year and a half since the last time I was in the hospital. I have never felt better! At a checkup two weeks ago, my doctors couldn't find a thing wrong with me or my kidneys. They don't know how to explain it, but I do!

I want to note quickly another food processing option that at a glance seems similar to juicing: the puree method, where a special machine whips whole fruits, vegetables, and even grains into liquids or creamy forms. But this process mixes a lot of air with the food, which is not welcome in the stomach. It does leave the fiber in, and fiber is good for you because it adsorbs and absorbs the enzymes or acids from the foods and liquids you drink. On the other hand, it leaves the fiber in—which makes the nutrients less accessible to your body. The creamy consistency also discourages chewing and encourages faster eating, thereby depriving food of the full complement of oral secretions necessary for full and proper digestion. Together with the large amounts of solid matter, this places greater stress on the digestive system than does juice.

So, while there may be some benefits to this method, don't substitute it for juicing. Avoid it altogether as you start on this program, and if you decide to add it later, don't use it at the same meal as juice.

GREEN DRINK

Here's a way to take what you get out of proper hydration, and what you get out of vegetables and vegetable juices, and go them one better: green powders. These are grasses, sprouted grains, green fruits, and green vegetables, dried and powdered and sold as supplements. They infuse your body with pure electrical energy and easily absorbed vitamins, minerals, and amino acids (the building blocks of proteins). Make sure you get a product that is organically grown.

As mentioned, you can add some to your vegetable juice for extra "oomph." We usually just add green powders to purified alkaline electron-rich water (often with pH drops) as part of our daily hydration. This green drink is made by blending one to three teaspoons into one liter (or quart) of water three times a day, for a minimum of three teaspoons into three liters of water daily, plus—since you want to get at least four liters of alkaline electron-rich water a day—some plain water in addition to the green drink. Make sure you avoid green powders with high-sugar fruits, algae, mushrooms, enzymes, or probiotics. The probiotics are bacteria and can ferment the green grasses in the formula, making it acidic.

Just keep your green drink in a water bottle so you can shake it up to keep the greens well mixed. Make up one bottle at a time, and use at room temperature. Your body has to work to warm up an iced drink or cool down a hot drink, so you can save it some stress this way.

Daily Hydration Schedule

- Upon rising: one quart/liter of alkaline electron-rich *salt* water. Add pH drops (ClO_2) or liquid sodium and/or potassium bicarbonate, then one tablespoon of whole, unprocessed mineral salts. You can add lemon or lime juice to taste if desired.
- Between breakfast and lunch: 1½ quarts/liters of alkaline electron-rich water with 1½ teaspoons of green powder and twenty-four pH drops (ClO_2) or liquid sodium and/or potassium bicarbonate
- Between lunch and dinner: 1½ quarts/liters of alkaline electron-rich water with 1½ teaspoons of green powder and twenty-four pH drops (ClO_2) or liquid sodium and/or potassium bicarbonate.
- Between dinner and bed: alkaline electron-rich water as desired, with lemon/lime juice, and eight pH drops (ClO_2) or liquid sodium and/or potassium bicarbonate per quart/liter.

Many people ask me about what good alkaline electron-rich water does since "everyone knows" it is just going into the highly acidic stomach. The problem here is not with water meeting acid; it is with what "everyone knows." There is no hydrochloric acid pouch in our body. The stomach wall makes sodium bicarbonate to alkalize the food, not digest it. For every molecule of sodium bicarbonate produced to increase the alkalinity of food a molecule of HCl is also created. HCl is a very strong and toxic acid. The HCl falls into the gastric pits of the stomach away from the food as the sodium bicarbonate rises to the top to contact the food for alkalizing. That is why after the food leaves the stomach, there is no sodium bicarbonate left—just the remaining HCl acid that has to be eliminated through the blood. Low-water-content, acid-forming foods like meats, eggs, and breads cause the release of larger amounts of sodium bicarbonate with an equal amount of HCl. High-water-content foods such as nonstarchy vegetables require much less sodium bicarbonate to alkalize the food, and therefore there is less HCl acid residue in the stomach left over after the food has exited. The result is no indigestion or risk of acid reflux, stomach ulcers, or even stomach cancer. Alkaline electron-rich water—being extremely high in electron content!—does not trigger the release of sodium bicarbonate and thus does not cause the creation of the acid HCl, so it does not interfere with the alkalizing of the food. In fact, alkaline electron-rich water, with its high concentration of electrons, helps the alkalizing of the food and also helps to neutralize the caustic acidic HCl, preventing the acidification of the blood and tissues. So drink up!

Chapter 8

·

Food Combining

To ensure thorough and proper alkalization of food in your alimentary canal, food combining is an important consideration. And there's a lot out there designed to help you understand and implement various food-combining systems. While the idea is key, however, the vast majority of available programs are usually confusing, often inaccurate, and tend to offer conflicting advice. And they are all too unnecessarily complicated.

I'm here to tell you it doesn't have to be that way. The thing to remember is that the human digestive system—the alkaline buffering system—is not designed to digest food but to alkalize the food in preparation for stem cell creation in the crypts of the small intestine. So avoid complex acidic meals or food that is difficult or impossible to make into an alkaline liquid. Different foods make different, specific demands on the alkalizing alimentary canal buffering system. That we are capable of alkalizing many different kinds of foods doesn't mean we can do so all at once.

Animal protein is highly acidic, and requires a lot of alkaline buffers. Most animal proteins exit the stomach still in acidic chunks rather than the proper liquefied state. Plant proteins, on the other hand, can be easily liquefied with the teeth. Most starches can be liquefied and alkalized with the teeth and in the stomach, so they enter the small intestines in a better state. The same is true for vegetables and fruit. Fats also are more easily alkalized, so they don't stress the system the way animal proteins do.

It doesn't take much to imagine that foods that require much different effort to alkalize do not do well when eaten at the same time. One will interfere with alkalization of the other, causing incomplete alkalization of both. Whatever is not efficiently alkalized by you can be biologically transformed into harmful microforms. It's another vicious circle: Compromised alkalization paves the way for negative microforms, and negative microforms further disrupt the alkalizing process. Poor food combining with acidic food is also a major cause of formation of sticky mucus, which is formed when the glands or cover cells secrete sodium bicarbonate to bind up dietary acids.

Take a minute to stop and think of all the American "classics" that combine acidic protein and acidic starch—meat and potatoes, fish-and-chips, chicken and rice, a burger and fries, a ham sandwich (or any kind of sandwich), to name just a few—and you'll begin to realize just how badly we abuse our alimentary alkalizing canals. Most of us don't even know what it would be like to have proper alkalization of food! But it is simple. Chew your food to a liquid state, mixing it with saliva and its sodium bicarbonate, then let the stomach and the pancreas finish bringing the pH of the food up to an ideal 8.4.

Combining sugar and starch, or sugar and protein, leads to the same kinds of problems. And just what is in the lunch boxes of the majority of kids today (I'd be willing to bet)? Peanut butter and jelly sandwiches! That manages to hit all the bases at once, guaranteeing an acidic digestion disaster.

Fortunately, the solution is simple: Mix no more than four foods, from no more than two types of food, at any given meal. For example, have steamed broccoli, and a mesclun and tomato salad with salt-marinated tofu or soba noodles, but not both (three vegetables, and one protein, or three vegetables and one complex carb). Choosing fewer foods provides the simplest load on the alkaline buffering system. With that in mind, and following the general principles of this program, if you use only one protein per meal, and only one complex carbohydrate per meal, you are most of the way there.

Lucia's Story

Because of my family history of sky-high cholesterol levels, and the terrible heart consequences, I'd always been careful about what I ate. As a home economist, homemaker, and mother of eight children, I was also careful about what I served my family. As my health deteriorated, with all kinds of symptoms bothering me, I experimented with different "healthy" ways of eating, constantly fine-tuning my approach.

I grew up eating well. My mother followed the FDA recommendations of the time, serving vegetables, whole grains, lean meats, and fresh fruits daily. Through my own early years as a mother, I moved to less meat, chose fresh vegetables—and usually served them steamed—switched to brown rice, and started to use natural supplements. I ground whole wheat myself and made fresh bread weekly. I eliminated sodas, simple sugar, processed foods, and milk. My health improved some, but not completely.

My health really began spiraling down after the birth of my eighth child, which required an emergency C-section and two blood transfusions far from home. As more negative symptoms appeared, and I felt my energy and vitality slowly ebbing, I worked harder to unlock what good nutrition could offer me. Food combining was one of the first things I explored, but my early results were discouraging.

I've tried different strategies over the years. I began by using the four basic food groups. A typical dinner was baked chicken, pan-fried potatoes, frozen broccoli, a canned peach with cottage cheese, and oatmeal cake. I experienced a full feeling afterward and felt as if I would like to lie down for a nice nap. And I continued to have hypoglycemia, high cholesterol, and sinus infections, among many other things. Next, I added more whole grains and fresh vegetables and cut back on meat, as suggested in the current FDA food pyramid. A typical dinner was brown rice and chicken casserole, fresh steamed broccoli, a slice of homemade whole wheat bread with butter, and homemade applesauce. My blood sugar stabilized, but I continued to have cravings as well as a wide variety of other health issues.

Next, I tried eating nothing but fruit and fruit juices from dawn until noon. The rest of the day I would be careful to have only one "concentrated" food (protein or fat) at a meal—and no more fruit. I ate meat, but never with a starch. The large amounts of fruit kept me craving sweets, and I experienced low periods every afternoon. I never felt energetic after eating meat. And I didn't find the food satisfying. So I went back to my previous diet—and gained more weight and added a host of health concerns.

And so it went until I learned about the Youngs' program, and the proper way to combine foods. The day I started eating alkaline and drinking a gallon of alkaline water with pH drops and concentrated green powder every day, my life changed. I immediately noticed a rise in my energy levels. The most important changes I made, besides getting plenty of good water, were to eat something raw at each meal, focus mainly on green vegetables, and use the more alkaline grains.

At first I wanted that feeling of having something stick to my ribs, but found that the high-water/low-sugar foods gave a sustained energy that I was not used to. Now dinner is typically a vegetable, soba noodles, and tofu stir-fry, or occasionally a small portion of grilled salmon, jasmine rice with almonds, fresh steamed asparagus, and some raw pepper strips. For lunch I almost always have a fresh salad built from spinach, dark green lettuces, avocado, cucumber, celery, carrots, radishes, pumpkin seeds, sprouts, a little baked tofu, and a dressing of lemon juice, olive oil, and spices. (For years I had cut out all fat/oil of any kind due to my cholesterol challenge. Nothing helped until I added liberal amounts of the good essential oils to my diet daily.) To that I add a vegetable and hummus wrap in a sprouted wheat tortilla, or a brown rice cake with almond butter. That follows a breakfast of steamed millet with avocado, tomatoes, and flax oil, or lightly steamed broccoli and buckwheat cereal. That usually keeps me going strong until well into the afternoon. I never feel low in the afternoon anymore.

Sometimes I snack on a handful of soaked almonds. Often I make a gently warmed vegetable soup with an organic vegetable broth, which I enjoy for breakfast, lunch, or dinner. These foods give me all the energy my body needs. The foods I crave now are healthy, alkaline foods that are high in water content and low in sugar.

I now understand that though we all have our genetic tendencies, we are not bound by them. The gene might be the bullet, but the trigger is our lifestyle. This lifestyle has proven successful for me and my family for over two years now, keeping us healthy, energetic, and satisfied. We find the food delicious and sustaining. I have enjoyed developing recipes that are as healthy and beautiful as they are tasty. I prepare alkaline meals for my family of five every day, and on Sundays, when the rest of our family and friends come to eat, I serve alkaline food for twenty or more. They've enjoyed it so much that my married children have adopted some of these principles for their own young families, and they've all enjoyed health benefits. I feel my quest for a truly healthy way of eating has finally paid off.

Pay careful attention to food combining in the initial weeks after a pH Miracle Whole Body Cleanse (see chapter 11). Once you're fully on an alkalizing diet, it gets simpler still. When you're eating mainly foods that are high in electron-rich alkaline water and low in acid sugar, you no longer need to worry about proper combining. You can't help but combine them properly, since you are, for the most part, limiting or eliminating the problematic acidic mucus-forming foods. The foods that have makeups most similar to that of our bodies (high water content, 70 percent or more; naturally occurring oils, 20 to 30 percent; low protein, 5 to 7 percent; and even lower sugar, 0.5 to 3 percent) all combine with one another with no problem.

When you are strong and symptom-free, you can indulge in more complex alkaline meals with no real harm. Still, at the beginning of the program, or if you are seriously ill, or if you just want to ensure you're on an ideal regimen, paying strict attention to the rules that follow will serve you well. (See the resources section for some books and charts with more details about food combining.)

FOOD-COMBINING BASICS

All you're trying to do is keep acid starch and acid animal protein separate, and keep acid sugars, including high-sugar fruit, away from just about everything. That's why, once you have fully made the transition to this program, avoiding acidic animal proteins, acidic sugars, and most acidic fruits, combining is not an issue. In the meantime, here are the official rules:

1. Low-sugar/high-water vegetables (or fruit) combine with everything. Eat them with protein, starch, or alkalizing cold-pressed oils—and with other alkalizing vegetables!
2. Eat mildly acidic starches with alkalizing vegetables or low-sugar fruit. Don't eat acidic starches (including starchy acidic vegetables) with animal protein, acidic fruit, or saturated oil. (For the purposes of food combining, "acid" is not necessarily the same as foods that make the body more acidic. The two most important examples of this exception are alkalizing lemons and tomatoes, which are themselves acidic but which actually make the body more basic because their alkaline mineral salts of sodium and potassium are more then enough to buffer the acidic sugars.) So when you do choose a grain (including bread or pasta) or winter squash or potato, eat it alongside alkalizing vegetables, and not with acidic fish, for example.

3. If you feel you must eat acidic animal protein, combine it with alkalizing vegetables or low-sugar fruit. Don't eat acidic animal protein with starch, or saturated oils. Alkalizing vegetable proteins combine with all low-sugar, high-water-content (electron-rich) vegetables and fruit, as well as with good alkalizing mono- and polyunsaturated oils. Here's the flip side of the point above: When you're having acidic fish, serve it with alkalizing vegetables but not an acidic grain. Get over paella (fish with rice); try fish on a bed of steamed alkaline greens, or atop a crunchy alkalizing salad.

4. Eat high-sugar acidic fruit on its own—if you eat it at all. Don't eat fruit with protein, starch, starchy vegetables (beet, potato, yam), or saturated oil. In fact, don't use high-sugar acidic fruit at all—with the exception of alkalizing lemon, lime, grapefruit, raw tomato, avocado, and red, yellow, green, and orange peppers—unless you are quite well, and then only in moderation and in season.

5. Eat healthy alkalizing mono- and polyunsaturated oils with alkaline vegetables and alkalizing fruit (tomato, avocado, red, yellow, orange, and green bell peppers, lemon, and lime). They also combine with acidic starches (which must be kept to 20 percent or less of your diet). Do not eat healthy mono- or polyunsaturated alkalizing oils with (saturated) animal fats or acidic proteins. Seeds, nuts, and avocado—all excellent sources of healthy alkaline fats—can be combined with alkaline plant or acidic animal protein, acidic starches, or even high-sugar (acidic) fruits. Don't douse your fish with oil or butter—use alkalizing lemon juice, salsa, or herbs instead—and you'll be all set.

Notable Exceptions: Avocado and Tomato

Avocado is actually an alkalizing fruit, but because it is low in sugar (acid) and relatively high in protein, it can be combined with alkalizing vegetables, even the acidic starchy ones, as well as with acidic grains. So I enjoy an avocado sandwich on yeast-free spelt bread, or avocado and tomato slices with lemon juice on jasmine rice.

Tomato, too, is a fruit. And although it is acidic, it has an alkaline effect in the body because of its low sugar content and high alkalizing mineral content. So, like the avocado, it can be combined as if it were an alkalizing vegetable.

Now, for the "whys" of those wherefores:

1. Most vegetables, and the few fruits we've mentioned, are your healthiest choices anyway, and the fact that they combine with any other healthy alkalizing choices just makes them even more ideal as the focus of your diet.

2. Acidic starch and acidic animal proteins are a bad combination, as explained earlier. Acids use up the sodium bicarbonate that is a component of saliva and is necessary for the proper alkalizing of food. Acidic starches, such as potatoes, bread, or pasta (and even whole grains), break down into simple acidic sugars in the body, so adding high-sugar fruits just layers sugar on top of sugar—and acid on top of acid. The combination creates enough poisons that it can actually shut down the immune system for five hours—or even longer. Oil slows digestion of acidic starch—though this won't be a problem if the acid starch is no more than 20 percent of your otherwise alkalizing meal. Mono- and polyunsaturated oils can neutralize acids, so don't avoid the healthy ones, like hemp oil, flax oil, fish oil, avocado oil, and olive oil.

3. When acidic animal protein is in the stomach, it creates more acid. When combined with acidic starches, the sugars in the starches make even more acid, leading to indigestion, heartburn, and gas—on top of all the other negative effects of a body that's too acidic. The same thing happens when you add more acid (including the acids created from high-sugar fruit). Oils slow the alkalization of animal protein, causing constipation and eventually acid reflux, heartburn, and gas.

4. Fruit—at least, the vast majority of fruit—is high in sugar and acid forming, so it is problematic even on its own. Combined with acidic protein, it is a recipe for excess acid (as well as indigestion and gas). Acidic starch and acidic fruit is just double the acidic sugar. In addition, they have vastly different liquefying times (acidic fruit is liquefied extremely rapidly), opening the door to fermentation right in your stomach and small intestine. Mixing acidic fruit with saturated or trans oil can lead to constipation and poor absorption of nutrients. Finally, while acid fruit are cleansers, vegetables are alkalizing builders of the stem cells, the blood, and then body cells. You unduly stress your body by asking it to do opposites simultaneously.

5. Saturated, acidic oil slows the liquefying of acidic animal proteins and acidic starch (though the latter will be a problem only if your acidic starches are exceeding that 20 percent of your diet).

> ### LEMONS AND LIMES: NOTABLE EXCEPTIONS
>
> Lemons and limes, or lemon and lime juice, are commonly thought of as acidic, but they actually have an alkaline effect in the body. So they do not fall under the warnings against combining with acidic foods, and can be used together with acidic starches, acidic proteins, or alkalizing mono- and polyunsaturated oils.

SEPARATING FOOD AND DRINK

One other combination you need to be aware of is food and beverages. Don't ruin an alkaline meal by washing it down with an acidic drink. Don't drink something acidic with an acidic food, either, or you will overwhelm your body's ability to buffer the acid. Cold acidic drinks are particularly troublesome, as cold shuts down the release of sodium bicarbonate from the cover cells of the stomach.

Drinking some electron-rich alkaline water (or other liquid) with acidic foods helps to buffer the acids and dilute acidic food chemicals. Or, if you're going to be having some acidic food, we recommend eating juicier alkaline food items first, such as alkaline vegetables and salads, to pave the way for heavier acidic items later in the meal. You may also find that a few sips of warm electron-rich alkaline water after a meal aids in buffering the toxic hydrochloric acid residues in the stomach. You can also take a teaspoon of sodium bicarbonate or mineral salts in three to four ounces of water to neutralize the toxic hydrochloric acid, settle your stomach, and help buffer the acids from the food ingested.

When you are eating a completely alkaline meal, however, you can drink alkaline water or alkalizing fresh juices with your other alkalizing food.

Part III

The
pH Miracle
Program

The chapters in this section provide all the details on how to embark on the pH Miracle diet and lifestyle program and how to incorporate it into your life, whether you choose to go all-out immediately to address an urgent situation, or take a more deliberate pace for permanent change. So right here we're just going to give you the four major steps of the program, without going into a lot of detail. We want you to see the forest before you get too involved with the trees.

The most basic outline of the program looks like this:

Step 1: Transition, for twelve weeks, gradually substituting for and eliminating acidifying foods, switching over to an alkaline diet.

Step 2: Cleanse, for one to four weeks, with some supplements and mild, natural laxatives.

Step 3: Strictly alkaline, for eight to twelve weeks, with additional supplements, including sodium bicarbonate or mineral salts. This means eating only alkaline foods. Your ultimate diet will be 70 or 80 percent alkalizing, but at the outset you're aiming for 100 percent. Essentially, you stick to high-water-content/electron-rich vegetables, mainly green ones, and have them raw as much as possible.

Step 4: Maintenance. Now you can proceed on to 70 or 80 percent of your diet being alkaline and adding the full range of healthy foods, including fatty fish, grains, soy, and starchy vegetables. You'll also add your full range of alkalizing supplements, including any you need to address specific symptoms.

For the purposes of writing a book, we've settled on general guidelines that everyone can follow. But truly the program should be individualized. Listen to your body and start where it is telling you that you need to be. Observe how it changes as you go through the steps and pace yourself accordingly. There's nothing magic about the timing of these four steps, and extra weeks here or faster progress there is all part of the experience, as long as you stay basically on track. The pH Miracle diet and lifestyle program works a bit differently for everyone who follows it, though the end result— radiant good health—is the same for all.

If you are very ill, you might start directly with step 2 to get the fastest results, and follow the strictest part of the program (step 3) for up to three months. Those of you who begin not too far out of balance may need only one month in step 3 before going with the fullest range of foods. It all depends on your progress.

You can also begin with a pH Miracle Whole Body Cleanse before you begin transitioning, if you want to give yourself a kind of jump start, but be sure to come back to the pH Miracle Whole Body Cleanse again as you are finishing your transition and ready to go ahead with the strictly alkaline diet. Some or all of the steps of the transition may take you longer than a week—go ahead and do what you need to do. It is a lifetime investment you are making, so doing it right is far more important than doing it quickly.

I've seen this program work, time and again, for seriously ill people—as well as for people who seemed pretty healthy in the first place. What works for one person, or even most people, however, may not do so for everyone. You must tune in to your body, its needs and responses, and take personal responsibility for it. Ultimately, no one knows more about you than you. This program is designed for people to manage on their own, but it is wise to seek input from knowledgeable practitioners if it seems appropriate. (If you find you are having trouble communicating your situation fully, you might ask the professionals you consult to have a look at this book.) In any event, you should consult a health care practitioner before beginning this (or any other) diet program or nutritional regimen.

Chapter 9

·

Transitioning

To be able to alkalize and liquefy your food more readily, you must take small bites. Quite literally, you should not bite off more than you can chew. So it is with making the transition to an alkaline diet. Ease into it if necessary, with a series of small victories, rather than trying to master the whole thing at once. Don't discourage yourself by trying to change too much too quickly. Make changes gradually. That is generally best for the body anyway, and increases the chances that you'll succeed in the first place and the chances that you'll stick with it for the long haul. (There is an exception for serious illness, when a drastic change may be just what you need—or there may be no time for a stepwise approach.) Moving toward an alkaline lifestyle is a process—not a single event or an overnight transformation. As you make your way "home," enjoy your journey.

Our family took more than two years to make the transition complete—and our youngest needed even longer in transition. (He is twenty now, and has been 100 percent alkalarian for years.) In part, that's because we were working out the system as we went along. On the other hand, we were already almost vegetarian, so the total change was not as dramatic as it might have been starting from a more typical American diet. Whatever the specific time frame that works for you, take it step by step, as we did, for clear—and lasting—results. Work through one transition at a time, allowing at least a week, and up to two to three weeks if you need to, to get acclimated at each step. Or take on a few together if that feels comfortable. Move on when you feel at home with them. Feel free to change the order of the transitions. You'll be building a solid foundation, then adding layer upon sturdy layer on top. So it'll be built to last.

Here's our very own twelve-step program.

TRANSITION 1: BREAKFAST

Probably the single biggest change you will make on this program is in what you have for breakfast. So it is as good a place to start as any!

Americans need to have a change of heart and mind concerning breakfast. Almost all of the conventional choices—eggs, pancakes, syrup, hot or cold cereals, fruit, juice, coffee, yogurt, bread products, sausage, bacon—make your body acidic or promote (or contain!) bacteria or yeast/fungus or other microforms. Many contain huge amounts of acidic sugars and simple carbohydrates, which acidify the blood and tissues, creating the environment that promotes the microforms. Others are dense sources of acidic protein (and, almost always, animal fat), which, in addition to being high in parasite activity, also promote microform overgrowth. And all these acidic foods are also very low in water content—and extremely constipating. It's no wonder laxatives are one of the best-selling over-the-counter remedies. On top of all that, we eat them in dreadful combinations (eggs and home fries, cereal and milk, toast and jam). What a way to start the day! Your body deserves to be replenished much more gently and wholesomely after the night fast.

So don't let the first meal of your day slow you down. This basically means making the same choices at breakfast that you would at any other time of the day. It may seem strange at first, but you'll be doing yourself a big favor by switching over to a soup, say, or a veggie wrap, or salad. Or how about a big plate of steamed broccoli? Or a colorful veggie juice? My (Shelley's) favorite is the Zippy Breakfast (see page 358) made with buckwheat (a seed) instead of a starchy grain. We need to learn from the traditions of some other cultures—for example, you'd be offered soup for breakfast in Japan. When we traveled in Israel, we were delighted to see tomato-cucumber salads as a part of every breakfast table. The American way—tremendous doses of sugar and protein (acids both), not to mention a big dollop of caffeine—might give you a short shot of energy initially, but over the long term the negative impact is drastic.

So begin with this new breakfast strategy, starting your day with an alkaline, low-carbohydrate, high-fiber, high-water-content, electron-rich—and delicious—meal. Try it even just for a couple of weeks if you don't feel ready to sign on forever. If you're like most people, you'll find your new breakfast provides a great amount of energy and burns longer into the midday without the drop in electron or electrical energy that so commonly occurs with an acidic starchy, sugary breakfast. Once you experience how good you can feel, I think it will be the junk food breakfast that seems strange.

TRANSITION 2: 70–30

This is another giant step: Build each meal to be at least 70 percent alkaline (and thus 30 percent acid). Better yet is 80–20, which is ideal, though 100 percent may be necessary if you are seriously ill. If you're already doing this at breakfast, lunch and dinner will be simple by comparison.

This is a visual measurement, not a measurement by weight or calories. Just give the vegetables the starring role on your plate, where acidic protein (like meat) or carbs (like pasta) might have been before. Make two or three alkalizing vegetables to go along with what you used to think of as your main dish. Or make a meal just out of these sides. Eat a big bowl of alkalizing salad or vegetable soup with each meal.

The earth is 70 percent water. Our bodies are 70 percent water. Make your plate match: at least 70 percent high-water-content, electron-rich, alkaline food.

TRANSITION 3: RAW

Cooking your food literally takes the life or electrical energy right out of it, and makes it void of electrons, so the more food you eat raw, the better. Raw foods are alkalizing and full of electrons or life energy, and so fit in that 70 to 80 percent we were just talking about. Ideally, all of that three-quarters of your plate is covered with high-water-content, electron-rich alkaline food—like having a huge salad with a side of brown rice or beans or pasta or tofu. And at least half that portion should be raw. (The other half should still be vegetarian and alkalizing, like lightly cooked soup, or steamed veggies, or stir-fry.) Start with that and as you get comfortable with the program work up to the ideal.

This is another reason big salads—and a variety of other kinds of salads—are such a great part of this program. Anything sprouted is ideal and full of electrical energy to run your body. With healthful dips and sauces to complement them, as a snack, appetizer, or side dish, raw electron-rich alkalizing vegetables are a wonderful, colorful, crunchy, and wholesome way to go. Make sure you include some each time you sit down for a meal.

Raw doesn't mean you have to have all your food cold. It is worthwhile to learn the difference between cooking and simply warming your food. When you do cook, do so as quickly as possible. For example, I am a big fan of quick steam-fry—it's like stir-frying, except you use a small amount of liquid instead of oil. And when I make a big pot of soup (which is often), I cook it just until it's done—and the veggies are still quite firm. In general, apply heat gently and in moderation. The thing is to not exceed 118 degrees F. (The simplest way to check is to stick your finger into whatever you are warming. If you can hold it in without pulling it out right away, you are in the right range. If you have to pull your finger out, the temperature is too high.) Avoid the burning, crisping, and browning that can convert otherwise healthy electron-rich alkalizing foods into acidic toxins. It is especially important not to heat oils. Steam your food rather than cooking it in oil. You can then apply liberal amounts of oil on vegetables after warming or steaming. Or use a nonstick cooking spray made of lecithin. It may take a little experimentation to get dishes just right, but the health benefits are worth it. Dehydrating your food is another way of preparing it for additional variety in texture and flavor without cooking it (see chapter 10).

When the weather is cold, warm cooked food might take a larger portion of your plate (keeping it alkalizing, though), while hot summer months bring more crisp, raw selections. Don't make this program so rigid it becomes a hassle. Keep it flexible and easy, and it will soon be something you do intuitively, rather than something you have to think much about.

TRANSITION 4: DESSERT

Phase out all acidic sugary desserts. One acidic sugary dessert can ruin even the best alkaline meal. At our house, we used to be stocked with ice cream and baked goodies like anyone else. First we switched to frozen yogurt and those granola-y "health food" cookies, then to Rice Dream bars. From there we went to simple fresh fruit.

Now that we're fully alkalized, for the most part we don't eat dessert. For us, a treat is a crisp, red bell pepper or thick slices of subtly sweet jicama. I realize that might be hard to imagine until you've reached the same place. But taste buds that may now be dulled by the effects of extreme acidic sugars and processed salt will come to appreciate the humbler sweetness of green alkalizing vegetables. A cookie or candy bar will seem much too sweet, even intolerable. You will see.

You may have some cravings until your sugar (acid) addiction wears off and your blood electron levels stabilize. Understanding why you get such cravings may help you ride them out. Find other things that will take the edge off, so you won't give in to early temptations. We have found when you crave acidic things such as sugar, alcohol, and tobacco, you are experiencing the body's need for alkalizing mineral salts. Take a pinch of whole mineral salts, or carry a small bottle of liquid salt with you and spray it into your mouth when cravings occur. The craving will go away in a few minutes. "Cheating" just makes the cravings last longer. However, if you do eat something not on your plan, waste no time beating yourself up over it. Just get right back to your alkalizing pH Miracle plan.

We do break down once in a while, like on vacation, but only when we are balanced and well. And then we eat dessert first, or by itself, in between meals, to avoid interfering with the healthy electron-rich alkaline foods we eat. And we always get right back in the game.

TRANSITION 5: MEAT

Getting meat out of your diet is painless when you go gradually. Cut back on and then get rid of the red meat first—beef, pork, lamb, and anything else you have. Make chicken the next to go, then turkey. Then comes ocean fish. You might want to include, as we do, the occasional fish on your menus. If you do want to have some animal protein occasionally, we recommend trout, sea bass, sole, tuna, swordfish, and salmon, as they are relatively safe, and are rich in alkalizing omega-3 oils fats.

Start with a vegetarian alkaline meal once a day, then twice, as you work your way to full-time. At the same time, experiment with building in more hemp meal and/or tofu, as well as raw nuts and seeds, including almonds, hazelnuts, pecans, and sunflower, pumpkin, flax, and sesame seeds. Almonds are especially good—substantially alkalizing and high in protein and calcium.

Be sure to steer clear of peanuts because of their high fungal content, however. And in general, avoid rancid nuts and seeds. If a batch of hulled seeds, such as sunflower or pumpkin, is sprinkled with broken or sick-looking seeds, don't eat it. It would be possible to remove the bad ones—in the unlikely event you had enough time and patience. If you get that rancid taste, an odd bitter sting at the back of the throat, get rid of the batch. Sesame and flax seeds, by the way, are almost always okay. Almonds and hazelnuts should either be shelled on the spot or have their brown protective skin intact. Do not use broken, gouged, or chipped nuts.

GO SOAK YOUR . . . NUTS

Soak nuts and seeds to activate their electrical potential or life force, eliminate acidic enzymes and enzyme inhibitors, and partially digest the protein, thus increasing their nutritional and hydrating potential by making all the good stuff they contain readily available to the body. Soaking also makes small seeds such as sesame and flax easier to chew, which you must do to release their electrical potential or electrons for energy.

Put nuts in a container, cover with alkaline water to one to two inches above the top of the nuts, and place in the refrigerator for an hour or two—for almonds, overnight. They will plump up, absorbing the water and the oxygen in the water. Then they will be ready to enjoy. Rinse them off and change the water every day. Keep them totally submerged. Eat them within two days, to prevent molding under the skin of the nuts.

TRANSITION 6: DAIRY

This step may actually be key to the first (breakfast), if you're one of the many, many people we talk to who can't think what to eat in the morning—or to give the kids—if not a bowl of cereal with milk.

The first thing to do is work on milk. Switch to hemp or soy milk (making sure to get one that isn't full of added sugars such as rice syrup) or rice milk (if you can find one that's not sugary). Move on to nut or seed milks, like hazel or almond. They are good sources of protein and calcium, and have that richness and creaminess that is so pleasing. You can dilute them to taste. They are good for adding texture in salad dressings or soups, or just to drink. (Though when it comes to something to drink, pure, electron-rich, alkalized water and fresh alkalizing vegetable juices are always your best bet.) I mostly use almond and sesame (aka tahini) milks, and occasionally cook with rice milk or coconut milk. You can make your own (see page 268). Or, for convenience, try a good ready-made almond milk, like the one from Pacific Foods (see the resources section).

After you've eliminated milk, other dairy products, such as cheese, yogurt, and ice cream, will be easy to cut out; you can find transitional substitutes at first and eventually go without. One of our new favorite breakfasts is Seed Pancakes with Coconut Whipped Topping (see page 356). It's so rich and creamy, you'll never miss the dairy!

EATING OUT

Some people worry that changing the way they eat will mean an end to socializing in restaurants. While it may be true that you'll have another transition to make, in the restaurants you choose or the dishes you order there, you are by no means stuck cooking for yourself in your own home forever. Many areas have vegetarian restaurants now (there are even a few featuring raw foods!), and more and more general restaurants are offering vegetarian and even vegan entrées. You'll be sure to find vegetarian options within Asian, Indian, and Italian cuisines. And most restaurants have salads or side dishes you can build a fine meal from if none of the featured entrées suits your needs. For example, you could put together a pretty good meal with a green dinner salad, an order of the vegetable of the day, and a side of black beans, brown basmati rice, or baked red potato. Of course, anyplace with a salad bar will do just fine, as long as you choose carefully to avoid the junk food and acidic salad dressings with vinegars and sugars. And don't be afraid to make specific requests—we do it all the time, and they are almost always graciously accepted. (Our most common requests are to hold the cheese, skip the bread, or leave out the mushrooms.) Most chefs are happy to do a basic vegetable stir-fry, if you ask for it. You can even follow the pH Miracle program at major national chains. If we are, for example, eating at the Cheesecake Factory, we order the avocado/sun-dried tomato egg rolls, roasted artichokes, and Thai lettuce wraps (with salmon substituted for the chicken), and perhaps one of the huge bowls of steamed broccoli and asparagus offered as sides. Of course, we do skip the actual cheesecake!

TRANSITION 7: YEAST

Bread is another tough one for a lot of families, but you must get rid of the yeast. At our house, we went first to yeast-free bread (your health food store will have some choices), then to rice crackers, then sprouted whole wheat tortillas. In the recipes section, you'll find some yeast-free breads and crackers you can make yourself (see pages 369–70). In addition to simple substitutions, you must also open up your thinking to meals that don't include bread or other yeast products. If you are one of those people who wouldn't know what to have for lunch if it didn't involve a sandwich, or breakfast if it didn't include toast, this may actually be the biggest challenge for you. Focus on what you *can* have, what is good for you, rather than what you *can't* have. The recipes section gives plenty of meal ideas, along with the recipes, to help you on your way.

During this transition, get rid of mushrooms, too—they are fungi, just like yeast.

TRANSITION 8: WHITE FLOUR

If you've eliminated yeast breads and baked desserts, you've most likely gotten rid of the major source of white flour in your diet. The other big hurdle is usually pasta. Most recipes will work well if you substitute cooked whole grains such as millet, spelt, quinoa, rice, and buckwheat. Try soba noodles (a favorite in our house), which are buckwheat, and satisfy the need for a chewy, warm food, especially in winter. We also love mugwort and wild yam soba noodles. If we use pasta other than soba, we try to make sure it is made with vegetables and without eggs—and serve it as a side dish, never a main course.

TRANSITION 9: WHITE RICE

Here's a simple one for you: Switch to brown rice. Or alternate, as we do, with white jasmine or basmati rice, which are natural white rices, or wild rice (or combinations). What we're really after eliminating here is all refined grains. You need to give the boot to anything that isn't whole grain. Best, as always, are sprouted grains. And remember, cooked grains belong in that 20 to 30 percent of your meal that is acid (except buckwheat, millet, quinoa, and spelt, which are not acidifying). The one starch you should abandon altogether, because of the high sugar and fungal content, is corn.

TRANSITION 10: ADDED SUGAR

Eliminating dessert might have taken care of a lot of this, but now it is time to scrub out the rest of the unnecessary sugars (acids). Check your cereal, bread, and anything you bought prepared. Don't rely on artificial sweeteners, because they all convert to highly toxic acids that can harm the brain. If you need a sweetener to help you transition while your taste buds adjust, try something natural like chicory root powder or stevia (made from a plant), which you can find at health food stores. There are several different types of stevia, some bleached, others in liquid form. We prefer raw green powdered stevia, which has had very little processing. You can find raw green stevia in some health food stores but you may have to special-order it, through the store or via the Internet.

TRANSITION 11: FRUIT

With the exception of the low-sugar fruits we keep talking about—tomato, avocado, lemon, lime—fruits are intense sources of sugar (acid), and must be eliminated if you are ill or have troublesome symptoms. Once you are in balance, you may still want to use them rarely and with care (and properly combined), as a treat. Fruits have nutritional value, but most have just too much sugar to use freely.

TRANSITION 12: CONDIMENTS

Most condiments are full of sugar, processed salt, or both. Or they contain fermented or acidifying ingredients. Experiment to find your favorite alternatives to ketchup, mustard, vinegar, mayonnaise, barbecue sauce, soy sauce, and so forth.

Your best allies are healthy mono- and polyunsaturated oils, lemons, limes, garlic, onion, ginger, spices, and, of course, healthy, whole mineral salts. The oils we like best are grape seed oil, flax seed oil, coconut oil, pumpkin seed oil, hemp seed oil, avocado oil, pomegranate oil, and olive oil. We use a lot of Essential Balance and Udo's Choice—combinations of healthful oils (see resources). All alkalizing oils should be added to food after cooking, since heating oil destroys its vital electrical energy or life force components. Better yet, use it with raw foods. Make salad dressings, for instance. (For times when homemade just isn't feasible, one salad dressing we like is Annie's Naturals Organic Green Garlic.) Rather than cooking in oil, steam your food and add alkalizing oil as you are serving it.

Lemon and lime add freshness and zest to just about any dish, and because of the low sugar content are alkalizing to boot. They also help stop sugar (acid) cravings. They are another key ingredient for many salad dressings. We put them in just about everything we make, right down to a glass of water. Garlic, onion, and ginger are all naturally antifungal and antiparasitic, not to mention their nice strong flavors, so include plenty of them, as well.

Getting creative with spices is going to be the key to making delicious meals that appeal to your taste buds. We love Spice Hunter brand spice blends, like Zip, which contains onion, paprika, chili pepper, cumin, garlic, jalapeño, coriander, cayenne, and oregano. They take a lot of the guesswork out, but leave the subtle, interesting combinations in (see resources). Experiment!

MARSHA'S STORY

Okay, I'll admit it. I used to eat bacon or sausage and fried or scrambled eggs for breakfast, with toast with jelly—or butter so thick I could see my teeth marks in it. Every day. I never gave it a second thought. And it only went downhill from there through the rest of the day.

It seemed like I was always sick with a cold or allergies, my skin and the whites of my eyes had a yellowish cast to them, and my eyesight was getting worse and worse. I was always tired, though I accepted the ebbing of my energy as part of the aging process. When I needed yet another, stronger contact lens prescription just three months after the last one (again!), it scared me enough that I decided to commit to changing my diet, adding more alkalizing foods and concentrated green powder and lots and lots of pure water.

I started with breakfast. I started using vegetarian burgers in place of the meat, and switched to soy margarine instead of butter. Then I learned to smash up tofu to look like scrambled eggs—I like them sprinkled with spicy seasonings. Then sometimes I'd put avocado slices on the plate next to the tofu scramble. Then I went on to having something totally different for me, such as soup, or avocado and cucumber over raw (not toasted) buckwheat.

Where I used to drink low-fat milk, I started with vanilla soy milk, or almond milk. Now I drink fresh vegetable juices or put green powder in my water, and use soy and almond milk only occasionally.

Just changing breakfast gave me much more energy. It also changed my long-standing habit of snacking starting by 10 AM. With an alkalizing breakfast, I'm not hungry again until lunchtime. Then, when I always had meat, poultry, or seafood (just like at dinner), I started using meat substitutes, and then extra-firm tofu. Now I mostly have beans or legumes stir-fried with broccoli or other vegetables along with a nice big salad. I've traded peanuts and peanut butter for soy nuts or almonds, and soy or almond butter. I use avocado as a base for creamy soups. I switched from vinaigrette on my salads to olive oil and lemon juice with seasonings.

My between-meals snacks have become celery, red, yellow, or orange bell peppers, baby carrots, or cucumber, with almond butter or hummus—where I used to have candy or chips. I still get to crunch and munch to my heart's content, and over time my huge sugar cravings have left me.

Since replacing meats and dairy three years ago, I haven't had allergies, a cold, a sore throat, or the flu. By flip-flopping my eating pattern to 80 to 100 percent alkalizing (where it used to be that much acidic!)—gradually, as I could manage it, not overnight—I gained more energy and stamina. I wake up earlier and stay up later, and my energy level is on an even keel throughout the day. The yellow tinge disappeared altogether. I lost—and have kept off—thirty-eight pounds. And my eyesight not only stopped deteriorating, it has actually improved. I've had two new prescriptions in three years now—this time less strong each time.

Once your transition is complete, and your symptoms (if any) are gone, and you are at a stable, natural, healthy weight, your body will be in appropriate alkaline–acid balance. Although you've done all this work because you are adopting a new way of life, not some short-term diet plan, we do want to note that a healthy, balanced body can withstand a certain degree of cheating. Not that we're recommending it, mind you, but we don't want you to think that the occasional sensational, acidifying indulgence will undo all you've accomplished. Though you'll have to be stricter in the beginning, that kind of treat here and there may be no problem at all for a balanced system. (We probably cheat once every other month or so.) And if it is a problem, now you know how to fix it. Remember, it can take up to twenty times the amount of alkaline food to neutralize a dose of acidic food, so you don't want to make your body do that often. It is the everyday bombardment of acidic foods that leave a body completely out of balance. Once you've gone through all these steps, and transformed the way you eat, you'll have gotten well. Now to stay well, of course you've got to continue on the path you've set so far.

Chapter 10

·

Putting It Together

The more you follow this program, the easier it becomes to follow. Your body adjusts to it, and so do you. It will come to seem second nature. Right now, though, you've got a steep learning curve. We're throwing a lot of information at you all at once, and you are probably looking at pretty significant changes in the way you live your life. Experience is the best teacher—but while you're gathering your experience, we want to give you some practical strategies for implementing this program. You'll learn here how to stock (restock, really) your kitchen, with food and equipment, as well as how to grow your own sprouts, and how to dehydrate foods. Finally, Shelley will share some of her secrets for using the program in your ordinary, everyday, no-doubt-already-busy life. Shelley will teach you that nothing tastes as good as good health feels.

STOCKING THE PANTRY

You're preparing to embark on the adventure of a lifetime—the adventure of a health-generating lifestyle. You have heard the science, and now you want to know how to continually live that science from the kitchen. When you take a look at what is in your house right now to eat, however, you're likely to face the grim reality that much of what you have isn't good for you after all, now that you understand the New Biology. You probably have a lot that is flat-out lacking in nutrition and fiber, and more that has a very acidic effect in the body.

To make it simple to follow this program, chances are you're going to need a makeover. But once you've transformed your kitchen, you'll find it easy, simple, and natural to follow the principles of a healthy alkaline diet. One key is to keep all the basic items you'll use a lot of on hand in your pantry and fridge, so you can prepare a delicious—alkaline—dish at the drop of a hat.

If you poked around my (Shelley's) kitchen for a few minutes, here's what you'd find:

- **Spices**. Just in case I can't get fresh ones, I keep dried spices, which I buy in bulk. I am always stocked up with garlic powder, onion flakes, cumin, basil, cilantro, cayenne pepper, turmeric, cinnamon, curry, and parsley. I also always have an alkalizing salt. I prefer pure mineral salts, Real Salt brand, Celtic Sea Salt (harder to find), Young pHorever pHlavor Salt from the Great Salt Lake, vegetized salt (which has dehydrated veggies in with the salt), Herbamare (sea salt and organic veggies), Trocomare (spicy, with sea salt, veggies, chili peppers, and horseradish), and Herby (quite hot because of the black pepper it contains). Beyond that, I like to use premixed spice combinations to take the guesswork out of things, avoid unnecessary clutter, and keep it simple! I'm a fan of the Spice Hunter brand (see resources). The combinations inspire me, too, be they Mexican, Italian, Thai, Jamaican jerk, Szechuan, pizza, curry, or Herbes de Provence. Not only that, you can make the same dish seem really different depending on what you shake over it.
- **Seeds**. I keep a supply of (raw) flax, hemp, chia, sesame, sunflower, alfalfa, and pumpkin seeds, as well as sprouting combinations. I also keep raw tahini (sesame seed paste) around.
- **Nuts**. I always have raw nuts on hand, too, usually almonds, hazelnuts, pine nuts, Brazil nuts, and macadamias, as well as fresh, seasonal pecans and walnuts and raw almond butter.
- **Grains**. I keep spelt, buckwheat, millet, kamut, quinoa, brown basmati rice, and amaranth handy, as well as unsalted brown rice cakes, quinoa and spelt pasta, buckwheat, rice and soba noodles, sprouted wheat tortillas, Lavosh crackers (made with tofu, and yeast-free), and flours (whole wheat, unbleached white, spelt, brown rice, rye, and millet in particular—soy and rice flour would be okay, too, as long as they are not stored for a long time). I also keep unleavened whole wheat bread (like Nature's Path Manna Bread) in the freezer (from the freezer section of the store).
- **Beans**. I usually have soybeans (sometimes known as edamame beans—look for them in the frozen foods section of your store), adzuki beans, lentils, mung beans, cranberry beans, black beans, black-eyed peas, garbanzos/chickpeas, pinto beans, and kidney beans. I almost always have hummus in my fridge, too.

- **Sea vegetables**. I often use nori sheets, dulse flakes, and arame, so I keep them around.
- **Tortillas**. Look for sprouted wheat varieties. Some wraps restaurants may sell you their tortillas. If you are able to set up an account (as a business) with the food manufacturing and supply company Sysco, you can get a variety of different-flavored tortillas—I like the spinach, garlic, onion, and pepper. Costco also sells tortillas, or you can make your own (see the recipe on page 370).
- **Healthy oils**. I always have a variety available, especially virgin cold-pressed olive oil, avocado oil (like Young pHorever Avocado Oil), grape seed oil, sesame oil, and flax seed oil, and a blend (like Udo's Choice or Essential Balance, under the brand name Omega Nutrition, or Arrowhead Mills). Hemp oil has quite a strong flavor, but I use it on occasion, too. Look for Essential Balance in the refrigerated section of your health food store, and keep it in your refrigerator or freezer. It is a wonderfully flavored oil combining organic flax, sunflower/safflower, pumpkin, borage, and sesame oils. It's the only oil organically processed, made from all organic seeds, and completely unrefined. It comes in a black bottle to keep light from damaging it.
- **"Milk."** For when I need it and don't have time to make my own, I keep almond, hazel, soy, or rice milks around.
- **Water**. I keep purified alkaline ionized electron-rich water in gallon containers. We have ionizers at several stations in our home, office, and guesthouses, providing freshly made electron-rich water.
- **Soy**. I always have some tofu handy, including baked tofu, and I often have soy burgers in the freezer (I like Boca Burgers, vegan variety).
- **Produce**. Since produce must be fresh, I obviously don't store it indefinitely—although the stuff that keeps, such as garlic, ginger (I keep a whole root in the freezer and grate it as necessary), onions, fresh and dried chili peppers, lemons, and limes, I buy enough of to always have around. And since I've always got something sprouting, I have a fresh harvest on any given day. (My favorite is a high-protein mix of mung beans, adzuki beans, lentils, peas, and sunflower seeds, and I often use a mix of alfalfa and other small seeds, too.) In my pantry, I'm never without sun-dried tomatoes packed in olive oil, roasted bell peppers packed in olive oil, and vegetable broth (make sure the one you choose contains no yeast).

Beyond that, I usually shop twice a week for fresh produce, and have a selection of fresh veggies and low-sugar fruits in the house at all times. You won't find them all at once, of course, but I often have baby field greens, dark lettuces, broccoli, spinach, kale, red and green cabbage, celery, carrots, cucumber, cauliflower, squash, zucchini, beets, radishes, avocado, tomato, bell peppers, chard, asparagus, green beans, leeks, and eggplant—basically, a variety of the foods eaten freely on this program. I always have some fresh herbs, especially parsley, basil, and cilantro, in my kitchen, and usually some fresh salsa (made with lemon or lime juice, never vinegar).

There are many, many more kinds of produce, of course, not mentioned here. Your selection should reflect your tastes, and your family's, as well as the recipes you use most often. Your kitchen won't look exactly like mine, but once it is well stocked, you'll find it is easy and natural to follow this way of eating. (Remember to read labels carefully to avoid hidden harmful foods, especially citric acid, sweeteners, artificial sweeteners, yeast, vinegar, peanuts, and corn syrup.) There's no need to go out and buy every single thing on this list at once. Start with a few items from each category and build up as you go along. Let it be an adventure to create a selection of alkalizing food choices for you and your loved ones!

THE RIGHT TOOLS

You can make a great alkalizing meal with just one good knife—and plenty of time. However, as any good carpenter knows, the proper tools do the job faster, easier, and with optimum results. Here is a quick look at the things I find are indispensable in my kitchen.

- **Good knives** are a must for cleaning, trimming, cutting, and chopping your veggies. I got along quite well with a three-piece starter set for years before investing in a larger set. I use them many times every day, and simply could not get by without them. If you've had poor-quality or dull knives, you'll be amazed by the difference a high-quality, properly sharpened knife can make. I'm a fan of Cutco knives, which come with a lifetime guarantee and hardly ever need sharpening.
- **A food processor** will cut your chopping, blending, and mixing time by as much as 90 percent, especially when you are preparing food for a crowd. I use a Cuisinart. I started with the standard seven-cup size, which is fine for everyday needs. (I use a sixteen-cup size now, when I'm preparing food for a lot of people at one time.) Look for one that comes with both sharp- and soft-edged S-blades, as well as shredding and slicing wheels. The sharp S-blade is useful for mixing, mincing, fine and coarse chopping, blending foods such as hummus,

emulsifying things such as salad dressing, and grinding dry ingredients including nuts, seeds, grains, and dried tortillas into powders.
I use the soft-edged S-blade to mix the dough for tortillas. And I
slice and shred all kinds of things—which I especially love because it
makes it easy to make beautiful salads.

- **A blender** is useful, too, for mixing, blending, and grinding. I use
  the Vita-Mix. It has a strong motor and a good variety of options for
  speed control (as well as reverse). The unique feature, and one I use a
  lot, is that if you leave it running longer, the friction it creates warms
  the food—so recipes like raw soups can be worked up very fast and
  then served immediately straight from the blender. (Of course, you
  can also serve them cold—just blend for a shorter period of time.)
- **Rice cooker.** Mine is almost always on the counter, full of freshly
  steamed brown rice, buckwheat, or other grain for my family to help
  themselves to at any time during the day. I use the Zojirushi brand,
  which will also cook legumes. Sometimes I start it up before I go to
  bed at night so we'll have warm rice for breakfast.
- **Salad Spinner.** I could not do without it (well, I'd never want to do
  without it). I use it all the time to wash and dry greens in a jif.
- **Mandolin.** This is great for doing extra-fancy cuts on veggies. Presentation is a key part of how you experience a meal, and this is a
  simple way to make dishes more elegant and visually appealing.
- **Saladacco.** I'm a fan of this small hand machine that can make angel-
  hair "pasta" out of vegetables such as squash. (I use yellow summer
  squash and zucchini, but any squash would work.) It also makes beautiful ribbon cuts that look like Hawaiian leis on such vegetables as
  beets and carrots.
- **Stainless-steel cookware.** I'm totally reliant on cookware made from
  high-grade surgical stainless steel. (I use Saladmaster brand; see resources.) The right stainless lets you heat your food up to 187 degrees
  without destroying its electrical charge or its vitamin and mineral content. And it won't leach poisonous substances into your food. Cooking in pots or pans made out of anything else can be hazardous to your
  health. Cast iron is highly porous, and the grease that gets into those
  pores will get rancid. Your body also can't assimilate the iron (ferric) that
  seeps from the pans into your food—you need the ferrous form—so the
  main nutritional reason to use cast iron is right out the window. Glass or
  enamel-coated pans generally have poor heat distribution so foods stick
  and burn, but worse is the fact that they contain lead. Aluminum is a
  very soft metal and undergoes an extreme chemical reaction with heat,

contaminating any food that comes in contact with it. Worse still are nonstick coated pans. When they scratch, chip, or flake, you get exposed to "resins . . . [that] may produce a condition termed polymer fume fever characterized by flu-like symptoms such as chills, fever, body aches, nausea and occasional vomiting" according to the Federal Aviation Agency Occupational Health and Safety Bulletin. Yum! And that's just the short-term effects! A chemical, C-8, used to make nonstick coating has been linked to birth defects in humans and to cancer in laboratory animals. The chemical is detectable in the blood for up to four years after exposure, and can show up in breast milk. Even lower-grade stainless-steel alloy chrome and nickel can bleed into foods containing salts or acids. That's why when I cook, I stick with the highest-quality stainless steel! I wouldn't risk my family's health on anything else.

Once you are committed to preparing mostly raw foods for your meals, you can really get into gadgets like these. Invest in them as you can, to make preparing your food simpler—and more fun (and sometimes prettier). Experiment, and enjoy.

SPROUTING

Sprouts, with their tremendous regenerating properties, are incredibly nutritious and alkalizing. All the wide variety of vitamins and minerals in a seed or grain explode when sprouted. Sprouting also takes starches, proteins, and hormonal agents in the seed and turns them into very alkalizing, easily assimilated, predigested proteins and subtle vegetable sugars. Finally, the phytochemicals that fight cancerous conditions appear in plants just as soon as they sprout. I think a person could live on sprouts alone with no (physical) problem at all.

So I keep plenty of fresh sprouts around all the time—I grow them. No green thumb necessary. Really. The process is simple. In no time at all, a pinch of seeds almost magically transforms into many times their original weight in fresh produce, sometimes in as little as two days.

Start with organically produced seeds. You can store seeds for sprouting for long periods of time (up to ten years if they are unopened, and one to two years if opened but kept dry and cool), so stock up and keep a variety on hand. Some of the easiest sprouts to grow are alfalfa, mung bean, chickpea, green lentil, sesame, sunflower, buckwheat, and wheat. The "Sprouting Guide" table provides basic directions for many common sprouts.

I soak the seeds overnight in purified ionized electron-rich alkaline water, until they're plump, then pour them into sprouting trays, let them drain, place the trays in a dark, warm cupboard, and rinse them twice a day. Actually, I keep the trays where we keep our water, so that when I get my first drink of the morning and my last one at night, I give the sprouts a drink, too, rinsing and draining them.

In two or three days, most sprouts will be ready to eat. Sprouts should be crisp and slightly sweet—never sour. If they are souring, as the store-bought ones often are, they have gone too long, and you should start again. Sprouts should never be browning or at all slimy. Store sprouts in the refrigerator in a glass jar or sealed plastic bag. They will keep for about a week.

You can also grow sprouts using quart jars with mesh rubber-banded over the top, or special sprouting jars with drainage lids, instead of the trays. Go with whichever method you find simplest!

I recommend kits from the Life Sprouts company to help get you started with sprouting (see resources). Most health food stores carry sprouting supplies, including seeds ready for sprouting.

SPROUTING GUIDE

Seed	Quantity	Soak Time (hours)	Rinse/ Drain (times daily)	Time to Harvest (days)	Height to Harvest (inches)
Alfalfa	2 T	6–8	2	3–6	1–2
Chinese cabbage	1 cup	6–8	2	3–4	½–1
Fenugreek	1 cup	6–8	2–3	3–4	½–1
Garbanzo	1 cup	16	2–3	3–6	⅛–1
Lentil	1 cup	8–12	2–3	2–4	½–1
Mung bean	½ cup	8–12	2–3	2–4	½–1
Peas	½ or 1 cup	8–12	2–3	2–3	½–1
Radish	2 T or 1 cup	6–8	2	3–4	½–1
Red clover	2 T	8	2	3–6	½–2
Sesame	¼ cup	8	2	1–3	0–1
Soybean	½ or 1 cup	16	3	3–5	½–1
Sunflower, hulled	½ or 1 cup	6–8	2	1–2	0–½

Ways to Use Sprouts

Sprouts are terrific raw, stir-fried, or steam-fried, on their own, or in sandwiches or salads, or sprinkled over soups. Try them all different ways—the more sprouts you get, the better. Everyone should make sprouts a part of their daily diet.

Almost any sprouts are good in salads, and I use them all the time in sandwiches and wraps, soups and juices, steamed dishes, and casseroles. They also make a great snack. Here are my suggestions:

- **Salad.** Alfalfa, Chinese cabbage, fenugreek, garbanzo, lentil, mung bean, peas, radish, red clover, sunflower.
- **Sandwiches.** Alfalfa, radish, red clover.
- **Juice.** Alfalfa, Chinese cabbage, radish, red clover.
- **Soup.** Garbanzo, lentil, mung bean, peas, soybean.
- **Casseroles.** Garbanzo, sesame, soybean.
- **Snacks.** Fenugreek, sesame, sunflower.
- **Steamed.** Lentil, mung bean, peas, soybean.

This is just to get you started! Use your imagination, experiment, follow your taste buds. Just keep eating sprouts!

DEHYDRATING

Using a dehydrator is a wonderful way to serve your food warm, but not cooked. It also makes it easy to keep fresh veggies in your pantry (once they are dried, fresh vegetables stored in an airtight bag or container will keep for at least a year in a dry, cool place). Food dehydrators are also useful for warming pâtés and loaf-type recipes before serving.

Dehydrated vegetables and nuts make great snacks and terrific garnishes. Enjoy them on their own, or with a favorite dip or pâté. They are very pretty sprinkled over soups, add texture to salads, and can accent any plate nicely.

Dehydrating most vegetables couldn't be simpler. You just clean and slice them (about one-quarter inch thick), marinate if desired, drain, and place on clean drying racks in your dehydrator. Dehydrate until all water is out of the vegetables and they are crisp.

You can do this with just about any vegetable. I especially like carrots, tomatoes, onions, celery, and bell peppers. For root vegetables such as winter squash, carrots, and yams, I like to marinate them for up to an hour in pure mineral salts, garlic, ginger, and spices.

Try dehydrating nuts, too. Start with soaked nuts. Marinate, as above, in a shallow bowl for one to twelve hours. Drain well, place in dehydrator, and dry until crunchy. Store in an airtight container in the fridge.

I use an Excalibur brand dehydrator because I like the way the air circulates throughout each tray, rather than just coming from the bottom up. The flexible, Teflex liners also make it easy to make batter-type recipes, such as Dehydrated Flax Chips (see page 375), and to lift off foods after they have dried.

TIPS AND TRICKS

Here are some of my favorite shortcuts for making and arranging alkaline meals quickly and easily:

• Keep a huge salad in the fridge at all times. I make one that will last about three days and fill it with such goodies as spinach, red onions, pine nuts, tofu cubes, shredded carrot and beet, radishes, and sunflower seed sprouts. Then I can grab a quick salad or fill a wrap quickly. It is also good to have on hand when kids come home from school with that ravenous appetite.

• Make enough of your favorite salad dressings to last all week.

• Use prepared spice combinations. I keep a selection in the pantry to add interest and variety to whatever dish I'm making.

• Keep a bowl of soaked almonds in the fridge. They are great for a sweet, crunchy snack, and on salads instead of croutons. They are also good for whipping up some nut milk in a hurry. Just cover raw nuts with plenty of water, soak overnight, and change the water daily. They'll keep for about three days.

• Mix up batches of your favorite spread, such as pesto or hummus, for use as a dip for raw veggies, a topping for steamed veggies, to spread on crackers, or to tuck into wraps. You can find some good ones at your local health food store, including dairy-less pesto, although you must always read the labels carefully so you know exactly what you're buying.

• Double or triple a cooked recipe and freeze for future meals or quick snacks.

• When soaking dried beans or cooking cabbage, add a dash of mineral salts to the water to make them less gaseous, reducing or eliminating the flatulence they can cause.

• Adding two tablespoons of pure mineral salts to the cooking water keeps broccoli and cauliflower crisp and preserves their electrical potential.

• Use a damp paper towel and a sprinkling of mineral salts to remove chlorophyll stains from your water bottle.

• Keep lemons and limes on hand to use as a vinegar substitute and to squeeze into your drinking water all day long. I use lemons somewhere in almost every meal I serve.

• Take a few packages of sprouted wheat tortillas and set them out to dry on your kitchen counter overnight. Or bake them in a low-heat oven, about three hundred degrees, for fifteen to twenty minutes until crisp but not browned. They should break easily, like a cracker. Grind them in your food processor or blender until they are like flour, to use when a recipe calls for bread crumbs or white flour. Store in an airtight container. They will keep for a few weeks in a cool, dry place (less in humid weather).

• Use your freezer to advantage. Store serving-size packages of nuts, herbs, and even good oils such as flax seed, so you'll have them when you need them (and they'll stay fresher, and defrost quickly). I keep a fresh gingerroot in the freezer; it's then easy to grate when a recipe calls for it. My favorite use for it, though, is to make fresh lemon ginger "tea" after a nice meal.

• Keep a rice cooker on the counter with a fresh batch of steamed legumes or grains for that 20 to 30 percent of your diet.

• Learn to do your own sprouting and keep fresh sprouts on hand for a great snack—or a nutritional booster to any meal.

• Be prepared for the desire for crunchy snacks by keeping healthy options easily available, such as baked sprouted tortillas, raw almonds (best soaked), raw veggies (one of our favorites is slightly sweet jicama sticks, which are good anyway, but can also help during sugar cravings), and baked tofu.

• Stock up on pure ionized electron-rich alkaline water—and drink up! When your meals are 80 percent alkaline, you may not feel a need to drink with meals, since most vegetables are already 70 to 90 percent water. But in between meals, drinking a lot of good water is one of the very best things you can do for yourself.

Chapter 11

·

The pH Miracle
Whole Body Cleanse

Our bodies, subjected as they have been to the typical American (acidic!) diet, could be designated Super Fund sites. They urgently need cleaning up from deadly toxic waste. Gradually transitioning to an alkaline diet may be the best way to make this a way of life rather than a short-term "diet" Band-Aid. But at some point, if you want to reap all the benefits of this program, you are going to need to clear out the old to make way for the new. As with a Super Fund site, you can't just plant new trees and build new houses—first you have to get rid of the sludge. You need to do a pH Miracle Whole Body Cleanse to rid the body of impurities, normalize digestion (the alkaline buffering system) and metabolism, and regain alkaline balance in the blood and tissues.

If you have an immediate, serious health concern, you may want to jump right into the program with a serious cleanse. Transitioning is all well and good if you have the option, but if you are plagued with negative (acidic) symptoms, more drastic action may be required. Otherwise, if you are taking your time making a transition, think about doing a pH Miracle Whole Body Cleanse as you near completion of your transition, so that afterward you can continue directly to a purely alkaline diet. Finally, even if you are planning a longer transition, you can begin with a cleanse as a way to sort of jump-start yourself. Of course, you can always do another cleanse after you're on a pure alkaline diet, anytime you want or need it. We like to do a springtime cleanse, just as the earth renews itself after a long winter.

A pH Miracle Whole Body Cleanse is something like a fast, but we think of it as a liquid *feast* instead because you sustain yourself on juices and liquid pureed food, not just water. On your liquid feast, you will be getting twenty times more nutrients than you would on your normal diet, because you are drinking your food in such concentrated form.

The length of a pH Miracle Whole Body Cleanse will vary from person to person, depending upon your current situation and how your body tolerates it. Typically, seven to twenty-one days will give you the results you want.

As you would with any fast, you should consult your health care practitioner before beginning a pH Miracle Whole Body Cleanse.

THE PH MIRACLE WHOLE BODY CLEANSE

The pH Miracle Whole Body Cleanse eliminates acid wastes and negative microforms throughout your body, detoxifying your blood, tissues, and the entire alimentary canal/alkaline buffering system. You have to get rid of the pollution that's built up in your body, and especially the colon, from eating all those poorly combined foods, processed foods, fried and overcooked foods, simple starches, and sugars. In other words, all those dietary and metabolic acids.

We recommend at least a seven-to-fourteen day pH Miracle Whole Body Cleanse—up to twenty-one days if you're seriously ill. (Seek supervision for an extended cleanse.) Seven days is good for everyone who can manage it. If you are not facing any particular health challenges and can't take much time out from your schedule, just seventy-two hours (three days) can still be beneficial—and can be done over a long weekend. The shorter cleanse is good for older people or children and teens. You can also use a brief cleanse to get yourself going after you've fallen off the wagon, or just to give your body a periodic break. Once you are fully transitioned, I recommend a liquid pH Miracle Whole Body Cleanse at least one day a month—twenty-four hours will do—just to give your body a break from solid food. However long you do it, a cleanse gives your body a good rest.

While you are on a pH Miracle Whole Body Cleanse, you should drink at least four liters a day of purified water with pH drops, with lemon or lime juice if you like. You can include, as part of or in addition to those four liters, six to twelve 8-ounce glasses of fresh green electron-rich alkaline vegetable juice, to help clear the acidic toxins out of your system and return your body to its alkaline design.

Try juicing cucumber, kale, broccoli, celery, lettuce, collards, okra, wheatgrass, barley grass, watercress, parsley, cabbage, spinach, alfalfa sprouts—just about any other green vegetable that appeals to you. The recipes section has many combinations to try, but here's one that's all green: one cucumber, one stalk celery, one-third bunch parsley, a handful of alfalfa sprouts, and some spinach leaves.

When you're juicing in general, you can use carrot or beet to sweeten the taste. But both contain sugar, which gets even more concentrated in the juicing process, so you always want to use them moderately. If you are dealing with an acute condition, you don't want to use them at all.

Some people, however, find plain green juices difficult to enjoy in the beginning. If that's you, you might try backing into a pH Miracle Whole Body Cleanse, so to speak, by starting out for a few days using carrot and beet, just to get used to drinking fresh vegetable juices, then weaning off the carrot and beet gradually, and upping the amount of alkalizing greens. (If you do choose to use it, take it easy on the beet at first—maybe half a medium-size beet a day to begin with—as it can add considerably to the bowel-cleansing effect of the juice.)

Make sure you always dilute the juice with alkaline water (whether or not you are on a cleanse)—ten times as much alkaline water as juice—and add four drops of ClO_2 or pH drops per cup. That will increase the alkalinity of your juice from 6.2 to 9.5.

LUCY'S STORY

I am the mother of eight children, so I need every bit of energy I can get. But at one (low) point in my life, I made a list of more than thirty chronic physical symptoms that were plaguing me, several of them debilitating. It spanned fibromyalgia, arthritis, difficulty breathing, and heart palpitation. Perhaps most concerning was my outrageously high cholesterol level. Concerning, but not surprising: My family is followed by the National Institutes of Health because of familial hypercholesterolemia.

My father died at forty-one of arteriosclerosis of the aorta. My father's father and two of my father's brothers died in their forties and fifties of heart disease. My two brothers have had heart bypass operations. My oldest sister had two heart bypass operations and a heart transplant, and passed away after a third heart bypass operation. My own cholesterol was usually around 425. When I gained well over fifty pounds over three years—at a time when I was eating less and exercising more than I ever had in my life—I knew I had reached a crisis point.

Thank goodness I finally found Dr. Young's program, which I feel has quite literally saved my life. I immediately started drinking a gallon of water with pH drops and concentrated green powder every day. A few weeks later I went through a cleanse with supplements and green juices for a week, followed by three weeks on green veggies transitioning into a diet that was 90 percent alkaline. Within weeks I was feeling more energy, sleeping better—and had lost twelve pounds. At the end of three months I had lost fifty pounds, and half of my thirty symptoms had cleared up. By the end of seven months, I had lost seventy-five pounds, and nearly all my symptoms had vanished. The low energy, flu-like symptoms, and general aches and pains of fibromyalgia slowly diminished. My feelings of anxiety and mental fog dissipated and I no longer felt fragile. I felt healthy and vital again! But what mattered to me perhaps most of all was that my cholesterol dropped 150 points, and my ratios were in the healthy range for the first time in my entire life (and without the negative side effects I experienced on all of the cholesterol-lowering medications I had tried). For the first time, I feel sure my heart is in this life with me for the long haul.

If you cannot make fresh alkaline juice, you can use the concentrated green powder mixed into water instead—one-quarter teaspoon per eight ounces of water—plus four drops of ClO_2 or pH drops. You can add the green powder to any or all of your four liters of water whether or not you are juicing. You can also take one to two capsules of green powder with your fluids and juices if you need the added convenience.

Instead of juice, particularly at your usual mealtime, you may prefer raw, pureed soup, like Popeye Soup, Broccoli Soup, Aspar/Zinc Soup, and Celery Soup (see "Soups" in part 4). You can also drink broth from soups like Healing Soup, and teas such as red clover, chaparral, pau d'arco, Essiac (a special blend of herbs), and raspberry leaf. Add three tablespoons of essential oils (cold-pressed flax, hemp, avocado, pomegranate, virgin olive, borage, primrose—or a blend, like Udo's) to your soups, or take it by the spoonful. Add four drops of ClO_2 or pH drops to your herbal teas.

Although many people have no trouble with the pH Miracle Whole Body Cleanse, it isn't always easy. You may feel some hunger. This is really just those greedy microforms screaming to be fed, so resist any urge to break your regimen unless you find you can't keep up with your daily routines. The initial hunger pangs are the worst, but once you are over the hump—usually, by the third day—you may actually experience an upsurge in energy and feel no need for solid food.

When hunger does strike, mineral supplements, particularly chromium and montmorillonite clay, may help (chapter 12). Also, try drinking lots of electron-rich alkaline water, or water with one-quarter teaspoon concentrated green powder per cup, to take the edge off. If you must resort to solid food, eat fresh, raw veggies or low-sugar fruit, like cucumber, tomato, celery, or avocado, or Healing Soup with the optional veggies added.

BASIC ALKALIZING SUPPLEMENTS

There's a whole chapter on supplements coming up, so here I (Rob) am just going to mention the ones that are particularly useful during a cleanse. Check out chapter 12 for details about the individual supplements.

Alkalizing supplements can maximize the effects of a pH Miracle Whole Body Cleanse and bring the body into balance more quickly, controlling dietary and metabolic acids and negative microforms. In general, alkalizing supplements should be taken with meals or drinks—one capsule three times a day, with meals. Liquid mineral colloids should be taken under the tongue, three to five drops three times a day, away from meals. (If you have been struggling with chronic or severe health problems, use up to six to nine times a day.) Wherever the directions are different for a particular supplement, I've noted this in the description. You could also follow directions on the package, but remember that less, more often, is better than more, less often. That is, taking one capsule six times a day is better than two capsules three times a day or three capsules two times a day.

During a pH Miracle Whole Body Cleanse, I recommend you take several things. The most crucial are pH drops (ClO_2 and sodium/potassium bicarbonate), alkalizing mineral salts, and concentrated green powder. Add four drops of ClO_2 or sodium bicarbonate per cup of pure water into all your pure electron-rich alkaline water. Mix one-quarter teaspoon of the concentrated green powder into eight ounces of pure electron-rich alkaline water three times a day, or take one capsule three times a day with a "meal" or drink. If you do nothing else in the way of supplements, do these.

Close runner-ups in importance are a multivitamin and a multimineral, with cell salts. Each capsule of the broad-spectrum vitamin should contain at least five hundred milligrams, and the multimineral five hundred milligrams. Among other things, nutritional deficiencies increase the toxicity of mycotoxins, so you want to be sure you get all that your body needs. The alkalizing minerals are particularly important because all other nutrients, including vitamins, proteins, antioxidants, amino acids, and carbohydrates, require minerals for normal biochemical functioning. So do all the alkaline buffers.

Finally, I'd also recommend liquid chlorophyll; glutathione; colloidal silver, copper, gold, titanium, rhodium, and iridium; and an antimycotoxin formula, ideally combining glutathione, N-acetyl cysteine, L-taurine, and organic sulfur.

PETE'S STORY

I was diagnosed with bladder cancer over three years ago, stage three (of a possible four)—not good. The doctors were worried that the malignant tumor could have spread to nearby lymph nodes and might have extruded through the bladder wall. It had definitely blocked one of the ureters connecting the kidney and the bladder. I underwent two months of chemotherapy, but I had such a severe negative response my wife thought I was going to die and my doctors recommended discontinuing treatment. Unfortunately, the treatment I had made it through had had no effect on the tumor. My doctors recommended removing the entire bladder surgically.

I was determined to fight the cancer, but I just couldn't believe radical surgery was my only choice. I set out to find out about my alternatives, and my search led me to Dr. Young. My blood turned out to be highly acidic, and live analysis of my blood showed my body chemistry to have a high degree of toxicity. My blood cells were a mess from years of eating garbage and ignoring my health.

I did a ten-day fast, with vegetable juices and soups, which, to my surprise, wasn't that bad. I started taking the recommended supplements, especially the pH drops and the concentrated green powder. After the ten days, I kept to vegetable meals, following the program to the letter. This was a radical change from my former diet, but I was determined to beat the cancer.

I told my doctors about my new approach, and although they were skeptical, they had nothing else besides drastic surgery to offer me, and agreed to monitor the tumor with intermittent MRIs. Many of my family and friends thought I was crazy. I had many tearful discussions with my wife, who was very supportive throughout, about which path to follow. One of my best friends accused me of trying to kill myself. But I remained steadfast. I would not vary my commitment to see this program through.

The first two months I lost between fifteen and twenty pounds, which confirmed my loved ones' suspicions, as I hadn't been overweight to begin with. But I felt better each week, with more energy and clearer thinking. I knew I was doing the right thing even before repeat blood analysis showed considerable improvement.

By three months into the program, there was no sign of any cancer spread, but my doctors kept suggesting surgical removal of my bladder. I was very opposed to that, naturally, especially now that I felt sure this program was working. I did agree to a diagnostic procedure, which revealed the tumor had not only shrunk, but also was suspended on a stalk to the bladder wall, no longer fully attached. The opening of the ureter was clear, and they were able to remove all of the old tumor during this procedure. The doctors took sections of muscle tissue of the bladder to test them for pathology (clear) and examined the ureter all the way to the kidney (also clear). There was no cancer in my bladder whatsoever, and only remnants of the carcinoma in the degenerated (and removed) tumor. I had won!

Amazingly, the surgeon still recommended removal of the bladder for what he called a "cure." I said thanks, but no thanks. I continue to get intermittent MRIs to monitor my bladder, but I know as long as I stay alkaline, the cancer will not recur.

A TYPICAL DAY ON THE PH MIRACLE WHOLE BODY CLEANSE

All the details may at first seem daunting, though you'll quickly get used to the routine. In the meantime, to help you sort things out, here's a typical schedule, which you can modify to suit yourself.

7 AM: Test the pH of your urine. If the urine pH is below 7.2, then take 2–3 teaspoons of sodium bicarbonate or mineral salts (sodium and potassium bicarbonate with magnesium and calcium carbonate) in 5–6 ounces of water.

7:15 AM. 1 liter pure water with pH drops (with lemon or lime juice if you like).

7:30 AM: Liquid colloidal supplements.

8:00 AM: Juiced greens and capsule supplements.

9 AM–noon: 1.5 liters pure water with concentrated green powder and pH drops.

Noon: Test the pH of your urine and saliva. If either is below 7.2, take 2–3 teaspoons of sodium bicarbonate or mineral salts (sodium and potassium bicarbonate with magnesium and calcium carbonate) in 5–6 ounces of purified alkaline electron-rich water.

12:30 PM: Liquid colloidal supplements.

1:00 PM: Raw soup or juiced greens and capsule supplements.

2–5 PM: 1.5 liters pure water with concentrated green powder and pH drops.

5 PM: Test the urine and saliva pH. If below 7.2, take 2–3 teaspoons of sodium bicarbonate or mineral salts (sodium and potassium bicarbonate with magnesium and calcium carbonate) in 5–6 ounces of purified alkaline electron-rich water.

5:30 PM: Liquid colloidal supplements.

6:00 PM: Soup or juiced greens and capsule supplements.

7–9 PM: Pure water with pH drops as desired (with lemon or lime juice if you like).

9 PM: Test the urine and saliva pH. If either is below 7.2, take 2–3 teaspoons of sodium bicarbonate or mineral salts (sodium and potassium bicarbonate with magnesium and calcium carbonate) in 5–6 ounces of purified alkaline electron-rich water.

WHEN WE SAY CLEANSE, WE MEAN *CLEANSE*

All this can have quite a laxative effect. Green juice alone can do it. This is the way your body physically gets rid of the acidic bad stuff. It doesn't just evaporate. This is just what you want: to make sure you get rid of the pollution that has built up in your body, and in particular in your small intestines and colon. Until you know your body's response to the program, it is wise not to have anything else planned so you can focus on the pH Miracle Whole Body Cleanse—and just stay fairly close to bathroom facilities. Be prepared to pay a visit to the bathroom at least six to ten times a day as the acidic toxins clear from your body.

If the program as described so far doesn't have this effect, you'll want to add a mild, natural laxative formula to your program. Look for one including magnesium oxide, magnesium carbonate, sodium bicarbonate, slippery elm, marshmallow, yellow dock, and gingerroot. Take four capsules every four hours. (See the resources section.)

Aloe vera juice is another cleansing aid. It helps break up pockets of undigested acidic animal protein, especially in the small intestine. Add one tablespoon of cold-pressed, whole-leaf juice to your green juice, or take with a "meal." Aloe vera juice is a mildly acidic product and is best not to be used on an ongoing basis. However, when a detox effort presents a substantial challenge, a few days of aloe vera can be helpful to break up hardened protein pockets, which need to be eliminated.

Remember, these products are designed to work! Don't be caught off guard, and by all means modify your approach if the results seem too vigorous.

For serious cleansing, acute or difficult conditions such as chronic constipation, diverticulitis, Crohn's, irritable bowel syndrome, or chronic diarrhea, you may want to add (or use instead) a lower-bowel-cleansing formula or other intestinal cleanser. Look for an herbal mixture containing cascara sagrada (more than in the mild laxative), turkey rhubarb root, psyllium seed, barberry root, gingerroot, fennel seed, red raspberry leaves, and cayenne. Take four capsules every four hours during the cleanse. Adults over sixty should take one to two capsules every eight hours. If you are having trouble eliminating, this lower-bowel-cleansing formula will get things going!

WHAT TO WATCH OUT FOR

During a cleanse, toxins are dumped from where they've been stored in the tissues into the blood so they can be eliminated. This means that for a while, your blood is actually dirtier than it started out. You may feel worse before you feel better. Different people experience varying degrees of unpleasantness, or none at all, during this "healing crisis," which may include nausea, weakness, dizziness, headaches, light-headedness, rashes, bad breath, flu-like feelings, and fatigue. (A note on rashes or other skin reactions: Do not suppress them with medications. At most, use a pure moisturizer or liquid vitamin E.)

When and if this happens, increase your daily alkaline water intake. Lots of alkaline electron-rich water with pH drops and fresh lemon or lime juice will help flush the toxins (and their negative effects) out quickly.

A healing crisis is actually a good sign. But it can be too intense, and therefore discouraging or even harmful. So monitor your progress closely. Some mild discomfort can be expected, but you should not experience undue discomfort. A healing crisis should be short-lived. If you experience an intense healing crisis, use the same dosages of all supplements but over a longer period of time in order to lessen the healing or detox crisis. If it does not subside within twenty-four hours, seek assistance from a professional health practitioner to find a way to do a cleanse that will work for you. Anyone with serious health problems should seek some professional supervision before beginning the pH Miracle program, including the Whole Body Cleanse. With guidance, you should be able to minimize or even avoid a healing crisis.

There is no medal for who can cleanse for the longest period of time, so do not push your body too hard for the sake of reaching a specific number of days. You should feel successful however many days you are able to cleanse. Each day you remain on it is one more day ridding the body of acid buildup. Each day after brings you closer to a fully integrated alkaline lifestyle.

OKAY, I'M CLEANSED. NOW WHAT?

You've removed the stockpile of acidic debris from your body of environment, diet, and metabolism, clearing the way for optimal health. The next step, after taking away what your body doesn't need, is to provide what it does need. If you give it the vital materials it needs to construct new and healthy cells, your body will heal itself and be restored to balance and harmony. This second phase should run for at least seven weeks, and ideally eleven weeks, after your cleanse is over (for a total of eight to twelve weeks, so adjust accordingly if your cleanse is more or less than a week).

A proper alkaline diet is essential here, no surprise. The key to this phase, as you go back on solid food, is reintroducing a still-limited range of healthy alkaline foods, as well as keeping clear of certain acidic foods. It's especially important to start with a high degree of conviction, commitment, and determination to follow your new and healthy dietary regimen. You want to get started off on the right foot!

You also want to keep your diet extremely low in starches, focusing on dark green and yellow vegetables; sprouted soybeans, seeds, and grains; nuts and essential mono- and polyunsaturated oils. At least 80 percent of it should be raw. The higher the level of electrons in your food, the faster you will repair and rebuild your body—and cooking destroys your food's natural electron concentration, or life force.

Continue with daily alkalizing green juices, but add some variety. Drinking juice just before a solid meal is good for digestion—supporting the alkalizing buffering system—but you should also have juice on its own.

Beyond that, for this phase you want to avoid (in addition to the unhealthy acidic foods described in earlier chapters) all complex carbohydrates, including high-carbohydrate vegetables (potatoes, sweet potatoes, peas, winter squash), all grains, and starchy legumes (meaning all of them, except soybeans and lentils), as well as fruit.

Otherwise, you want to eat as laid out earlier in this book, focusing on alkalizing vegetables, especially green and yellow vegetables, and including healthy mono- and polyunsaturated oils, low-acid sugar fruits (tomato, avocado, lemon, and lime), soybeans, tofu, lentils, and raw seeds and nuts (of the healthy types), preferably soaked. Think vegetable soups, steam-"fried" vegetables, and lots of salads, with liberal amounts of flax, hemp, avocado, and olive oils (added after any cooking).

If your pH Miracle Whole Body Cleanse was shorter than seven days, or included some solid foods, you might want to proceed with even more than 80 percent of your diet being alkaline for these eight to twelve weeks.

During this phase, the principles of proper food combining are crucial (see chapter 8).

BRINA'S STORY

I had sixteen inches of my intestines cut out when I was twenty-six. The diagnosis was irritable bowel syndrome and possibly Crohn's disease. The doctors were not exactly positive about my prognosis, and told me I'd need to be on medication for the rest of my life.

I refused to believe I had to live with this condition, so I went to the book section of my local health food store and started reading. What I found there changed my life. I started to heal by eating a mostly raw, alkaline diet. But it wasn't until I discovered Dr. Young's program that I truly experienced my own pH miracle. The cleanse is what made all the difference. I started a ten-day liquid feast as soon as I finished reading about it. While I was resting my intestines by not eating, I was able to feel my intestines—and it felt like there were open wounds all along their interior walls. I've read that it only takes two weeks for every cell in the intestines to be replaced. I didn't have to wait even that long: On the fourth day, in what seemed to be only an instant, I felt the wounds were healed. All the pain was gone. And it has never come back for going on eight years now.

ADDITIONAL ALKALIZING SUPPLEMENTS

At this point, you should continue with the supplements already begun and add a few more. Again, you'll find more information on supplements in Chapter 12, so here I'm only going to mention the ones that are particularly helpful in this phase. The two most generally applicable supplements are alkalizing mineral salts of sodium and potassium bicarbonate and magnesium and calcium carbonate; and an anti-yeast formula containing glutathione and/or N-acetyl-cysteine. Beyond that, depending on your situation, the following optional supplements can be necessary or valuable: an alimentary canal acid absorber mix of montmorillonite clay and psyllium seed powder and an antiparasite formula containing black walnut hulls. You may also want to use pomegranate seed oil and avocado oil, and vitamin D.

MOVING FORWARD

Congratulations! Now you're ready to move on to the full program, assuming you've made good progress to this point. You can add one serving per meal, properly combined and not to exceed 20 percent of your diet, of the following foods: starchy vegetables (peas, red potatoes, winter squash, sweet potato), legumes, and organic, unstored whole grains (millet, spelt, buckwheat, kamut, quinoa, brown rice, and wheat). And that's it. You're alkaline.

As you add foods after a pH Miracle Whole Body Cleanse, carefully observe your body's reactions. If any symptoms return, a longer period of totally alkaline meals may be in order, until more healing takes place.

At this point you can add additional alkalizing supplements to address specific symptoms (if any remain). You'll read more about how to do that in chapter 12.

SECOND NATURE

All this may seem a little overwhelming at first. That's normal when you're faced with a lot of new information. Don't be discouraged. Take some time to familiarize yourself with these alkalizing concepts. Don't be intimidated. Remember how complicated driving a car was in the beginning? Now it's so natural that your mind can move through many other thoughts quite smoothly while the once new and seemingly complicated behavior has become second nature and automatic. The same will happen as you gain experience with your new pH Miracle lifestyle.

The combination of cleansing when necessary or beneficial and a good diet is designed to keep your body in balance over the long term. It will restore pH balance, stop overgrowth of negative microforms, and heal the damage resulting from the acidic toxins they emit. I do want to note, however, that as far as this biochemical approach can take you toward wellness, you cannot overlook the environmental, intellectual, psychological, emotional, and spiritual factors that also influence your overall well-being. To truly achieve optimal health, you also need to break the pattern of negativity that feeds sickness and disease. The acidic diet you're leaving behind is just one example. You also have to deal with chemical exposure, prescription or recreational drugs (including cigarettes and their nicotine), and, less obviously, negative thoughts, words, and deeds.

The more closely you adhere to the guidelines in this chapter—and in this book—the better your results will be. You should begin to experience success quickly, so I want to caution you against believing that just because you are better, you are truly well. Especially for those who have been struggling with health challenges, this may be unfamiliar territory. Relief of your symptoms is all well and good, but when you persist with the program into a completely alkaline way of eating, you'll experience total wellness that might be beyond what you can imagine while you are plagued by symptoms.

Healthy alkaline living should be instinctive, but clearly somewhere along the way humans have lost the ability to sense it. At this point, extraordinary means are required for its recovery. Fortunately, you hold those means in your hands right now. But what you all must do is get your health under control—then get past it. Don't let it become an obsession. Don't become its slave. A healthy alkaline body and mind put you in a position to better serve the universe. So they are worthwhile aims, certainly. Just don't get so absorbed in attaining them that you miss out on the unpredictable play of Life!

Chapter 12
·
Alkalizing Nutritional Supplements

Even if your diet were ideal, we'd still recommend supplements. Today's food is a mere nutritional shadow of what it once was—and should be. It is grown with artificial fertilizers in depleted soil and sprayed with pesticides to within an inch of its life. It is harvested early and shipped long distances, and it languishes in trucks and warehouses and on shelves, losing nutrients and electrical potential with every passing minute, for far too long before it ever reaches your kitchen. There are exceptions, of course, but the general picture is grim.

And even if you had a perfect diet of perfect food, your body is so physiologically assaulted by an acidic environment that you'd need alkalizing supplements just to compensate. The average person is exposed to five hundred acidic chemicals a day. (And that's not even taking into account what we knowingly put into our bodies when we eat poorly.)

So in this chapter, I (Rob) am going to detail for you the daily alkalizing supplements I recommend for everyone, as well as those aimed at particular symptoms. You'll see some of the supplements discussed in the chapter on the pH Miracle Whole Body Cleanse covered in more detail here, as well as additional suggestions.

START WITH THE RIGHT PRODUCTS

There are many good products out there, but still you must choose your supplements carefully. Steer clear of anything with added sweeteners. Make sure to get products with no alcohol, glycerin, citric acid, or sugar—four acid ingredients that many companies use as preservatives. Some supplements are contaminated with yeast and fungus, or their spores, and thus are counterproductive at best, and downright harmful at worst. Stay clear of products that contain algae, mushrooms, enzymes, or probiotics. You should check with any company you buy from to find out if they are sensitive to this issue and what safeguards they have in place. For my money, if they aren't checking on it somehow, that's not a company I'd buy from. Some reliable, high-quality brand names are Source Naturals, Soloray, Innerlight Inc., Young pHorever, pH Miracle, and Nature's Way.

DOSING

You can always take supplements according to the instructions on the packaging. I'll give you my guidelines here. For the recommended supplements that come in capsule form, take 1 or 2 capsules at least three times a day. (So, that's up to a maximum of 3,000 mg per ingredient per day, though most you'll be using in combinations so you won't reach the maximum for any one ingredient, and you shouldn't try to.) The liquids, except $NaClO_2$ or sodium chlorite or potassium hydroxide, you should take under your tongue, 3–5 drops three times a day. With either form, in serious conditions, you can increase the frequency (keeping the amount the same) to six to nine times a day. Where dosing directions are different, I've noted that in the description.

The standard capsule size in the supplement industry is 500 mg. They may contain up to 500 mg of a single ingredient, or a mix of ingredients (some of which may be inert) up to a total of 500 mg per capsule. Liquid colloidal preparations should contain 5–10 parts per million (ppm).

I am not actually picky about how much exactly you get of any one ingredient within this framework for capsules and liquids. Most of what I'm recommending comes mixed with other things, and you'll certainly want to take advantage of combinations to keep the total number of capsules you take within reason. The combinations (at least from the good companies) mix ingredients that complement one another, so if you get 25 mg rather than 50 mg of one thing, you're probably getting an extra 25 mg of something else that works similarly in the mix. There is general agreement on what level of each ingredient is effective, and most manufacturers use roughly the same amounts. If you look at all the options on the health food store shelf, you'll see there's at least a loose consensus about how much you should take. Anyplace where the specifics matter, I've spelled that out in the descriptions below.

Keep in mind that the doses given here are generalized, and based on a body weight of 154 pounds, or 70 kilos. Everyone's body chemistry is unique, and you may require a greater or lesser amount than what is suggested depending on your weight, body type, health challenges, genetic constitution, and sensitivity. If you're lighter or more sensitive to supplements, stay on the lower end of the range I've provided. If you're heavier or not seeing the results you want, move to the higher end. You'll find what is right for you. Listen to your body.

As with any nutritional supplement program, you should consult your health care practitioner before you begin taking anything.

LIQUID COLLOIDS

Much of what I recommend is in colloidal, or liquid, almost homeopathic form. Colloids are the smallest biological form of any matter, and are small enough to pass through membranes. Nutrients in this form need no digestion; they bypass the alimentary canal and are easily absorbed and ready for use by the body. There is no need to waste energy converting them into a usable form, as with standard supplements. This is particularly important if you have an illness, as that will further compromise your digestion (alkalizing buffering system), increasing the risk of leaving you malnourished and anemic just when you most need alkalizing electrically active nutrients.

Although they are generally absorbed more quickly, liquids are not necessarily superior to other forms. But they are almost always a good idea. If you use both liquid and capsules, you'll give your body a range of benefits.

Liquid colloidal supplements can be taken anytime, though you should use them apart from meals, with doses spaced out over the day. Place drops under the tongue, rather than swallowing them, for rapid, direct absorption into the bloodstream. You can also take them through your nose with a nebulizer. You can take one supplement right after another this way, though you should leave fifteen-second intervals between them. Or put them all into a few ounces of pure water and drink your "colloidal cocktail" slowly. Or nebulize them at about 5–10 ml per treatment. Any way you do it, you are aiming for 3–5 drops three times a day. Keep in mind that taking less, more often, is better than taking more, less often. That is, 3 drops five times a day is better than 5 drops three times a day.

USING SUPPLEMENTS

When you are shopping for supplements, you may not always be able to find the exact combinations described here. I've generally listed the ingredients in the order of importance, so although I'm a big believer in the power of the combinations, you'll get most of the benefit out of a blend with at least the first couple of ingredients here.

Later in this chapter, we'll get the specific supplements targeted to specific symptoms and conditions. I want to start, however, with the basic things everyone would benefit from taking daily, such as vitamins and, especially, minerals. Nutritional deficiencies can cause their own problems, of course, but on top of that they also increase the toxicity of mycotoxins. And in a vicious cycle, mycotoxins interfere with nutrient absorption, creating deficiencies. Minerals are especially important because without them, vitamins and alkaline buffers cannot function. Plus, minerals are what our soil—and thus our food—lacks. Low- or no-impact exercise flushes dietary and metabolic acids out of our bodies, but with them go some alkalizing minerals. Furthermore, specific to our purposes here, detoxification (as with the pH Miracle Whole Body Cleanse, or just shifting to an alkaline diet) requires extra mineral nutrients, especially the mineral salts of sodium, magnesium, potassium, and calcium.

If all the information that follows seems like too much, remember that you can make quite a lot of progress using just concentrated green powder and alkalizing pH drops along with a alkaline diet. A multivitamin and a multimineral formula compose the next basic layer. Beyond that, the benefits are laid out here to help you decide what is best for you (working along with a health care provider). All the alkalizing supplements here complement the dietary changes you are making, support you while you are making those changes, and protect you when you don't eat right. They are invaluable if you are facing particular acidic symptoms. But you have to determine what works best for you—including how many supplements you can manage.

THE ALKALINE STARS

Here's what everyone should take daily. If you remember the COWS plan from chapter 5—(chlorophyll, oils, water, and salts)—this is going to look very familiar. The same four things that are the foundation of your diet form the basis of your alkalizing supplement program, with the addition of a multivitamin and a multimineral supplement.

C Is for Chlorophyll, and Concentrated Green Powder

Supplement what you get through the plants you eat with concentrated green powder or liquid chlorophyll. You can take them separately, or use them to boost the effects of juiced greens. (Just don't use *instead* of juicing.) If you aren't accustomed to the taste of vegetable juice, you may find that a mint-flavored liquid chlorophyll smooths it out quite a bit. (Be sure to avoid the preparations with added sugar or glycerin, which is especially common if mint is added.) Add 1 teaspoon liquid chlorophyll per eight ounces of pure water. You can find liquid chlorophyll at your local health food store or online (see resources). There are many brands, but the best are Young pHorever, World Organics, Innerlight, and DeSouza's.

Ideally, at least 3 of the 4 liters of water you drink should also have a teaspoon of liquid chlorophyll or a powdered concentrate of vegetable and fruit greens and grasses mixed in. Many different companies make this kind of supplement, and many different concentrated green powders are on the market. Single-ingredient powders (just wheatgrass or alfalfa, for example) may be easier to find, but you should look for a mixture of green grasses and vegetables and fruit, which are easily assimilated and rapidly alkalizing, and combinations that are naturally rich in fiber, which bind with and remove toxins from the body. The key ingredients are (organic) wheatgrass, barley grass, and kamut grass. They should be mixed with a variety of green vegetables such as broccoli, kale, and spinach—the exact ones are less important than simply getting a wide variety. A formula containing avocado and cucumber, rich in alkaline salts, which can bind mycotoxins and take them out of the body, would be an excellent choice. Sprouted ingredients such as hemp and soy are good, too, as the sprouting phase is when a plant is at its nutritional peak.

Green powder is nutrient-rich (including easily digested protein) and helps to gently transition your blood and tissues from acidic to alkaline, reaching a natural, ideal pH balance. It is the primary food supplement for building healthy blood.

A concentrated sprouted organic wheat (wheatgrass) supplement is another excellent source of concentrated chlorophyll. You can also take capsules, in the usual way. Look for a combination with 25–50 mg of each ingredient, for a total of 500 mg per capsule.

O Is for Omega-3 and -6 Oils

Omega-3s, especially, are absolutely crucial to your health, so you should supplement what you get in your diet from fish, seeds, and oils.

Long-chain polyunsaturated omega-3 oils can chelate or buffer environmental, dietary, and metabolic acids. Omega-3s and omega-6s are normal parts of human cells, and are especially abundant in brain cells, nerve synapses, visual receptors, adrenal glands, and sex glands. They protect the heart, inhibit cancer cells, and provide a range of other health benefits besides.

Omega-3s protect the heart in a variety of ways. They help disperse saturated fatty acids, which like to stick together, thereby avoiding lumps of fat in the blood that dampen electrical charges. They keep blood platelets from getting too sticky, resulting in lower likelihood of clots that can cause heart attacks or strokes. They lower triglycerides by up to 65 percent. They lower cholesterol and low-density lipoprotein (LDL). They lower very low-density lipoprotein (VLDL) by half. They also convert the harmful VLDL into LDL, which is particularly helpful to people with diabetes. High triglyceride levels, and especially LDL and VLDL, are associated with cardiovascular disease: high blood pressure, atherosclerosis, heart and kidney failure, stroke, and heart attack. Furthermore, our bodies make prostaglandin PG3 from EPA. PG3 helps prevent strokes and heart attacks, lowers high blood pressure (by blocking the production of pressure-raising PG2s found in meat), and prevents pathological blood clotting in the lungs and blood vessels.

The omega-3s eicosapentaenoic acid (EPA) and docosahexaenoic acid (DHA) are antimycotoxic, lowering levels of repair proteins (a sign of mycotoxins in the blood) in the arteries. Repair proteins are also involved in the development of atherosclerosis, so lowering them is a double bonus.

Omegas can help:

- Lower blood pressure, blood cholesterol, and risk of stroke and heart attack.
- Normalize fat metabolism in diabetes and decrease the amount of insulin diabetics require.
- Prevent liver damage due to alcoholism, reduce withdrawal symptoms from quitting an alcohol addiction, and help with a hangover.
- Contribute to building a prostaglandin that helps some schizophrenics.
- Cause weight loss by increasing metabolic rate and fat burnoff.
- Relieve premenstrual breast pain and PMS. Borage oil together with

vitamins and minerals has been shown to bring improvement in almost 90 percent of patients.

- Prevent drying and atrophy of tear and salivary glands (Sjögren's syndrome).
- Prevent arthritis in animal studies.
- Improve the condition of hair, nails, and skin.
- Improve some types of eczema.
- Slow or stop the progress of multiple sclerosis, especially if begun soon after initial diagnosis. (Fish oils have been used with equal effectiveness.)
- Help treat nerve degeneration (diabetic neuropathy) in Type 2 diabetes, when sugar and saturated fats are removed from the diet as well.
- Kill cancer cells (cells infested with mold and mycotoxins) in tissue culture without harming normal cells; animal studies have shown EPA and DHA to inhibit the growth and metastasis of tumors.

Another beneficial omega, the omega-5 CLA appears in rare plant form in pomegranate seeds (CLA is commonly found in meat and dairy), so the seeds and their oils are very good for you.

Cold-water fish are good sources of omega-3s, and their oils in supplement form are a good choice. There are plant sources as well, if you wish to avoid all animal products—including from flax, hemp, walnut, and soybean oils. Note, however, that the body converts the omega-3s found in plants into the forms found in fish, a several-stage process that requires *work*. So if you have a weakened system, it may be better to take the preformed (animal) omega-3s.

Omega-6s are found in the seeds of borage, primrose, sunflower, and black currant, as well as in fish oils. Gamma-linolenic acid (GLA) is the primary one. Borage seed oil contains up to 24 percent GLA, evening primrose oil about half that. Borage also contains about 34 percent linoleic acid, another omega-6. Safflower has 79 percent, sunflower 69 percent, almonds 26 percent, pumpkin seeds 42 percent, and canola 28 percent. Hemp oil has an ideal ratio of three parts omega-3s to one part omega-6s—just as fish oils do.

EPA and DHA are found in cold-water fish and other northern marine animals. Trout, salmon, mackerel, sardines, tuna, and eel are the richest sources of omega-3 fatty acids. For those who wish to avoid animal products, there are plant sources for a precursor to EPA and DHA, another omega-3 called alpha-linoleic acid (ALA), including flax, hemp, walnut, and soybean oils.

Get at least 3,000–4,000 mg daily of each omega to help the body buffer acids and maintain its alkaline design. Make sure the supplements you use are fresh. Checking is easy: Break open a capsule and take a whiff—there should be no "fishy" odor.

W Is for Water—Alkaline Water

Water is not a supplement in and of itself, of course, nor should it be: Water is absolutely central to good health and in no way "supplemental." But the best ionized, filtered, alkaline, electron-rich water *is,* all by itself, a potent antioxidant, much more powerful than taking a vitamin C tablet, for instance. Furthermore, water is the delivery system for two of the most important components of this program—green powder and alkalizing mineral salts.

S Is for Salts and Sodium Bicarbonate

Whole, unprocessed mineral salts are antioxidant, antibacterial, antifungal, antitoxin, anti-inflammatory, and anticarcinogenic. They are immune enhancing. Taking them daily helps reduce dietary and metabolic acidity and slow down or reverse the processes of aging and decay in the body. Mineral salts reduce high blood sugar, cholesterol, irritation, inflammation, and bone loss. They improve digestion, especially as it becomes slower and less complete with age, and help your body alkalize food.

Mineral salts can be used to detoxify and purify the body from the buildup of dietary and lifestyle-produced acids. Regular use improves overall health and energy and reduces fatigue. Mineral salts also help increase endurance, stamina, and speed, and so are useful not just for daily life but also for athletic performance of any kind. Mineral salts release oxygen in the body, fighting microforms (including Candida) that thrive in the absence of oxygen, chelate foreign material, and neutralize acids. Salts help your body stay alkaline.

For supplement use, you want a combination of chlorine dioxide (ClO_2) or its precursor sodium chlorite ($NaClO_2$), magnesium carbonate ($MgHCO_3$), potassium bicarbonate ($KHCO_3$), and calcium carbonate ($CaHCO_3$), in roughly even amounts. Your best bets will be mineral salts from the Great Salt Lake, the Dead Sea, the Celtic Sea, or the Himalayas. We have our own formula called Young pHorever pHour Salts, and you can find something along the same lines at your health food store. Another option is Innerlight's 4 Salts powder or capsules, available online. Tri-Salts is another product that has just the magnesium, potassium, and calcium carbonates, but no sodium. You can use that, or a similar formula, if you can't find all four together, adding in whatever is missing separately. You can use sodium bicarbonate (see below) to fill in sodium. If even that is out of reach, you can just get some good sea salt and eat as much of the darkest green foods you can manage.

The best way to get your mineral salts is to stir up your own salt solution: Take 1 teaspoon in one 8-ounce glass of alkaline water, three times a day. With liquid mineral salts, add 15 drops per liter or quart of water—and drink four of those liters/quarts a day. For smaller servings, add 4–6 drops to 8–12 ounces of water. Or follow the directions on the label of the product you are using.

SALT THERAPY

You may wish to take more alkalizing mineral salt, or use it differently, if you are facing any of the symptoms on the following list. Though I've recommended doses, be sure to monitor your urine pH while using salts. It should be between 7.6 and 8.0 if you are dealing with minor symptoms, or between 8.0 and 8.4 for serious health challenges—and adjust your salts intake accordingly. And remember, salts are for use this way only when you are committed to an alkaline diet.

- For weight gain that comes from metabolism decreases and thyroid production decreases that come with aging, take 1–3 teaspoons of salts in 4–6 ounces of water.
- For indigestion, acid reflux (heartburn), or nausea, take 1–3 teaspoons of salts in 4–6 ounces of alkaline water to buffer dietary acids and excess HCl. You can also take it just before an acidic meal to buffer or chelate food acids.
- For constipation, take 1–2 tablespoons of salts in 1 liter of alkaline water first thing in the morning, on an empty stomach. You can do this anytime you need or want to clean the alimentary canal and flush the bowel. Use mineral salts such as magnesium carbonate or magnesium oxide to break up undigested proteins in the small intestine.

- For pain and swelling due to injury or lactic acid buildup from exercise, take 1 tablespoon of salts in 1 liter of water.
- For psoriasis or other skin irritation or inflammation, spray liquid colloidal mineral salts directly on the skin. You can make this liquid colloidal mineral salt spray by adding 1 teaspoon of Himalayan or Real Salt, or a combination of the four alkalizing mineral salts, to 4–6 ounces of water.
- For rheumatism or joint pain; insect bites; blisters; wounds; poison oak, ivy, or sumac; or other skin irritations or imbalances, take a brine bath in a tub full of hot water with 5–6 tablespoons of mineral salts stirred in. (Or use Epsom salt.) Anyone interested in healthy, beautiful skin can benefit from a similar soak, which pulls acid from the skin and lets salt's healthy minerals penetrate your skin to promote natural cell growth in your skin cell layers.
- To prevent muscle cramps add 1 tablespoon of mineral salts to 1 liter of alkaline water and drink three times a day.
- To slow the bone loss that increases with age and can lead to osteoporosis, add 1 tablespoon of mineral salts to 1 liter of alkaline water and drink three times a day.
- To clear sinus congestion, spray salt solution directly in the nasal passages. Add 1 teaspoon of mineral salts to 4–6 ounces of alkaline water and mix. Take this mixture and put into a neti pot or a nose spray applicator and infuse the solution slowly into your nasal passages. (See resources.)
- For lung congestion, add 1 tablespoon of mineral salts to 1 liter of alkaline water and drink three times a day.
- For hormone or endocrine system problems, add 1 tablespoon of the four alkalizing mineral salts to 1 liter of alkaline water and drink three times a day. A healthy endocrine system runs on electrons transported on the backbone of mineral salts. Salts counter age-related hormone issues including loss of muscle mass and skin tone, and decreased sex drive, in both men and women.
- For sleep problems, including sleep apnea, add 1 tablespoon of mineral salts to 1 liter of alkaline water and drink three times a day. Salt is a natural hypnotic.
- To counteract allergy symptoms, add 1 tablespoon of mineral salts to 1 liter of alkaline water and drink three times a day. Salts act as strong natural antihistamines.

- To maintain your libido and fight erectile dysfunction (ED), add 1 tablespoon of mineral salts to 1 liter of alkaline water and drink three times a day. Salt increases oxygen circulation, which improves ED.
- To prevent varicose veins and spider veins on your legs and thighs add 1 tablespoon of mineral salts to 1 liter of alkaline water and drink three times a day.
- To stabilize blood sugar levels, add 1 tablespoon of mineral salts to 1 liter of alkaline water and drink three times a day.
- To stop cravings, including for cigarettes, alcohol, coffee, tea, or chocolate, spray liquid colloidal mineral salts in your mouth. You can make your own salt solution with 1 teaspoon of the four alkaline mineral salts, Himalayan Salts, or Real Salt in 4–6 ounces of water.
- To combat acne, spray liquid colloidal mineral salts directly on the skin. You can also make your own salt solution with 1 teaspoon of the four alkaline mineral salts, Himalayan Salts, or Real Salt in 4–6 ounces of water.
- For athlete's foot or other fungus, spray liquid colloidal mineral salts directly on the affected area. You can also make your own salt solution with 1 teaspoon of the four alkaline mineral salts, Himalayan Salts, or Real Salt in 4–6 ounces of water.
- For motion sickness, spray liquid colloidal mineral salts directly in your mouth. You can also make your own salt solution with 1 teaspoon of the four alkaline mineral salts, Himalayan Salts, or Real Salt in 4–6 ounces of water.
- For a sore throat, spray liquid colloidal mineral salts to the back of the mouth. You can also make your own salt solution with 1 teaspoon of the four alkaline mineral salts, Himalayan Salts, or Real Salt in 4–6 ounces of water.

You can also use salts in specific ways to support and enhance athletic endeavors:

- To increase energy and reduce fatigue, take 1 teaspoon of salts in 3–4 ounces of alkaline water.
- To increase stamina, endurance, and speed, take 1 tablespoon of salts in 1 liter of water an hour before exercise or an athletic event.

- To increase sprint speed (running or swimming), take 1 tablespoon of salts in 6–8 ounces of water one hour before the event.
- During marathons or any extended athletic event, take 1 tablespoon of salts in 6–8 ounces of water every hour.

Sodium bicarbonate ($NaHCO_3$) has long been well known and widely used—often under its most familiar alias, baking soda, or sometimes bicarbonate of soda. It occurs naturally in many mineral springs, and is also produced artificially. Much of the hundred thousand tons a year produced worldwide has aluminum added, so you have to be careful in selecting a safe, pure version. Check the label. One good choice is Bob's Red Mill brand, which is plain baking soda, uncontaminated by aluminum.

I recommend baking soda to everyone—1 teaspoon of baking soda dissolved in four to sixteen ounces of water two to three times a day. (Up to 1 tablespoon if you are struggling with a serious health challenge.)

Broad-Spectrum Multimineral Formula with Cell Salts

Look for a combination of a wide variety of minerals and trace minerals, plus the twelve cell salts. You should get 1 mg each of the cell salts (mineral salts, also known as tissue salts, which are at the foundation of every cell, and without which we would die). They are potassium sulfate, magnesium phosphate, sodium chloride, sodium phosphate, sodium sulfate, calcium phosphate, calcium sulfate, calcium fluoride, ferric phosphate, potassium chloride, potassium phosphate, and silica. Those should be mixed in with the macro minerals, including calcium, magnesium, manganese, zinc, and iron, plus all of the trace minerals—of which there are about eighty-seven. The wider variety you get, the better, but in case you can't find all eighty-something, be sure to get phosphorus, potassium, zinc, selenium, copper, chromium, and iodine. Each capsule of the multimineral formula you choose should be 500 mg, as most are.

Broad-Spectrum Multivitamin Formula with Cell Salts

Here again, look for a wide variety of vitamins, ideally combined with cell salts (same as above). At minimum, it should have vitamins A, thiamine (B_1), riboflavin (B_2), niacin (B_3), choline (B_4), calcium D-pantothenate (B_5), pyridoxine hydrochloride (B_6), biotin (B_7), inositol FCC (B_8), folic acid (B_9), cyanocobalamin (B_{12}), vitamin C, vitamin E, and PABA.

Vitamin D₃

Most people are deficient in vitamin D, and it is so crucial to good health in so many ways, I recommend to everyone taking 2,000 IU daily. Choose the D_3 form; it's the most potent. (People challenged by bone density loss should use much larger doses; see page 205.)

Magnesium

Magnesium is one of the four major alkaline buffers of the body. It is also essential for maintaining a healthy body temperature at 98.6. You'll get some magnesium carbonate in your mineral salts, but I also recommend 500 mg a day of magnesium chloride.

Potassium

Take 1,000 mg of potassium chloride at least once a day, in addition to what you will get in your mineral salts.

THE SUPPORTING CAST

If you are ready to expand your use of nutritional supplements, the next place to look is at the list of supplements most useful during a cleanse. They form a core alkalizing supplementation program. (They are listed here in alphabetical order.)

• **Antimycotoxic buffers** include superoxide dismutase (SOD), catalase, glutathione, glutathione-S-transferase, glutathione peroxidase, and methionine reductase. These are not digestive enzymes; rather, they chelate (bind to) acids, allowing them to be excreted from the body. These powerful antioxidants are neutralizers of dietary and/or metabolic acids, essentially "mopping up" excess dietary and metabolic acids and so preventing damage to healthy body cells.

• **Caprylic acid** controls negative microforms and their toxins. It is an antifungal saturated fatty acid approved by the FDA in 1984 for sale over the counter. Studies have shown that patients treated with caprylic acid have completely eliminated fungus from their stool. It can also bring about a remission of symptoms in fungus-related health problems, and appears to be safe and effective with no serious side effects. The most effective caprylic acid formulations are those designed to be released in the colon, where most fungus resides. Along with being effective in eradicating fungus, caprylic acid is also useful after treatment for gout, indigestion, yeast infections, toe fungus, and rashes, as well as for prevention. Caprylic acid almost always comes in a formula combined with:

• **Flavonoids** from antioxidant fruits and vegetables. These are potent acid neutralizers. Quercetin, hesperidin, curcumin, luteolin, proanthocyanidin, naringenin, catechins, and artichoke extract are among those found to be effective.

• **Glutathione**, a super antioxidant, helps the body repair damage from stress, pollution, infection, and damage due to dietary and metabolic acids. It buffers acidity in the cells to help maintain the alkaline design of the body. It is also antiviral, antimycotoxic, and detoxifying in general, and prevents and calms inflammation. It plays an important role in metabolism.

Glutathione is especially valuable to anyone dealing with the symptoms of anemia, impaired glucose tolerance or diabetes, atherosclerosis, lung congestion and inflammation, herpes, hearing loss, poor sperm motility, cancerous conditions, Parkinson's, cataracts, or acute or chronic joint or muscle pain. Glutathione also supports the immune system. A botanical extract of glutathione from the avocado plant is showing promise in clinical testing as an adjunct to cancer therapies.

Glutathione is not an essential nutrient—the body can build it on its own, given the correct resources. It can be synthesized from the amino acids L-cysteine (see below), L-glutamate, and glycine—essentially, from protein.

Most Americans get less than 100 mg glutathione daily via diet, but we'd benefit from several times that. Supplements are commonly found in doses ranging from 50 to 2,000 mg daily. The liquid version we sell contains 430 mg per dose. You should take glutathione three times a day. Choose your supplement carefully—many glutathione supplements are obtained from yeast fermentation and must be avoided. There are healthy sources available, though. Ours, for example, is extracted from avocados. Using avocado oil will also add some glutathione (along with other beneficial components) into your diet.

• **N-acetyl cysteine**, a form of protein, controls negative microforms, and is a powerful antimycotoxin. It provides excellent protection against a broad range of toxic hazards (including the toxins acrolein, in barbecue and cigarette smoke and auto exhaust; paraquat, an herbicide; overdoses of acetaminophen, the pain reliever in Tylenol; halothane, an anesthetic; and the side effects of the anticancer drugs Adriamycin and cyclophosphamide). Studies show that N-acetyl cysteine can also bond to toxic heavy metals such as lead, mercury, and cadmium and escort them out of the body. But perhaps its most valuable function of all is that glutathione (see above) can be derived from it.

N-acetyl cysteine is a normal component of the human body, but to receive its maximum benefits you'll need supplements. Take 500 mg three times a day in capsule form; for a liquid version, take 1 teaspoon three times a day.

An Antimycotoxin Formula

To detoxify mycotoxins and expunge acids from the body, look for a combination of glutathione, N-acetyl cysteine, L-taurine, and organic sulfur, all of which are excellent at binding to toxins and escorting them out of the body. The usual dose applies: 1–2 capsules, three times a day, though if you are using more than one of these individually, you should take less of each, say around 1 capsule three times a day.

• **Noni fruit concentrate,** which is antifungal and antiparasitic. It works by activating phytonutrients and allows the body to renew its cells and rebuild healthy blood and tissue. It also improves alkalizing of food in the alimentary canal and absorption of nutrients, and helps cells use protein. Noni regulates the health of cellular proteins, as they are used in the creation of different body chemicals. Noni fruit has been used traditionally throughout Polynesia for a wide range of symptoms, including digestive problems, intestinal parasites, skin disorders, allergies, arthritis, and diabetes. The active ingredient, xeronine, is also found in papaya, and is physiologically active in trace amounts. Minuscule amounts occur in practically all healthy cells of plants and animals. Noni fruit also contains significant amounts of xeronine's precursor, proxeronine.

Don't worry, noni is a very bitter—low-sugar—fruit. As a result, though, many supplements are unfortunately full of added sugar or other sweetener. Be sure to steer clear of those! You also want to avoid any pasteurized noni products. Most likely you'll find noni as a powder, in capsules. You may also be able to find a liquid colloidal preparation, which would be ideal.

• **Pine bark extract**. One of the most valuable bioflavonoids is pine bark extract, which helps bind up acidity, thereby reducing inflammation (aches and pains) in the body. It has been shown to bind directly with the body's connective tissue, maintaining and repairing it. Pine bark extract is an exception to the rule in that even if it comes in normal-size capsules, most products contain just 25–50 mg of the stuff, which is fine. You still want to take 1–2 capsules, three times a day.

• **Rhodium and iridium**, which are minerals that come in colloidal form, provide nourishment to cells that have been damaged by mycotoxins, allowing them to recover their ability to communicate with one another effectively.

DNA conductivity was increased ten thousand times when a rhodium atom was added at both ends of the strand. Of course, this was done in a lab, and it has not been determined that the body does this. But it does show that the superconductive (allowing electrical current to flow without resistance) potential of a metal can be biologically active. US Naval Air research has shown that cells in living tissue communicate with one another in a superconductive fashion, but the identity of the superconductors was not determined. While there is still much we need to understand about the process, clearly these conductive metals are effective in stimulating electrical impulses at the cellular level, inducing the flow of electricity in and among cells.

• **Silver** supports the body's own natural defense system, and is a powerful natural alkalizer. It assists in the organization of cells that make up new tissue. Look for a liquid colloidal preparation.

BOB'S STORY

I was lining a water storage shed with highly flammable materials, on the roof doing fire watch while my partner was inside working. The pump attached to the truck was grounded improperly, causing static electricity in the lining of the hose, which combusted in a large explosion. My partner was burned over 90 percent of his body, and died in the hospital four hours later.

The flames shot up through the skylight, through which I was gazing, so I received a flash burn. I was blown off the roof and landed on the ground, my face and hands badly burned. I was taken by air ambulance to the hospital burn unit.

My head was swollen to twice its normal size, my eyes swollen shut, my face black and crisp. My nose had more or less disappeared in the swelling, so breathing tubes had to be inserted into my nasal cavities. My ears were severely burned, my fingertips charred and numb, my fingernails melted.

I was told I had second- and third-degree burns on my face and third-degree burns on my hands. The head of the burn unit told me I would be in the hospital for two or three months and would need many skin grafts, especially to my hands. He said he thought I would lose my fingertips and my ears.

The very next day, my mother brought me colloidal silver, with directions to use it externally and internally as frequently as possible, because it assists in growth of new tissue. She had learned from Dr. Young that silver's negative electrical charge counters the positive charge of a damaged body area, bringing it back into balance and enabling the body to regenerate and heal itself. Mom sprayed undiluted colloidal silver onto the burned areas, and I took it by drops under my tongue. I also took cat's claw, germanium, flax seed oil, and vitamin C, as Dr. Young recommended, and, once I was well enough to eat, lots and lots of greens. As soon as I was off intravenous feeding, my mother brought me wheatgrass juice, green juices, and concentrated green powder to bolster my nutrition and healing.

My mother applied the silver many times a day. It was absorbed into my skin instantly. It felt cool and tingling and loosened the tension on my face, hands, and fingertips. The tips of my fingers and the skin under my nails started throbbing and tingling. The staff said it was because my nerves were healing and the blood was circulating.

After only one day of treatment with silver, it was obvious that healing was happening very rapidly. New tissue and skin grew back at an accelerated pace. The swelling of my head diminished rapidly, and the breathing apparatus came off almost immediately. The plastic surgeon told me I was healing twice as fast as any burn patient he'd ever seen in his long career.

When I told him it had to be because of what my mother was giving me, and the alkaline diet, the doctor asked to see what I was using. He read the ingredients and said he didn't see anything wrong with using it (in fact, the healing salve used by the burn unit contained silver), though he noted that the hospital could not be held responsible if anything negative occurred, since it was not a hospital-prescribed medicine.

I still have my fingertips and my ears. I had one skin graft on each hand, but my own skin grew back so fast with the help of the silver that the grafts were useless and actually fell off! I was out of the hospital in two and a half weeks—not two or three months! What most amazed me was that my new skin looked better (smoother) after it healed than it had before I was burned.

The burn unit staff marveled that they had never seen anything like my recovery. The nurses asked if they could use my pictures to show to other burn patients, to help explain the healing process. I was happy to say yes, but asked them to tell them about the colloidal silver, too, and the greens I was getting. They said they'd do their best.

I know I am truly blessed to have healed from these terrible burns with no damage—and no scars.

• **Undecylenic acid**, made through vacuum distillation of castor bean oil, is another fatty acid proven to eradicate or devolve yeast and fungus and counter their toxins. Listed in the US Pharmacopeia for use as a topical antifungal, undecylenic acid can also be used orally for treatment of psoriasis, neurodermatitis, and intestinal fungus. Some studies have shown that undecylenic acid is even more effective than caprylic acid.

Undecylenic acid is almost always sold combined with caprylic acid (above). Look for a formula that contains 25–50 mg of each.

CATHERINE AND CHERYL'S STORY

When my daughter Cheryl got so sick that she had to be hospitalized and put on antipsychotic drugs so strong they came with a possibility of causing permanent nerve damage, the doctors admitted they weren't even sure what was wrong. Schizophrenia? Bipolar disorder? A psychotic episode? I knew we were really in deep when one of the many, many doctors I consulted in my search for something better for Cheryl—a psychiatrist so well known that if I used his name, you might recognize it—told me, "They'll give her condition a name and they'll give her a drug, but they don't really know what they're doing or what they are talking about." This from a man whose business it is to give these things a name and prescribe a drug, who in fact has gotten famous for doing so! He suggested I find a residential facility and check her in for at least a year—in part to get some rest for myself!

I wasn't about to send Cheryl off into the hands of still more doctors and psychologists, none of whom seemed to have a clue what was really going on or what to do about it that might actually be productive. I turned my search to "alternative" medicine, and found a psychiatrist who deals with depression and mental illness through nutrition. Through my own research, I had already started Cheryl on an all-organic, high-protein diet and approximately two hundred supplements a day. This new doctor agreed with that approach, and added weekly B_{12} shots. Cheryl seemed to be getting better.

Eight months and six thousand dollars into this regime, Cheryl was still having violent mood swings and depression, and she finally slipped back into psychosis. She ran away and it was a year before we could get her back into the hospital again. I had to smuggle supplements in to her in plastic containers—as "malteds," ironically. No supplements were allowed for the mentally ill patients—only dangerous antipsychotics, and as much sugar and caffeine as they liked. And don't even get me started on the food. I could never approach the subject of nutrition with her doctors, never mind tell them she was taking hundreds of vitamins a day. When Cheryl was released from the hospital faster than many other patients, many of whom were less ill than she was at the outset, the doctors attributed her rapid recovery to their new wonder drug.

After she was released, I took her to Mexico for live cell therapy to the tune of fifteen thousand dollars. It allowed her to get off the drugs, but it didn't stop her mood swings or depression. She cried almost every day from May to September. So did I.

Throughout all this, my own health seriously degenerated. I had been neglecting my body, and the incredible stress took its toll. I was swollen all over (from yeast, I now know). I had pain all over my body. My vision was often so bad I could hardly see. I had no energy to speak of.

Finally, I ran across Dr. Young. Both Cheryl and I had live blood analysis and learned about the parasites in her blood that cause anxiety and depression. We learned about this program, and I knew that, at last, we had found the solution.

We both did the cleanse and started taking several antifungal/ antimycotoxin formulas, including colloidal caprylic acid, undecylenic acid, germanium, and N-acetyl cysteine, as well as rhodium and iridium for the brain, multivitamin with cell salts, L-taurine, and omega-3 oils, then continued to the full diet.

Cheryl's depression stopped. Her mind is clear. She laughs regularly.

I am ecstatic. My "baby" is well. My health is better than it's been in years. My mind is clear and keeps getting clearer. I am more perceptive, visually and mentally. My skin feels wonderful and I can see my cheekbones again for the first time in twenty years. I have greatly increased energy and a general sense of well-being.

Our kitchen is filled with bowls of sprouts of every variety. We are eating almost totally raw, and she is concocting many wonderful and some, shall we say, "interesting," recipes. We hope to be starting an "Un"Cooking class soon. Cheryl has a vision of opening a "Diet Center" based on the principles of *The pH Miracle*, where people can come and get well. Thanks to this program, I know whatever her dreams, she'll be able to make them come true.

THE CAMEOS

The following nutrients, also in alphabetical order, are helpful for bringing your body back into balance. Once you are there, they are optional, though you'll do well to continue with them.

All these would be great on their own, but they are often found in combination formulas as well. When you are evaluating products and various combinations, these are some of the most beneficial ingredients to look for:

• **Butyric acid**, another short-chain saturated fatty acid, helps chelate mycotoxins that increase low-density lipoproteins (LDL cholesterol). It is healing to the mucous membranes of the stomach and small and large intestines. It can, for example, repair the damage *Candida albicans* creates in the intestinal walls. Butyric acid also boosts immune function by detoxifying the lymph system of yeast and fungus and their associated mycotoxins. Butyric acid, which comes as a liquid, alone, or with other antifungals, can be hard to find. As long as you are getting caprylic or undecylenic acid, you don't have to worry about getting butyric acid if you can't find it.

• **CoQ10** is one of the three strongest and most versatile antioxidants in the body. It increases cellular energy, reduces toxic acid levels in cells, and protects the heart and brain against dietary and metabolic acids.

• **Gallium** helps form antitumor compounds. It has specific areas of activity in the human brain and has been reported to reduce the rate of brain cancer in laboratory animals. British research shows that pregnant women taking supplemental gallium reduced the rate of brain cancer in their children. Take 3–5 drops of a colloidal preparation three times a day, or follow package directions.

• **Garlic extract** improves the alkalinity of the body and also increases HDL cholesterol while lowering total cholesterol. Garlic has been widely used in health and medicine for centuries. For example, both the Roman poet Virgil and the Greek physician Hippocrates mention it as a remedy for pneumonia and snakebite. Though it is silent on the snakebite issue, modern science does tell us that garlic is a good antifungal and antibacterial agent and inhibits yeast and mold as well as fungus and bacteria. It has been shown to be effective against the bacteria *Staphylococcus aureus* and *E. coli*, in particular, as well as on *Candida albicans*. Of these three common organisms, Candida has been shown to be the most sensitive to garlic juice.

Even small amounts of garlic are effective, but the chemical component that is most therapeutic (allicin) also gives garlic its strong odor. So beware of the "odorless" formulations (though they may still provide benefits to cholesterol levels and fat metabolism).

Garlic supplements are particularly important if you don't like the taste or smell of garlic, and so aren't getting it in your regular diet.

• **Organic germanium** is a metallic element that helps eliminate yeast and fungus, thanks to its promotion of increased production of interferon, which has antitoxic and antiparasitic activity. It also enhances metabolic chemical reactions based on oxygen (which, in the human body, is most of them). Organic germanium also stimulates electrical impulses on a cellular level, helping the body discharge certain unwanted electrical fields and allowing much-needed current to flow through. In other words, it helps establish the desired electrical balance. That's crucial because electricity provides fundamental organization and control in the body—like a framework for all other processes. Germanium capsules generally contain just 25–50 mg; if you get a combination, look for that much germanium.

• **Gold** supports the body's own natural defense system. It has been used successfully to treat arthritis, skin ulcers, burns, certain nerve-end operations, various types of punctures, obesity, and inoperable cancer, but fell into disuse with the advent of antibiotics and other (toxic) drugs. Gold is a conductor of electricity, which may help in cellular communication, metabolism, and regeneration. Research has shown that gold has the potential to repair damaged DNA. Gold can have a psychological balancing and harmonizing effect, easing depression, seasonal affective disorder, melancholy, sorrow, fear, despair, anguish, frustration, and even suicidal tendencies. The preparation of gold to look for is expensive jewelry. Just kidding! Seriously, the colloidal form is what you need. Use 3–5 drops three times a day, or follow package directions.

• **Olive leaf extract** acts against morbid microforms, is an excellent antimycotoxin, and has antibiotic properties. It also benefits the cardiovascular system by protecting HDL cholesterol ("good cholesterol") from oxidation. Botanists believe it is the chemical compound oleuropein's presence throughout the olive tree—in the wood, fruit, leaves, roots, and bark—that protects it from insects and bacteria. Furthermore, calcium elenolate, made from one of oleuropein's breakdown products (elenolic acid) is a major destroyer, or growth inhibitor, of many kinds of microforms. Another byproduct, aglycone, has a similar inhibitory effect. Olive leaf extract acts against various fungi, as well as salmonella and *Staphylococcus aureus* bacteria. You can use olive leaf extract on its own, though you should note that this is another exception: Solo capsules will contain just 25–50 mg of olive leaf extract, and that is just fine. You should look for similar amounts in each 500 mg capsule of a combination.

• **R-lipoic and R-dihydrolipoic** are two of the most potent and versatile antioxidants in the body. They exist in our every cell and tissue. They strengthen immunity, improve energy in cells, protect brain cells against neurotoxicity, and remove excess heavy metals, like mercury. A number of studies have shown that they can lower blood sugar levels in people with diabetes, and prevent diabetic complications (especially cardiovascular and neurological problems).

• **Thioctic or lipoic acid** chelates mycotoxins collecting in the liver and normalizes liver enzymes. It has also been shown to remove mercury, arsenobenzols, carbon tetrachloride, and aniline dyes. Experiments demonstrate a vast increase in oxygen supply and use with lipoic acid treatment. This liquid can be another tough one to find. Your best bet may be as a combination with caprylic or undecylenic acid, and again, if you are getting one or both of those two, this one is not crucial.

• **Rare metals including osmium, ruthenium, palladium, and platinum,** as well as the gold, gallium, rhodium, and iridium discussed above, have extraordinary electrical conduction properties. These are electrostimulators, but with a different specialty than gallium: increasing the ability of DNA to conduct electricity and enhancing communication among cells. They also stimulate metabolism.

Research at the Bristol-Myers Squibb labs indicates that using precious metals in the presence of cancer can correct altered DNA. Scientists coupled these elements with the cells via a transfer of light—encoded bursts of ultraviolet laser light. Electrons that flow through a superconductor pair off and convert into light. Superconductors assist light transfer, and gallium, gold, rhodium, iridium, osmium, ruthenium, palladium, and platinum increase the light found in the human body.

Choose a colloidal preparation and take 3–5 drops three times a day, or follow package directions.

EDNA'S STORY

All I wanted to do was sleep. I would sit in my office and find I could not stay awake. I'd go home at night and fall asleep on the floor until it was time to go to bed. I was not functioning well or doing the work I needed to do. I couldn't even attempt to exercise. I was stressed and pale, enough so that people would ask me if I was okay.

I was ready to try anything, so when live blood analysis was suggested to me I thought that, eccentric as it sounded, I'd just go and see what it was about. Knowing what I know now about what I was (and wasn't) eating, I shouldn't have been surprised that the analysis showed acute yeast/fungus imbalance, adrenal stress, and irregularly shaped red blood cells.

I went on a cleanse with supplements and juiced green vegetables. After three days, I added all sorts of vegetables, and turkey and fish. I ate stir-fry for dinner, nibbled on carrot and celery sticks for lunch, and had vegetable juice for breakfast.

I started taking vitamin B_5, beta-carotene, a multimineral, pH drops, undecylenic and caprylic acid, bromelain, citron, chromium, vanadium, omega-3, borage and fish liver oils, colloidal silver, and a few herbal combinations with at least another twenty ingredients. I couldn't believe how many pills I had to take! By the time I took my supplements and a little juice, I would be full.

I stayed on this regimen for two months with no cheating. Gradually, I felt better and better. After the first week, the color returned to my face and I had more energy. I slept better at night. The most important thing to me was that I could go home and prepare dinner for my family of nine. Along with feeling better and having more energy, there was another benefit: I lost sixty pounds. My husband says that even my eyes are brighter.

I went shopping and bought a dress with a straight skirt. I haven't worn a straight skirt in twenty years. My closet was crammed with clothes from size eight to eighteen, and I just cleaned out everything above my current size: nine!

At my follow-up blood test, I was pleased to actually see my improvement on the monitor screen. This time I had perfectly round red blood cells, and the fluid was free of most bacteria and had very little yeast.

I really do enjoy what I eat now. Before I would never eat raw nuts or avocado. They tasted awful to me. Now my taste buds have changed, and even vegetables taste sweet! Tomatoes are a real treat for me.

This program brought back my sense of well-being and allowed me to lose weight I haven't been able to lose any other way. It literally saved my health.

ADDRESSING SYMPTOMS WITH SUPPLEMENTS

Beyond the alkalizing basics, the correct supplements can also be powerful tools in clearing up specific symptoms. You can add the supplements below to the routine you've already established for yourself, thereby tailoring it to your specific situation. Use them until you leave the acidic symptoms behind, taking them occasionally as necessary for prevention thereafter. If you need the same supplement for more than one condition, don't multiply the dose—but do use the highest dose given.

Adrenal Stress

Symptoms include insomnia, fatigue, low blood pressure, poor circulation, feeling cold all the time, getting light-headed when standing, arthritis in joints and back, drowsiness or sleepiness in the afternoon, and chronic pain. You have four options, which you can take together:

- With each meal, take 2 capsules of an **adrenal formula** including glandular adrenal and calcium D-pantothenate (vitamin B₅).
- Take 3–5 drops under the tongue, three times a day, of an **antimycotoxin formula** containing glutathione, N-acetyl cysteine, L-taurine, and organic sulfur. Caprylic and undecylenic acid, pine bark extract, and grape seed extract would be good additions.
- Take 3–5 drops under the tongue, three times a day, of a formula containing **chromium** and **vanadium**.
- Take 3–5 drops of a liquid **B complex,** three times a day, under the tongue.

Bone Loss

Bone loss leading to osteoporosis and/or fractures can be prevented with the right nutrients.

Vitamin D regulates calcium metabolism and helps prevent and heal the progressive bone loss that can lead to vertebral and hip fractures. The body uses vitamin D to grow and continually remodel bone.

Many studies, including a recent meta-analysis published in the *Archives of Internal Medicine*, demonstrate a decreased risk of bone fracture in older adults taking vitamin D supplements at sufficient levels. (Vitamin D also has anticancerous properties.)

You can get vitamin D in green fruit and veggies, and cod liver oil, but most of the vitamin D you get (aside from supplements) is produced by your own body when it is exposed to sunlight. Most of us, women especially, would benefit from supplementation as well—the majority of people are vitamin-D-deficient.

There are many forms of vitamin D; the two major forms are D₂ (ergocalciferol) and D₃ (cholecalciferol). They are known collectively as calciferol. Vitamin D₃ is more potent than D₂, so that is what I recommend you look for in a supplement. Take 50,000 IUs of vitamin D₃ daily if you already have lost bone density.

I would also recommend 500 mg of **magnesium chloride** and 2,000 mg of **potassium chloride** daily.

Congestion or Other Sinus Symptoms:

Experiment to see which methods work best for you:

- Dissolve 2 capsules of an **anti-yeast formula** in a bottle of saline solution (available at pharmacies). Spray into your nostrils at least three times a day, following package instructions.

- Use 3–5 drops of **colloidal silver** or **liquid pine bark** extract three times a day, under the tongue. Or use 1 or 2 drops in each nostril once or twice a day. If you can't get liquid pine bark extract, use the powder mixed with pure water.
- Dissolve ½ teaspoon of **mineral salts** or **sodium bicarbonate** in 4–6 ounces of purified water in a neti pot or squeeze bottle to rinse and clear the sinuses.
- Add 3–5 drops of **NaClO2 (sodium chlorite)** to 8 ounces of pure or alkaline water and drink three times a day.
- Use **seed oils**, such as flax seed oil and borage oil, in capsules as you would any supplement. Or take 1 teaspoonful three times a day. Or use more in your diet!

Sinus symptoms should steadily disappear on their own as toxins are cleared from the body and good digestion is restored.

Diabetes and Other Pancreas Problems

These issues may include hypoglycemia and hyperglycemia.

- Look for a **pancreas formula** including glandular pancreas, uva ursi, dandelion root, parsley, gentian root, huckleberry leaves, raspberry leaves, buchu leaves, saw palmetto berries, kelp, and bladder wrack. Take 2 capsules with each meal.
- Take 3–5 drops of **liquid** or **colloidal chromium** and **liquid vanadium** before each meal, under the tongue.
- **Chromium**, a mineral, is a co-factor that facilitates the binding of insulin to glucose and thus reduces blood sugar levels and acidity. When chromium levels are low, HDL levels fall and insulin resistance develops. (Triglycerides and total cholesterol both rise as well.) Chromium supplementation has been shown to improve insulin receptor function. Studies indicate that acidic glycation by-products (hemoglobin A1c) were reduced and glucose returned to normal in most people who took chromium. (Their total cholesterol fell, too.) Take 1 teaspoon of liquid colloidal chromium three times a day.
- **Vanadium** helps to uptake the chromium to help in making effective glucose and insulin interactions. Take 1 teaspoon of liquid colloidal vanadium three times a day with liquid chromium.

- **CoQ10** has been shown to lower blood glucose by 30 percent in diabetics. It also cuts ketone bodies (potentially poisonous acids produced by the body when metabolizing fats for energy) as much as 30 to 59 percent. Take 1 teaspoon of liquid colloidal CoQ10 three times a day.
- **Cinnamon extract** (or methylhydroxychalcone polymer, if you prefer) chelates and buffers the acids that cause Types 1 and 2 diabetes. A study published in the *American Journal of Clinical Nutrition* demonstrated that taking cinnamon extract enhanced sugar uptake and reduced the need for insulin in people with diabetes. Take 1 teaspoon of liquid cinnamon extract three times a day.

Eye or Ear Problems

These may include cataracts, glaucoma, redness, blurred vision, poor eyesight, ringing in the ears, earaches, soreness or swelling of the ears, eardrum damage, hardness of hearing, and (in rare cases) loss of hearing. Use 1 drop of **colloidal silver** topically (directly in the eye or ear) three times a day.

Gastrointestinal discomfort

To relieve intestinal gas (flatulence), enteritis, colic, and heartburn, look for a **digestion formula** including papaya leaves, peppermint leaves, gingerroot, catnip, fennel seed, and saw palmetto berries. Take 2 capsules with every meal. You then have two other choices:

- Take 1–2 capsules of **noni fruit concentrate** before meals with a small amount of water and 1–2 capsules of an anti-yeast formula containing undecylenic and caprylic acids, and **herbs that aid in digestion,** half an hour after each meal.
- For digestion of fats, with each meal, 1–2 capsules of noni fruit concentrate and an **antimycotoxin formula** containing N-acetyl cysteine, L-taurine, and organic sulfur, at least, and perhaps caprylic and undecylenic acids, pine bark extract, and grape seed extract.

Infectious and Degenerative Symptoms

These may include AIDS and cancer. Try **colloidal formulas of osmium, ruthenium, and palladium; co-enzyme Q1** (CoQ1, also known by the

acronym for its hugely long chemical name, NADH); and the anti-yeast
undecylenic and **caprylic acids**.

Joint and Muscle Pain

You have four options:

- Take 3 capsules of a **calcium** and 4 capsules of **marine lipids/borage oil formula** with each meal. To make sure it combines properly, take the oil with meals made up of vegetables or vegetable juice.
- Take 3–5 drops of **colloidal calcium**, **colloidal boron**, and an **anti-mycotoxin formula** (with N-acetyl cysteine, L-taurine, and organic sulfur, and perhaps caprylic and undecylenic acids, pine bark extract, and grape seed extract), three times a day, under the tongue.
- Take a **joint and muscle formula** including colloidal glutathione (3–5 drops, three times a day, under the tongue), calcium and magnesium (2–3 capsules three times a day, with meals), and zinc (2–3 capsules three times a day, with meals). For acute or chronic conditions, use 4–6 capsules three times a day.
- Take a **formula containing the herb yucca,** which reduces inflammation, soreness, and swelling.

Liver Stress

The liver, which filters toxins from your body, should itself be detoxified at least three or four times a year. Look for a **liver formula** combining glandular liver, dandelion root, red clover, chapparal, yellow dock root, cascara sagrada bark, licorice root, sarsaparilla root, celery seed, burdock root, echinacea, Oregon grape root, stillingia, prickly ash bark, buckthorn bark, cayenne, kelp, and wild yam root. Take 2 capsules at least half an hour before each meal (three meals a day), with an 8-ounce glass of pure water, for a total of 180 capsules in thirty days. This approach can also help in cases of hepatitis, cirrhosis, and jaundice.

GLANDULARS

Glandulars, such as glandular liver, here, glandular lung, below, and others in this section, are in fact animal products, usually from cows. They are used in the formulas specifically to act as messengers of sorts: They carry nutrients to specific areas. That is, they bring nutrients to the part of the body the gland came from. For example, when researchers tag the formula above with radioactive isotopes and then follow it through the body, they can observe it going directly to the liver. You can get similar products minus the glandulars if you want to be scrupulous about avoiding animal products, though they won't be as targeted.

Lung Problems

These may include pneumonia, asthma, bronchitis, croup, tuberculosis, colds, flu, hay fever, and emphysema. Look for a **lung formula** including glandular lung, pleurisy root, wild cherry bark, slippery elm bark, plantain, mullein leaves, chickweed, horehound, licorice root, kelp, cayenne, and saw palmetto. Take 2 capsules with each meal. You can also use 5–10 drops of **colloidal silver** or **pine bark extract** in a respirator. You can buy a respirator at your local drugstore. Add water and colloidal drops and it creates a mist in the air for you to breathe in, which is great for lung or nasal congestion.

SHIRLEY'S STORY

I finally went to the hospital just after Thanksgiving. I just couldn't seem to get rid of what I thought was a terrible cold, and had been coughing almost continuously day and night for about a week. So the doctors admitted me for tests. At first they thought it was pneumonia. Then the lung specialist thought it was another kind of infection in my lung. The medication he prescribed seemed to help, and I went home after a few days.

Just before Christmas, my doctor called to ask me to return for more tests after the holidays. Back in the hospital, the doctors found two "spots" on my liver, and a very low sodium count, and they told me they suspected I had cancer! The next day, they found a mass on my lung. Then a CT scan found a tumor on the right side of my brain and another behind my left eye. They finally traced the origin of the cancer to my bronchial tube.

The doctors told my daughters—but not me—that I had small cell cancer, a very aggressive form. If I took chemotherapy, I'd have two to three years to live. Without it, I'd be looking at six months. The doctors asked my daughters not to give me the particulars about how long I had because they didn't want me to lose hope.

I had my first chemotherapy treatment, which took three days. I then started radiation treatments for the tumors in my head—fifteen treatments over three weeks.

In the middle of all this, my daughter came to stay, loaded down with bottles of pills and books and tapes about Dr. Young's principles. She totally changed my diet and started me on a bunch of supplements. She kept about ten little brown bottles of what she called colloids on my dressing table and gave them to me before and with meals, as Dr. Young recommended, until I learned how to take them myself. I began to notice a different sensation in my head as well as in my chest.

After about two weeks of my daughter's pH Miracle treatment, I had my first appointment with my doctor since leaving the hospital. He told me my blood work came back normal. Seeming a little confused, he asked if I had had radiation to my chest. I hadn't. He told me that the mass in my bronchial tube was gone—and that if the cancer was not in the place of origin, it was probably nowhere else to be found in my body!

For the second time talking with my doctors (after my diagnosis), I couldn't believe what I had just heard. It took a few hours for it to really sink in. What a weight had been lifted off my shoulders—and my family's! How we celebrated!

Still, I took two more chemotherapy sessions (I guess my doctors couldn't quite believe it, either). My blood work continued to come back close to normal, which is highly unusual. At my next doctor's appointment, a month after the last checkup, I got astounding results from my CT scan: The tumors in my head were definitely gone! My doctor discontinued my chemotherapy and told me to check in with him in another two months. His last words are still ringing in my ears: "Whatever you're doing, keep on doing it!"

Lymphatic Blockage

You have two options:

- Take 1 capsule in the morning and another in the evening of a **lymphatic formula** including fish liver oil, beta-carotene, dandelion root, eyebright, marshmallow root, licorice root, and parsley.

- Although this is not a supplement, it is a very helpful approach to lymphatic blockage, so I wanted to include it here: a series of at least twenty-four lymphatic massages—massages that move the lymphatic fluids and help to move toxins out of the lymph nodes by stroking with the hands in the direction of the lymphatic vessels—no downward movements. Lymphatic massages proceed from the feet to the legs to the torso toward the heart, from the lower back to the upper back over the shoulders toward the heart, and from the fingers to the arms to the shoulders to the heart. Consult a massage therapist experienced in this area. Regular massage therapy can also be very beneficial. Even easier, perhaps, is daily dry brushing of the skin. Simply get a skin brush at a natural food store or body shop and brush away, wet or dry—but always toward the heart.

TAISHA'S STORY

I'd been under extreme stress for a long time, and it started to take a physical toll, including high blood pressure and erratic heartbeats and fibrillations. I've also struggled for years with a very painful left breast and lymph node in my left armpit, and very low energy that rendered me dysfunctional to a large extent.

The pain became progressively worse, and I discovered a lump in my left breast. Wisely or unwisely, I chose not to have a mammogram, opting to honor my intuition and beliefs instead. I wasn't prepared to have a biopsy, needle biopsy, drugs, surgery, chemotherapy, or anything that might further endanger my life, so the mammogram wouldn't have served a useful purpose anyway. I realized I was taking a risk, of course, but I wanted to give my body the best chance of being healed in a natural and holistic way.

I started taking colloidal silver after a friend told me he had learned from Dr. Young about its being a broad-spectrum natural antibiotic that fights yeast, fungus, parasites, and viruses. I also learned about the herbal tea Essiac—according to the article I read, President Kennedy's personal physician had cured himself of cancer by only taking Essiac. I took the colloidal form rather than having to use the tea. Then from Dr. Young I learned about iodine (for my hypothyroidism), the anti-yeast/fungus combination of caprylic and undecylenic acids, and pine bark extract.

> To my amazement and delight, four days after starting to take the Essiac and caprylic acid, my lump had totally disappeared! My energy level is definitely improving. I'm still struggling with some health problems, but I realize this is a process, and as I embark on an alkaline diet like the pH Miracle, and get more rest, I know my health will get better and better.

Parasites

Take an **antiparasite formula containing black walnut hulls**. Take 4 capsules three times a day for ten days, then break for four days. Repeat this cycle at least six times. Although you can get black walnut hulls alone, I prefer one of the combinations that include it.

Reproductive Organ Disorders

You have two options:

• Take 3–5 drops **colloidal rhodium** and **iridium** three times a day, under the tongue.

• *For women:* Look for a **female tonic** including glandular ovary, glandular uterus, black cohosh, licorice root, raspberry leaves, passionflower, chamomile, fenugreek, black haw bark, saw palmetto berries, squaw vine, wild yam root, and kelp. Take 2–3 capsules with each meal, and 3–5 drops **colloidal calcium** and **colloidal boron** three times a day under the tongue. Take a **soy sprouts formula** (made by dehydrating say, twenty ounces of soy sprouts into one ounce of the supplement via low-heat dehydration), 3–5 drops three times a day with meals. You can also use progesterone cream as directed on the package.

• *For men:* Take 1–3 capsules of a **men's formula** including glandular prostate, parsley, saw palmetto berries, corn silk, buchu leaves, cayenne, kelp, and pumpkin seeds with each meal, and 3–5 drops each of **colloidal zinc, colloidal vitamin B$_6$**, and a **liquid amino acids formula** (look for, among others, lysine, methionine, arginine, leucine, tyrosine, tryptophan, and phenylalanine), three times a day, under the tongue.

Thyroid Problems

Look for a **thyroid formula** including kelp (to deliver iodine), gentian root, saw palmetto berries, cayenne, and Irish moss. Take 1–2 capsules with each meal.

Toxic Stress (Oxidation and Mycotoxins)

Try colloidal or liquid vitamin C, echinacea, glutathione, calcium, boron, silver, lithium, selenium, pregnenolone, pine bark extract, fish liver oil, beta-carotene, dandelion root, eyebright, marshmallow root, licorice root, parsley, N-acetyl cysteine, L-taurine, sulfur, caprylic and undecylenic acids, grape seed extract, and a multimineral. A soy sprouts formula is another natural source to buffer acidic hormones in men and women.

Weight Control and Fat Metabolism

You have several options—you can mix and match:

• Take 1–2 capsules of a **multivitamin** and 1–2 capsules of **a mineral formula** daily. Getting your nutrients in a capsule that is predigested saves energy, and there will be little or no acid produced in getting the nutrients.

• Take 2–3 capsules of **pine bark extract** one hour before each meal and 3–5 drops of **colloidal chromium** and **vanadium** three times a day, under the tongue (use capsules if you can't find it in colloidal form).

• Take 1–2 capsules, three times a day, with meals, of a **pituitary/thyroid formula** containing kelp, gentian root, saw palmetto berries, cayenne, and Irish moss.

• Take a **liquid amino acids formula** (look for, among others, lysine, methionine, arginine, leucine, tyrosine, tryptophan, and phenylalanine), 3–5 drops under the tongue, three times a day.

• *For women:* **Colloidal calcium** and **colloidal boron**, 3–5 drops each, three times a day, under the tongue, and 1–2 capsules of a **women's formula** including glandular ovary, glandular uterus, black cohosh root, licorice root, raspberry leaves, passionflower, chamomile, fenugreek, black haw bark, saw palmetto berries, squaw vine, wild yam root, and kelp.

For men: **Colloidal zinc** and **colloidal vitamin B$_6$**, 3–5 drops each, three times a day, under the tongue.

- A formula containing the fat **lecithin**.

- **Citron** or **garcinia cambogia**, an alkaline bitter fruit, helps in reducing acidity and thus the need for the body to retain fat.

- Here's another one that isn't a supplement: Follow the diet portion of this program strictly! Your weight will naturally control itself once you are eating alkaline. You will also find drinking 8 ounces of dark green vegetable juice six to eight times a day, as in the first part of the cleanse, helpful.

Supplements are powerful allies in this program. They will maximize the results you get from the pH Miracle Whole Body Cleanse and an alkaline diet. But there is no such thing as a magic bullet—no one thing is going to solve all your problems for you, or keep you healthy forever. And as powerful as they are, they are no match for that great scourge—the typical American diet. If you don't change the way you feed your body, any nutritional supplements you take will be overworked. The combination—lifestyle, diet, and supplements—is the key.

Chapter 13

·

Alkaline Exercise

Exercise makes you breathe. It makes you sweat. It pumps your lymph system. And in doing so, it is an invaluable component of getting and staying alkaline. That's because the power of exercise to cleanse your body, eliminating acids and all kinds of toxins, is just as important as its ability to build strength and enhance flexibility. It is just as important as the cardiovascular benefits and the support of the bones and joints and the stress busting and the mood stabilization. It is just as important to clear acids from the body as it is to boost metabolism, or to improve blood pressure, triglycerides, and insulin levels. That's why we've included an exercise plan as an integral part of the pH Miracle program.

The key thing is to get exercise. But you also have to make sure it is the right *kind* of exercise—and the right amount. Too little, too much, or the wrong kind, and you'll make yourself more acidic.

LOVE YOUR LYMPHATIC SYSTEM

You can burn calories with pretty much any form of exercise. But burning calories is *not* the most important thing about exercise. Sweating is. Perspiration moves acids out of your body through the pores in your skin (thirty-five hundred of them per square inch!). In fact, sweat is one of the main ways your body has of eliminating acids. Moving your body enough to break a sweat pumps the lymphatic system, which serves to remove toxins and acidic wastes from body tissues and fluids and release them through the skin. Sweating opens up your pores, which allows both liquid and gaseous acids to pass through. If you are exercising enough to sweat, you are also exercising enough to increase your breathing, and respiration is another key way for acids and toxins (in gas form) to leave the body.

The lymphatic system is a secondary circulatory system that runs parallel to the blood system, composed of a network of lymphatic nodes, capillaries, and vessels that carry a clear, alkaline fluid called lymph. (The spleen, thymus, appendix, tonsils, and bone marrow also contain lymphatic tissue.) Its purpose is to move fluid away from the tissues back into the blood, and to move acids, wastes, bacteria, and other toxins out of the body. The lymph also delivers nutrients to the cells, and helps exchange oxygen and carbon dioxide. The lymphatic system supports the immune system by moving white blood cells around the body.

You have lymphatic vessels pretty much anywhere you have blood vessels. They are lined with a thin, smooth wall of muscle. There are hundreds of lymph nodes spread out along these vessels, with particular density in the neck, armpits, and groin. Lymph moves through the vessels into the lymph nodes to be filtered, but it doesn't have a large built-in pump the way your circulatory system does (the heart), so it requires pressure changes to stimulate the flow of lymph. Those pressure changes occur through deep breathing and muscular activity. In other words, exercise is what you need to activate your lymphatic system, and you need to pump your lymphatic system to get and keep your body alkaline.

If the lymph slows down or stagnates, you'll have poor circulation, and fresh oxygen and fuel can't get to the cells. The cells themselves will bathe in acidic, rather than alkaline, fluids—fluids that may have toxins and debris in them without the lymph system functioning to pull them away. Your body won't work as efficiently, and you'll feel you have no energy. You'll have systemic and/or localized pain due to acid buildup. You'll retain fluids—one of your body's strategies for neutralizing acid. And you'll be wide open to degenerative disease.

These are the far-reaching effects of a lack of exercise and a lymph system that doesn't get properly "pumped." Acid foods, sugar, and toxic chemicals cause lymph problems, too. Acidic waste from chemical reactions in the cells, from breakdown of tissues and cells, and from any acidic by-products that can't be cleared by the bloodstream, can block your lymphatic system. Emotional and psychological issues can have an effect, too. (See chapter 14.) Unmanaged anger, stress, fatigue, or emotional shock can slow the lymph system.

CHOOSE AEROBIC EXERCISE

The wrong kind or amount of exercise, however, can actually block your lymphatic system. Lack of regular aerobic exercise has that effect, and so does overexercising. Anaerobic exercise (more about which in a minute) is also a problem. What you need is aerobic exercise—in moderate amounts. Aerobic exercise is any exercise that increases the body's use and flow of oxygen—*aerobic* means, literally, "with oxygen." The increased oxygen demand is what causes the familiar increase in heart rate and breathing.

Many types of exercise are aerobic. Whether or not a particular exercise is aerobic often depends on how it is performed. Generally, aerobic exercise is exercise of moderate intensity done for a relatively long period of time. Jogging several times around the track at a reasonable pace? Aerobic. Jogging full-out so you can't carry on even a small conversation with your running partner? Not.

ANAEROBIC EXERCISE

Exercise that causes the body to incur an oxygen debt, however—exercise that is *anaerobic,* "without oxygen"—shuts down the lymphatic system and will make the body more acidic. What enables the body to make any movements at all is the electrical potential or free electrons that every cell in the human body requires in order to function properly. We recharge our bodies with electron-rich alkaline foods, drinks, and sunshine. Without those electrons, we couldn't power any exercise at all. When electrons are consumed for energy, this creates acidic by-products, which vary somewhat depending on the source of the food or drink we are obtaining our electrical potential or electrons from. As long as the body is taking in plenty of oxygen, carbon dioxide—a less toxic acid—is released through the lungs as the body extracts energy via respiration. But without sufficient oxygen—in anaerobic conditions—the metabolic process shifts from respiration to fermentation, and the more toxic lactic acid is formed and expelled into the tissues. The classic example of anaerobic exercise is weight lifting (especially when you tend to hold your breath). But anytime you exercise to the point where you are gasping for oxygen, you are doing anaerobic exercise—even if it's a type of exercise we tend to think of as aerobic. Cycling? Generally aerobic. Cycling up long hills? Anaerobic.

Anytime you do any kind of exercise to the point of exhaustion, you have crossed the line into anaerobic exercise. That is, anytime you feel exhausted, and have soreness or pain in your muscles—that's the lack of oxygen talking. Exercise exhaustion can be a whole-body phenomenon, or it can be just in a particular muscle or group of muscles. When you feel that burning sensation in your muscles, you are overexercising. Your muscles are exhausted, and they are not getting enough oxygen. More serious exercise exhaustion can give you tightness in the throat, reduced peripheral vision, light-headedness or dizziness, and, at the extreme, feeling faint, weak, or ready to pass out. Certain types of exercise can be very exhausting if not done right, and you should be especially conscious of avoiding exhaustion when you are doing long-distance running or swimming, intense weight lifting, and Spinning. Otherwise you'll be getting more acidic rather than more alkaline.

FAT VERSUS SUGAR

Any metabolic acid can cause aches and pains, but lactic acid is the one usually causing the aches and pains you feel during and after exercise—the muscle aches you get after a tough or unaccustomed workout, for example. Lactic acid is very toxic. It is always found in greater concentrations in the body wherever there is irritation, inflammation, or pain (as well as in and around cancerous tumors). And it's a sign your cells are primarily breaking down to release needed electrons for increased demands for energy. The waste product of this cellular breakdown is increased amounts of an acid known as sugar.

When your body accesses electron energy from fat, however, twice the amount of energy is released—and just half the acid waste as compared with obtaining electron energy from carbohydrate or protein. Proper aerobic exercise—paired with a proper alkaline diet—allows your body to access electrical energy in the form of electrons from fat. You'll increase your electrical energy, strength, and endurance and move acids out of your body at the same time!

When you are exercising anaerobically, your sugar acid levels will increase and you'll feel light-headed or dizzy. You'll be able to hear yourself breathing, as you inhale and exhale through your mouth rather than your nose, and you'll be unable to carry on a conversation while exercising. Your muscles will be tight, your fists balled up, and your brow furrowed; you may have a knot in your throat. Your sweat may smell like ammonia. Your peripheral vision may narrow, and you may feel disconnected with your environment, even to the point where you don't hear your feet hitting the ground when you're running, for example. Your thinking may become cloudy, and you may become agitated or anxiety-ridden. Your hands or feet may tingle or be cold, or you may have burning sensations there or elsewhere in your body. You may experience systemic or localized pain. In short, you're not going to feel good! The signs are pretty much the same when you are over-exercising, or exercising to the point of exhaustion.

How you feel when you are exercising aerobically and moderately, and accessing your electron energy needs from fat, is a whole different ball game. You'll feel peaceful, grounded, connected to your environment, even euphoric. You'll think clearly. You'll breathe quietly and easily, through your nose, and be able to chat while exercising. Your facial expressions will be relaxed and happy, and you will feel more flexible. All your senses will be enhanced. You feel no pain: you're in the zone.

Pain when you exercise is a sure sign that you are oxygen-deficient and producing increased metabolic acids (lactic acid and sugar) rather than accessing your electron reserves—and acidifying your body. You are stressing, rather than strengthening, your body. So be sure to keep your exercise pain-free, fully electron-charged from alkaline foods and drinks, and aerobic. If at any point you do feel pain or discomfort while exercising, stop immediately and hydrate with an electron-rich alkaline green drink with pH drops or good alkaline water to restore alkalinity and to increase your reserves of electrons.

GET THE AMOUNT OF EXERCISE THAT'S *JUST RIGHT*

Like Goldilocks, you shouldn't settle for exercise that's too much or too little. You need to get the type and amount of exercise that's "just right." That means at least twenty to thirty minutes a day of activity. If you don't exercise every day, acids will build up in your tissues. But you don't have to do it all at once; if it works better for you to break it into ten- or fifteen-minute sessions, go right ahead. In fact, exercising more often is better than exercising for longer periods of time in one go.

You should always consult with your doctor before beginning a new exercise program, particularly if you've been a bit of a couch potato. Once you've been cleared for takeoff, start with a variety of low-impact aerobic exercises, like brisk walking, cross-training or elliptical machines, easy jogging, swimming, biking, or—our personal favorite—rebounding (bouncing on a mini trampoline). Mix it up with more static exercise like yoga, Pilates, and certain types of weight training. Add in passive exercise in the form of whole-body vibration, sauna, and massage.

For the core, specifically aerobic, portion of your exercise routine, ideally you'll first do a brief warm-up, followed by at least twenty minutes of moderate to intense exercise involving large muscle groups, ending with a short cool-down period. (Warm-up and cool-down simply comprise the same exercise you'll do for the heart of the workout, but with the intensity dialed way back, to ease your body into and out of it.) Your best overall pace is one that will ensure that you break a sweat within ten to fifteen minutes, but is never painful.

All this presupposes you're eating an appropriate amount of healthy al-kaline food for your body weight. If you're following the pH Miracle plan, your body will be getting the electron energy or fuel it needs—no more, no less—which allows you to streamline your workout this way. If you eat more than you should—or more acid than you should—you need more exercise.

SWEAT MORE, WEIGH LESS

If you are exercising moderately but not sweating, or not sweating much, try the following strategies to get the acids flowing out of your body:

- Make sure you are drinking the amount of water recommended in chapter 7. Build up to it gradually if necessary.
- Drink at least one liter of green drink at least thirty minutes before exercising.
- Exercise more often or for longer periods of time. Do thirty min-utes instead of fifteen, or do your fifteen-minute routine twice a day.
- Try adding passive exercise: Take a thirty-minute infrared dry heat sauna at 140 degrees F. You *will* sweat! Be sure to hydrate yourself with green drink.
- Dry brush your skin daily to open pores. You can do this in the shower after a workout.
- Take an Epsom salts bath to open the pores and draw out acidic toxins.
- Have a lymphatic massage (see page 225) twice a week.
- Begin a daily routine of stretching, breathing, and isotonic exercise—or yoga, which is all those things.

DO YOUR AEROBIC EXERCISE *JUST RIGHT*

When you are doing aerobic exercise, it's important to keep the intensity moderate so you don't cross over into anaerobic, sugar-producing exhausting exercise. What that means varies a bit depending on the person, and the exercise, and the conditions of the day. So there's not some hard-and-fast rule to follow to do this right. But just a little monitoring of your body will guide you. We've already mentioned that you want to be able to hold a conversation while exercising—in other words, to have enough breath to do so. You want to breathe in through your nose and then out through your nose. This will force you to breathe more deeply and to expand and contract the diaphragm. Ease up if exercise ever becomes painful or even uncomfortable. And make sure you *sweat*. Beyond that, there are just a few specifics we think will help you stay in the right range.

Walking

Go far enough, or long enough, to break a sweat. That may be about twenty minutes for a man, but thirty minutes for a woman. Be sure to breathe in and out through your nose, expanding and contracting your diaphragm (your stomach should extend out and then in).

Jogging

Jogging should always be pleasurable, and never painful—and you should be able to breathe through your nose throughout. If you begin to experience any pain while jogging, slow down and walk for a while until the pain subsides.

Cross trainers

These are also known as elliptical trainers. Start out on the lowest settings, and do at least thirty minutes a day.

Rebounding

This is the most efficient workout you can do. To get the same effect of fifteen minutes on your rebounder, you'd have to do thirty to forty-five minutes of walking or jogging over hilly terrain. For our money, rebounding is the overall best form of low-impact aerobics. (For more information on rebounding, see *The pH Miracle for Weight Loss*, which contains detailed information on the benefits of rebounding, and a full rebounding workout.)

STATIC EXERCISE

You can do static exercise every day. We recommend yoga, Pilates, stretching, and weight training.

Yoga

Yoga is an excellent form of exercise because it emphasizes balance, strength, flexibility, and stamina all at once. And though some classes focus pretty much exclusively on the physical, many contain an element of philosophy and/or spirituality. Pretty much anywhere along that spectrum will be good for you, as long as the specific approach appeals to you. Just check out any given class before making a commitment, to ensure a good fit. We practice and teach a form of traditional and kundalini yoga we developed called Younga Yoga, which combines isotonic stretching, static contraction, and repetitive movements with rapid breathing in and out through the nose.

In almost any variety, yoga is a discipline for the mind and emotions as well as the body, and, in fact, aims to integrate the three into a unified whole. Furthermore, the breathing exercises involved improve circulation and oxygenation, especially when used in conjunction with stretching and static exercises. Best of all is "breath of fire"—short, rapid breaths through your nose. (You can use the breathing you learn in yoga to enhance any type of exercise you do.) Yoga is an excellent stress reliever, besides reducing physical tension in the body. It can boost self-esteem, improve concentration, and increase your sense of overall well-being through calming the nervous system. I recommend at least thirty minutes of it every day.

Pilates

Pilates also aims to integrate mind and body, as it works the muscles, including the often overlooked deeper muscles, and focuses on core strength (around the abdomen and back). Pilates techniques, which emphasize efficient and graceful movement, are designed to improve alignment and breathing, and increase body awareness, by simultaneously stretching and strengthening the muscles.

Stretching

Stretching helps acids taken up into the connective tissues to be quickly removed from the connective tissue and eliminated. Just as squeezing releases water from a wet sponge, stretching forces acids out of the connective tissues and into the interstitial fluids to be taken up by the lymphatic system.

Weight Training

This can be an excellent form of exercise, but it must be done correctly or it will do more harm than good. In general, you must be sure to keep it pain-free. The macho "no pain, no gain" mantra is not just a myth, it's also downright harmful. You can increase muscle size and strength without it.

You need only eight exercises for a full body workout—if you do them the right way. For each of eight exercises, do one repetition. At the point where your muscle is fully flexed, hold for at least fifteen (and no more than thirty) seconds. Return to the starting position—and go on to the next exercise. Do this three times each week, and that's it. Eight exercises, one time, for a total of roughly two minutes, and you're done. Actually, make that four minutes, since you should be on the rebounder bouncing for fifteen seconds after you finish each move to disperse any residual acid that may have been created. (A similar stint on a whole-body vibration machine, or a bit of stretching, would do the same.)

PASSIVE EXERCISE

Several passive forms of exercise are also excellent for moving the lymphatic fluids, reducing acidity in the body. These are good options for people who, for whatever reason, can't exercise sufficiently. For the rest of us, they are a good supplement to our regular exercise. You might not get *all* the benefits of aerobic exercise or weight training, but then, most passive exercise is more luxurious. How does a massage or sauna sound, for example? And one passive exercise (whole-body vibration) can be combined with more familiar forms of exercise for a complete, balanced workout. Here are the best passive exercises to help you lower your acidity and stabilize your sugar levels.

Deep Breathing

Deep breathing helps release acidic toxins from the body by increasing lymphatic flow. The first organ that lymph and its toxins reach upon being deposited into the bloodstream is the lungs; deep breathing helps to expel the toxins, taking some of the stress off your lymphatic system. Deep breathing is done by taking long deep breaths through the nose and then releasing the air slowly back out through the nose. I would recommend taking breaks for deep breathing throughout any form of exercise you do.

Acupuncture and Acupressure

These modalities create positive energy fields at the points needled or pressed, increasing blood flow and facilitating healing and regeneration of stressed areas of the body (which could include the pancreas).

Infrared Sauna

Infrared sauna (dry heat sauna) with its radiant heat causes a profound sweat, flushing toxic acids and heavy metals from the body. Infrared saunas heat the objects in them—your body—rather than just the air, the way ordinary saunas do. The steam or wet heat of regular saunas can carry negative microforms like yeast and molds that you breathe in. Dry heat in an infrared sauna is much more comfortable, as well, the way Phoenix at a hundred degrees is bearable and Miami at the same temperature is a misery. There are a host of other benefits. A dry heat infrared sauna also:

- Speeds up metabolic processes, including those in the pancreas.
- Inhibits the development of negative microforms.
- Creates a "fever reaction"—rising body temperature—which removes acidic wastes.
- Normalizes the number of white blood cells.
- Exercises the heart.
- Reduces blood pressure.
- Dilates blood vessels.
- Relieves pain.
- Speeds healing of sprains, bursitis, arthritis, and circulation problems in the hands and feet.
- Increases blood circulation, and thus the removal of acidic toxins through the pores of the skin.
- Promotes relaxation and creates a sense of well-being.

So look for an infrared sauna; some gyms and spas are installing them. We recommend thirty minutes in the sauna at 140 degrees. Remember that sweating depletes the body of beneficial minerals, too, so replenish with an alkalizing green drink with pH drops before, during, and afterward.

Massage

Massage of all types (from acupressure and ayurvedic to Thai and water) helps calm the central nervous system, stimulate blood circulation to the tissue, promote relaxation, reduce muscular tension, and relieve stress. Improving blood circulation in the body brings fresh oxygen and nutrients to the cells while removing toxic, metabolic, acidic waste products from the cells. Where areas of the body are tight and tender, circulation may be impaired, and acids may stagnate.

Lymphatic Massage

Also known as lymphatic manipulation, this treatment focuses on moving lymph through the body, thereby speeding up the elimination of acids, waste products, and other toxins.

The strokes used in lymphatic massage are always oriented in the same direction that the lymph drains—toward the lymph nodes and the heart. The pressure of direct touch and the gentle, rhythmical sequence of movements pumps the lymphatic system much the same way exercise does. Applying pressure to the lymph nodes pushes the lymph therein toward the heart; when pressure is released, the node expands, pulling lymph into it, increasing lymph flow throughout the body.

This kind of gentle massage improves circulation and relaxes muscles, reduces pain and swelling, strengthens the immune system, balances hormones, tamps down overactivity of the sympathetic nervous system, and improves digestion, increasing absorption and use of nutrients. And, of course, it is a great way to relax and a terrific stress reducer. Not to mention that being cared for and cosseted provides a feeling of well-being. A lot of these same benefits accrue no matter what kind of massage you get, but no other type will do as much to circulate the lymph.

Shelley has studied lymphatic massage with a person trained by the originator of the method, and practiced it for more than eighteen years. She's had excellent results, though they are even better when combined with nutritional therapy. I only wish we were as attuned to the power of lymphatic massage in this country as they are in Europe, where most insurance plans cover it fully, and doctors routinely write prescriptions for it.

You'll get best results from regular massages from a practitioner with specialized training in lymphatic massage. A series of at least twenty-four lymphatic massages, two to three times a week, will give you your best chance of moving the lymphatic fluids, and moving toxins out.

A word of warning: If your body is very acidic, you may feel sluggish, foggy, achy, fatigued, or nauseated after a lymphatic massage. Some people get a headache. These are symptoms of detox, and they are normal as the acids that were stuck in your body are processed. Have a green drink to facilitate the process, get plenty of rest, and you'll feel good within twenty-four hours.

Self-Massage or Body Brushing

Using a brush on dry skin can provide many of the same benefits as lymphatic massage. Always rub toward the heart. Work the area immediately around the lymph node first, applying pressure toward the node, and work your way out. Or simply get a skin brush at a natural food store or body shop and brush away, wet or dry—but always toward the heart.

Whole-Body Vibration (WBV)

WBV is at once a type of massage and a form of exercise. It's recently been gaining in popularity, building on a background of use by elite athletes, universities, physical therapists, and some spas and fitness centers to become a trend among celebrities and their trainers and moving from there increasingly into the mainstream.

A WBV machine is essentially a platform to stand on, with a motor underneath to vibrate it, and some kind of handle or railing you can hold on to to stabilize yourself. You stand or sit or lie (this is the "passive" part) on the platform while it gently vibrates. The vibration generates systematic involuntary muscle contraction throughout the body. That is, it puts almost every muscle in the human anatomy into training. In fact, it exercises every *cell*. The stimulation from the vibrations generates accelerated forces on the muscles (more muscle fibers are activated this way than by normal, conscious muscle contractions). It also pumps the lymphatic system. And it does all this with minimal stress on the joints and ligaments.

BENEFITS OF WBV

Years of solid science and peer-reviewed research papers have laid out the many health benefits of WBV. WBV:

- Removes excess acid from connective tissues and muscles.
- Improves blood circulation and lymphatic drainage.
- Increases metabolism; burns fat; decreases production of fat cells; prevents weight gain.
- Raises energy levels.
- Increases muscle strength and tone. (You can increase your muscle strength up to 50 percent this way in as little as three weeks.)
- Increases flexibility and range of motion (these are the first effects you are likely to see).
- Improves balance and coordination.
- Improves stamina, speed, and mobility.
- Builds bone density and fights osteoporosis.
- Improves posture.
- Decreases cellulite and boosts body's natural collagen production, toning and tightening skin.
- Increases production of regenerative and repair hormones.
- Boosts levels of testosterone.
- Decreases levels of cortisol (which is released under stress).
- Reduces back and joint pain.
- Decreases blood pressure.
- Elevates serotonin and neutrophine levels, improving mood and increasing the sense of well-being.
- Ensures delivery of oxygen and nutrients to the cells.

WBV was first studied by a scientist working with Soviet cosmonauts in an effort to prevent muscle and bone loss during their time in space. The astronauts did vibrational training sessions before leaving for missions, which increased their bone density, flexibility, and strength. And when they returned from their mission, they had less bone and muscle loss than previous crews had with the standard preflight training (which included weight training).

The vibration re-creates some of the strain of weight necessary for bones and muscles to grow. In a weightless environment, astronauts' bodies don't get that. And here on earth, if we don't exercise our bodies, our bones and muscles don't get enough stress to trigger bone and muscle development, either. The extreme case of this is what happens when we are bedridden, and our skeletons and muscles don't even have to do the work of carrying around our body weight: dramatic loss of bone density and muscle tone and strength.

When you stand on a WBV platform, the pleasant vibrating action runs up your whole body from the feet. The vibration stimulates receptors in the Achilles tendon that stimulate nerve receptors, which track up to the cerebellum—the part of the brain responsible for balance. The brain then tells your muscles to actively contract to maintain your equilibrium, thus creating a workout that is as therapeutic as it is muscle toning.

The intensity and direction of the vibrations are essential for safe and ef-fective WBV. Look for a machine where the table moves back and forth ap-proximately eight degrees, or four degrees up and four degrees down. This mimics your own natural walking gait. (WBV machines where the table is stationary and vibrates only up and down rather than back and forth can be harmful when used for more than a minute at a time.)

When you find the right machine, I recommend staying on it for up to ten minutes at a time. Start out at four to five vibrations per second (four to five hertz) for several weeks. This level of vibration is good for releasing acids out of the tissues and is an excellent warm-up for other exercise, such as jogging or weight lifting. It is also a good way to release any tightness or soreness in your muscles.

If you increase the vibration to fifteen to twenty hertz for just five min-utes, you simulate jogging or running—the equivalent of an hour of jog-ging! (Do not use vibrational frequencies of more than twenty hertz for more than one minute.) If you do ramp up this way, be sure to go back down to four to five hertz vibration as part of your cool-down. In total, you should do no more than ten minutes at a time on WBV machines (and again, only on the machines that vibrate horizontally—no more than one minute on machines that vibrate vertically).

You will probably feel awkward your first few times on a WBV machine, or you might feel a slight dizziness or light-headedness from the release of acids from the connective tissues into the bloodstream, but as you gain experience your body will adapt to the vibrations. You can use the WBV machine every day, ideally two to three times a day. (Multiple sessions on the WBV machine are especially good when you feel stiff or sore.) We add vibration on to our other exercise routines, but you can actually substitute it if you like. We use it every day, especially to warm up for our daily morning run, since it loosens and stretches out the muscles.

Some people use WBV by just standing or sitting on the platform—truly passive exercise. But you can intensify the effects (and make your exercise time that much more efficient) by performing pretty much any exercise from a typical gym workout while on a WBV machine. You can do static or dynamic movements. You can kneel or lie down. You can place your hands or other parts of the body on the platform to change the emphasis.

Chapter 14

•

Motivation—How to Get It, How to Keep It

These, then, are the practical steps involved in switching your body over to a new way of living, eating, and thinking. Breaking it down this way, taking it slow rather than making an overnight switch, is all many people need to get started. They get the why, then the how . . . and they are on their way.

But there are a number of internal processes that happen alongside the practical preparations, and they can be stumbling blocks for some people. The people who are off and running have probably already dealt with various motivational issues, and they may not have even been conscious of the process. For the rest of us, here's a quick look at some of the issues that have to be considered in order to allow for a change like the pH Miracle to happen.

For starters, here's the whole process: awareness, investigation, knowledge, potential, motivation, action, patience, results. You have to start with awareness. Maybe you looked in the mirror one day and realized, "Whoa! I'm getting fat!" Or you recognized that you just don't feel as good as you used to. Or you decided once and for all that you were sick and tired of being sick and tired.

That awareness pushed you into investigation. You saw your doctor, called a diet center, bought this book. You started to look into how and why you got into the situation you are in, and how you can improve it or get out.

That is, you developed knowledge. In this case, you learned about acids and bases, yeasts and fungis, mucus and mold, and what it all does to your body—and the options for preventing all that damage and restoring optimal health. Maybe you saw a healthy change work in someone else's life. In short, you identified the potential benefits. That inspired motivation and self-confidence, which moved you into action, and with patience (and perseverance) will lead you to the results you desire.

Jo's Story

I spent a lot of time and energy seeking the perfect physique. I was obsessed with working out and running. I ate a strictly low-fat diet. Now I know that I was practically living on sugar, but back then I felt that the carbohydrates I was consuming were the only way to get the energy I needed for my thirteen- to fourteen-mile runs. But as time went on, instead of increased energy, I found that fatigue, irritability, and depression had become a part of my life.

In a way, I wasn't surprised, as I'd watched several people in my family struggle with mental disturbances. Part of what I witnessed was how they deteriorated as a result of the drugs they took that were supposed to help them, so I refused drug treatment myself. But I didn't want to keep on living the way I was.

Fortunately, that's when I found the pH Miracle program. I came to realize my fatigue and depression were just expressions of the way I was eating, living, and thinking, which was upsetting my body's chemistry. When I cleaned up my blood through diet and lifestyle modifications, everything changed. I no longer suffered from depression and mood swings. My whole attitude became positive as I reclaimed the vibrancy and passion for life I once had as a young person. Talk about motivation!

Still, like most people I have my moments of weakness, when thoughts of doughnuts and bagels dance in my head. I occasionally indulge in whatever my taste buds ask for. The big difference is, now it is because I just want something different—not because I'm desperate for a sugar fix! Anyway, sweets just don't taste as good anymore. I'm more likely to want vegetables and green drink now, and my yearnings for junk food are few and far between.

When I think back to how sick and tired I was before this program, it is easy to stay motivated. And then there's the way my husband looks at me in a tight pair of jeans! Among other things, I know he's motivated to stay healthy, too. It's a matter of choice—quite a simple choice, actually, once you fully understand it, simple to make and simple to keep.

You might be anywhere along this spectrum right now. If you find you are stuck, take a look to identify which phase it is, exactly, where you break down. Maybe you're motivated, but haven't organized to take action. Maybe you took action, but lost patience and never saw the results that would have come. But there are no magic bullets or instant solutions! Maybe you investigated, but didn't really "get" the answer . . . you missed a few details . . . or need to review a bit . . . you haven't yet truly developed knowledge. Maybe you are waiting for knowledge to somehow drop into your lap out of the clear blue sky, and haven't undertaken any investigation. Maybe you haven't even had that initial realization that something must change, and you're waiting for that awareness.

Wherever it is that you find yourself stuck, pick it up from there and follow through to the end. Conscious effort is usually all that is necessary to jump-start the process. And remember, as you go through this process, anytime you have trouble you can come right back here to find out where you are stuck. Maybe you will do great eliminating acidic meat and dairy and added sugar, but just can't let go of the fruit. Even for that kind of detail, this process will help you work it out. You should expect there to be more than one hurdle that you have to clear to win the race!

Some people will take these steps out of order. And that's okay. The most common variation is to start with the action, even if you haven't developed the knowledge or really don't quite believe the potential. In that case, just try the program out. See how it goes. Take a trial-and-error approach, and a wait-and-see attitude. For some people this is the most persuasive approach of all. If you try the program, and you start to get results, then you will truly recognize the potential, experience the knowledge, and recommit to investigation and action, with renewed patience, and, in the end, even better results.

So if you're one of those we haven't yet convinced, consider taking a chance, trying it for yourself. You may be the only one who can convince yourself. No one's making you take a loyalty oath for a lifetime on the program as a prerequisite. So go ahead. You've got nothing to lose by trying—and everything to gain.

Motivation is so important—and sometimes so difficult—that we want to devote this chapter to exploring it. You must always stay focused on your motivation—and the results you want to see happen—as you begin to make these important and healing changes. If you forget why you want to make the change, the risk is that you'll start to view the program as a kind of deprivation, rather than the gift of life and health that it is. You have to be specific about your motivation to make this program a new way of life, not just a temporary patch. That focus will be helpful when you crave foods that aren't good for you, or when well-meaning friends or family want you to indulge with them. If you stay focused on your own motivations, goals, and intentions, and gently but firmly turn down foods that could contribute to your condition, those around you will eventually understand and respect your choices. (And when they see your results, don't be surprised if they want to know how to do it themselves!)

DISCOUNTING

Some psychologists talk about levels of "discounting" when it comes to problems, a process of not seeing reality clearly enough, ignoring the importance of some aspect of a problem or situation. Discounting can harm you and hold you back. If you cross the street without looking both ways, you are discounting several things such as your health, life, family and friends, various responsibilities, finances, consideration for motorists, and so on. The higher the level of discounting, the more potentially serious a problem might be.

The first or highest level of discounting is to deny the *existence* of a problem. We see this with addictions like alcoholism all the time. But we may be discounting the existence of any number of problems—not just addictions. For example, many people consider as normal the long list of symptoms that plague so many of us, like excess weight, fatigue, skin problems, anxiety, depression, allergies, irritability, the flu, indigestion, headaches, PMS, high blood pressure, yeast, food cravings, and getting one or two colds a year. These problems may be typical. They may even be statistically average. But they are *not* normal in a healthy body. Calling them normal is *discounting* the existence of a problem. If you don't admit to yourself that excess weight or headaches or indigestion are a problem, then you are certainly not likely to address them.

The next level of discounting is to admit the existence of a problem but to deny that it is important. "Yes, I get very tired all the time, but it's no big deal. I just take a little nap during the day and I'm fine." The next level of discounting is to admit that a problem exists, and admit that it could be a

serious sign of something, but to discount that there is much that anyone
can do about it. "Yes, I'm forty pounds overweight, and yes that's probably
making my heart work too hard, but half the world is overweight and doctors admit they have very little success in helping people lose weight and
keep it off. In the long run, people just can't change certain things."

The final level of discounting is to admit the existence of a problem,
admit that it could be important, admit that some people can change, but
conclude that *you* cannot change. "Yes I know that many people have given
up this terrible and dangerous habit of smoking, but I've tried everything
and I can't do it." Or, "Yes, I know that my terrible indigestion is bad for
me, that it could lead to other problems, and that being on pills for the rest
of my life is not a good solution. I have one friend who gave up coffee but
she has more willpower than I do. Besides, when I go out with people, I just
can't find anything good to eat that's supposedly healthy. So what can I do?
I just get so tired of beating my head against the wall!"

News flash! There are solutions to life's problems, and there are many
positive ways to approach them. This new updated version of *The pH Miracle* clearly shows how *you* personally can solve both the little health problems
and the big health problems. Meanwhile, you can eat plenty of delicious
food and regain a feeling of health that you have not experienced for many
years. But you cannot discount *at any level* the reality of whatever it is that
you are dealing with. In order to be motivated to make the changes, you
first have to be realistic about the existence of problems, their level of se-
riousness, and the fact that there are solutions you can implement in your
own life.

MAKE A COMMITMENT

Starting on this program is making a commitment to yourself, your life,
your health, your well-being. We recommend a five-step approach to making sure you honor that commitment—and honor yourself.

Step 1: Define and Record Your Motivation

The first step in focusing on your motivation is to state the change you
want to see in your life. Identify it as specifically as you can, in the form of a
desired outcome: "I want to be free of my headaches so I can enjoy more activities with my family"; or "I want to be slim"; or "I want to have the energy
to enjoy life, my family, and my work"; or "I want to be really well." Someone with acute illness might simply say, "I want to live!" Even someone who

is presently healthy has a motivation, perhaps, "I want to prevent and avoid illness and enjoy a long life." Once you are clear on what your motivation is, write it down. Note your reasons for change, and the benefit to you and others. Seeing it in print makes it somehow more real or more serious.

Step 2: Set a Realistic and Appropriate Plan

In order to make change that is effective and lasting, we must be honest with ourselves. Seriously consider exactly what will have to be done to make your motivational idea a reality. Take into account just where you are starting from, and plan the specific steps you need to take to get you there. Make sure to keep it reality-based. If you plan too much too soon, you'll defeat yourself before you are even out of the starting gate. If you oversimplify, giving in to wishful thinking, you'll never get results.

Include a time frame in your plan, but remember that the ultimate blue ribbon doesn't necessarily go to the first one over the finish line. Pace is vital. This is more like a marathon than a sprint.

Break each new behavior change down into steps. This program should be an exciting process, not an overwhelming, overnight challenge.

The more imbalanced or sick you are, the more reason you have to find motivation, and the more commitment is required to find balance and wholeness. If you are very far from where you live, you won't be able to get home by going only halfway back. If you've got garbage in your house that is attracting flies, you can't get rid of the flies by taking out half the garbage. In this vein, you're not going to shed long-standing health concerns by planning to go off coffee or candy while staying on bread and fruit. You might indeed see some improvement—you just shouldn't confuse that with really getting well. (We might add that unless you are acutely ill, you do want to avoid extremes. More extreme measures may be needed for extreme problems, however.)

A more realistic plan would go something like this: "I will take the next six months to do all I can to eliminate my headaches. I will make two major transitions each month, until I've made all the necessary changes to bring my body back into a state of balance." You would then spell out the specifics appropriate to you and your situation, such as, "I will start drinking fresh green vegetable juices and try an alkaline meal at least three times a week," and "I will eliminate all added sugars for one week, then phase out the high-sugar fruits until I reach a state of balance," and "I will drink four liters of properly prepared electron-rich alkaline water a day, including one mixed with green powder."

Write your plan down. Do it now, while you are thinking about it and this is all fresh in your mind! Then make sure to keep it where you can see it.

This book lays out the basic steps, in a reasonable order. But individuals will work it in their own way and must take personal responsibility for themselves and their results. You are unique, and the most anyone else's program can do is give you a good foundation. You have to build your own house. This is your chance to customize the design to make sure you are comfortable in your new home—and to maximize your success.

Step 3: Practice Your New Habits

Whatever your plan is, start to do it. Practice having a totally alkaline, electron-rich breakfast at least three times a week, then five, then seven. Practice going without a heavy, acidic sugary dessert after dinner. Practice skipping the acidic alcoholic beverage before or with dinner. Practice choosing an alkalizing vegetarian entrée in the restaurant.

Practice is repetition, and repetition of any skill increases your ability in that skill. As you practice these new, healthy habits, you will develop a skilled, intuitive way of feeding your body what it needs without feelings of deprivation. Instead of thinking about what you can't have, you will feel blessed with your growing awareness of the great abundance available to you.

Step 4: Evaluate, Review, and Reward Your Progress

Monitor your symptoms. (Remember, all symptoms are caused by over-acidity.) Write down your symptoms, and any changes in them, so that you can go back and review if you run into a plateau. Seeing the changes you have experienced will help you visualize the excellent benefits that are still within your reach. Are the symptoms diminishing, or have they gone? Do you feel lighter, brighter, more energetic? Have you lost some weight? Do your clothes fit better? Write it down. Note who made a comment about how you were looking better or noticed a change in you. Ask yourself if you stayed with your plan, and if the same plan is still the appropriate one for you. If you're having trouble making the change, reevaluate your goal. If it seems too harsh—or too lax—adjust it (within the bounds of appropriateness to your condition) so that it is more reasonable for you to achieve. And to the extent you did what you set out to do, reward yourself. Actually, the best reward for bringing your body into alkaline balance will probably be simply the disappearance of acidic symptoms. If you desire a reward beyond that, be careful to avoid the common tendency to make food a reward— especially unhealthy acidic food. Buy yourself a new pair of pants for your new size. Make time in your schedule to do something you love but rarely get to do—read a book, take a bubble bath, listen to a favorite piece of music. Get a great lymphatic massage or a relaxing spa treatment. Treat yourself to a class that's always intrigued you. Hang new art in your home. Choose something that nourishes your new self as your new pH Miracle diet nourishes your new and increasingly healthy body.

Step 5: If You Fall Off the Wagon, Simply Get Back on Again

Feeling guilty or down about your mistake is a waste of time, a drain of energy—and will only cause more acidity. Forgive yourself and just start moving forward again. Restate your motivation and goals.

If you find yourself having a very hard time staying on the program, and giving up too easily or too often, you may be running into the fact that eating is, for most of us, not just physical—it is also highly emotional. Many times, we use food for comfort in response to stress, when what we really need is to find a way to relieve the stress permanently. We need to understand why we turn to food for comfort, and where else we might get that comfort. If exploring that is more than you can do alone, or if you feel deep emotional wounds, we encourage you to seek a good counselor to help you shed some light on the dark areas. Sometimes a lifetime of events have welled up within us and we need help in releasing emotions that slow down our progress in other areas of life.

MICHELLE'S STORY

Besides working full-time and being the mother of three great kids, I've been something of a professional patient for my entire adult life. It started very young, with chronic upper respiratory problems two to three times a year until the age of ten. From there the list just goes on: two serious bouts of pneumonia, chronic gastrointestinal problems, menstrual disorders, serious concentration and information-retention problems, adrenal/thyroid problems, fatigue, dizziness, hiatal hernia, anemia, hypoglycemia, muscular skeletal disorder, pituitary dysfunction, severe nervous tension, on-and-off addiction to prescription amphetamines (doctor's orders), an eating disorder that required hospitalization, and depression.

I've taken two hundred prescription medications—not to mention what I tried over the counter—but nothing worked. Now I know why. But at the time it was all I could do to find the strength to go on and act as if everything was fine.

So maybe you can understand why it almost seemed like good news when my doctor suggested a total hysterectomy when I started to suffer severe ovarian dysfunction. "Fine," I said. My mom died young of ovarian cancer anyway. I thought the hysterectomy might solve all my health problems. Maybe they all stemmed from having a bad hormonal imbalance.

After the surgery my doctor came in and said he thought he'd found the reason I'd suffered all the abdominal discomfort—my uterus was the size of a large cantaloupe. *Great!* I thought—with the cantaloupe out, surely my troubles would end.

And my abdomen did feel better. But that was about it. I still had an array of the same old problems. One doctor told me that women tend to get depressed and suffer gastrointestinal problems and that I should just learn to live with it. He offered me hormone replacement (which only made me feel worse) and noticed some Candida around my nails for which he prescribed Diflucan.

An allergist told me I was antibody-deficient, and referred me to another doctor who put me on more Diflucan. It didn't help much, and I worried about the potential for liver damage.

I found a doctor who had me try all kinds of new medicines, with no luck. Then he recommended surgery to remove a portion of my large intestine. What a catastrophe that turned out to be! I had so many complications, infections, and antibiotics my planned four-day hospital stay stretched into seventeen. Need I say that as soon as I got out of the hospital and started really eating again, all my symptoms returned?

I went back to pretending everything was fine, with the help of occasional amphetamine prescriptions to keep me going. But I knew this was all wrong. You shouldn't need drugs of any kind on a daily basis. And you certainly shouldn't feel rotten all the time (with or without the drugs). I developed two new symptoms: My hearing was becoming muffled and I was losing the vision in one eye. I lost it completely one night after eating a piece of cake! When my bad days really started to outnumber the good, I made a New Year's resolution to get myself well.

My first real clues came from a book I found in the health food store. I started doing my own research, but when I looked for a doctor to work with me I was told over and over again that this was a bunch of loony hogwash.

Then my cousin told me about Dr. Young. As I learned about the pH Miracle program, right away I felt he was talking about me and my problems. I knew, finally, that this wasn't all in my mind—and that there was a solution. I was also glad to realize I wasn't alone. You can't imagine the burden that was lifted from me that day.

Within a week of starting on the program, my energy picked up. My digestive system became more comfortable. The most major change was the clearing of my "brain fog." I gained alertness, and my concentration level was 100 percent better. (I was able to sit down and write this!) My sore, bloodshot eyes completely cleared up. My skin, hair, and nails were glowingly healthy. I can't remember a time when I actually felt entirely well like this, but now I am ready for a long future of it.

WHAT YOU THINK, MATTERS

For this program to work for you, there must be a change in the way you eat and live. Perhaps most important, there may need to be a change in the way you think. There are a handful of commonly harbored—but dangerous and self-destructive—attitudes that prevent people from finding the wholeness and healing this program provides. I want to review them briefly here, so that if one of them rings a bell for you, you can take a second look at your stance:

- *This condition runs in my family, so there's nothing I can do about it.* This attitude, like Michelle's (see the box), prevents you from taking personal responsibility for your own body and your own health, and therefore from taking steps to control, eliminate, and prevent the disease. As we said earlier, this type of thinking discounts the fact that you can change . . . regardless of what happened to other family members. You can personally take steps to control, eliminate, and prevent the disease. Certain apparent weaknesses or predispositions to symptoms may be inherited, but there is always much you can do to foil fate. Avoiding this sort of resignation or discounting is the first step. Genes never tell the whole story (and usually, you don't even know if you have the genes in question anyway). Even if you do have the genes, there's always something you can do to lessen, put off, or curb a condition. (And your genes will also become healthier when *you* become healthier!)

- *My doctors say they've done all they can.* Michelle had to overcome this one, too (see the box). What she came to realize is that no matter how wonderful your doctors, if you are still struggling with acidic symptoms, not everything has been done. But the more important point here is that the ultimate responsibility for your health and your body lies with you, not with any doctor. And you are the best judge of what is working and what is not, and what feels right trying and what doesn't.

- *One way or the other, I'm going to die when it's my time, so I might as well enjoy myself and eat anything I want in the meantime.* Whether or not you believe your days are numbered by some higher authority, you have the power to fill whatever time you have with misery thanks to careless abuse of your body—or to enjoy every last minute you have in excellent health. Death may not be something to fear, but the greatly diminished quality of life that usually precedes it is.

- *I'll just pray for healing. God will heal me.* There is nothing to contest that faith and prayer can heal us, and we do believe in miracles. But to ask for healing while refusing to cooperate in every way we can to heal ourselves is, to our minds, a futile attempt at becoming whole. Also, requesting wholeness while knowingly facilitating the disease process sounds like, "Help me, even though I won't help myself."

THOUGHTS AND EMOTIONS

Those who wish to regain their health or prevent health challenges must be properly motivated to address the issue on all fronts, including eating, drinking, and *thinking*. This is not just a diet; the true pH miracle is a *lifestyle*.

The eating and drinking part is actually sometimes the easiest. The "thinking" part includes your thought processes, belief system, psychological health, emotional well-being, personal level of consciousness, and an entire host of attitudes, feelings, and behaviors.

Emotions can cause even more acid than food and drink. Powerful negative emotions come from all sorts of places and in all shapes and forms.

They can include thoughts, feelings, experiences, conscious and unconscious memories, and dreams. Any of the many and various problems in living can cause emotional trauma. They all come under the umbrella of "stress." And stress causes significant amounts of acid to be dumped into your body.

The great majority of people, even people in the most profound medical crises, can return to an excellent level of health if they conscientiously work to rebalance the body's original alkaline design. Conscientiously changing their eating, drinking, and lifestyle, and carefully following the pH Miracle program, they can and will be successful. They can return to a level of health they have not experienced for many years, a level of health they never even quite imagined.

But a small percentage of people fail to find full good health despite working hard to change their unhealthy eating and drinking habits. They share one crucial trait in common: They are challenged by psychological, emotional, behavioral, or spiritual problems that, perhaps, they do not fully address, and in any case do not fully resolve. Where they fall down is at the "thinking" part of the pH protocol. Their patterns of thinking, ruminations, and emotions aren't addressed in enough detail. Unhealthy beliefs, attitudes, biases, value systems, or a diminished level of consciousness hold these people back. They seem unable to bring an end to ongoing guilt, grief, blaming, resentment, anger, self-pity, fear, anxiety, feuding, self-loathing, mistrust, greed, false pride, spiritual confusion, and so on. Perhaps they need professional guidance to deal with whichever of these issues dogs them, but do not seek it. The stress of all this adds significantly to the acid in the body, and not even an alkaline diet can fully balance it out.

When physical health challenges are accompanied by serious emotional and psychological problems, you must somehow address them. Despite what you may be thinking, it is not always a "shrink" that provides the answer. There are many ways to relieve stress and begin to reduce this part of the acidic overload. Of course it's true a well-trained and experienced psychologist, psychotherapist, or psychiatric social worker can make a critical difference. But so can a minister, priest, rabbi, or other spiritual adviser with years of experience and wisdom. A good book can set you on the right path. Reading the works of great thinkers in the realm of intellect and spirit is an excellent way to change your mind-set and quietly challenge the type of thinking that keeps your body mired in an acidic lockstep. (Some of our favorite books are by David R. Hawkins, MD, PhD, who writes about the body/sense/mind/intellect/spirit continuum so clearly that simply reading his work will immediately raise your level of consciousness.) You may want to study the stories of miracle workers, saints and mystics, religious martyrs, past-life experiences, near-death experiences, people who apparently died and came back to life, and the lives of Great Spiritual Souls such as Jesus, Mother Teresa, Gandhi, Mohammad, Joseph Smith, Brigham Young, and Shirdi Sai Balba. As you become more aware of how higher consciousness actually operates, it helps you leave behind some of those thoughts and behaviors that pull you down. Higher consciousness equates to more peace and alkalinity for the body. Lower consciousness equates to more turmoil and the creation of unwanted acid.

To fully experience the pH Miracle for yourself, you must explore, pursue, investigate, read, inquire, and search for answers that set your mind at ease. Why do bad things happen to good people? What are we to learn from accidents, devastating illnesses, or setbacks in life? How is it that some people seem to be able forgive and forget or simply turn the other cheek? How can you learn to do that? What does it mean when people say, "Expect a miracle"? What does it mean when people say, "There are no mistakes in life"? These are questions that everyone must answer for themselves. Look for ways to answer. Develop understanding.

To gain or regain your ultimate goals in health and wellness, your motivations must reach out far enough to encompass the broadest possible spectrum of the world around you. You must strive to eat the foods that bring healthy physical and mental processes to your life, drink the fluids that help to cleanse and purify your body, create the thoughts in life that allow you to forgive yourself, cut others some slack, look only for the good in every situation, and bring peace and understanding to yourself and those around you.

The value of change is the result. In this case, the peace and harmony that can arise from embracing the change of this program as part of everyday life are yours for the asking. You've made it this far because you want the best for yourself and those you love, and by following these steps you'll be whole and strong, and able to enjoy the best this world has to offer. If that's not motivation, we don't know what is.

Part IV

pH Miracle Recipes

Choosing the Right Recipe

I'll let you in on a secret: Before I (Shelley) understood about how foods heal, I never really enjoyed cooking. It was just another time-consuming chore that made a mess—and had to be done all over again just about as soon as you got it all cleaned up. I felt as if I was stuck in the kitchen when I would much rather have been out there in the rest of the world. But now that I realize how great an impact what we eat has on our health and well-being, I love to create healing meals. And I treasure the tangible nurturing that feeding my family represents. I still want the process to be efficient, though! I like to spend a little time preparing a meal—and a lot of time relaxing and enjoying every mouthful (and enjoying the company of my family, which is also part of the healing power, if you ask me!).

I also want to create something I'll want to eat—and that my family will enjoy, too. So this section is composed of the recipes I use that keep us all happy. I'm not too long in the kitchen, we all eat healthfully—and we love what we eat. We eat heartily, too, I might add, since some people seem to think at first that this way of eating is "for the birds," or "rabbit food." All of these dishes celebrate variety, texture, and out-of-this-world flavors at every meal. It is never boring. (All this and they are easy on the pocketbook, too. It doesn't cost any more to buy organic ingredients than it did to pay for meat, cheese, candy, beer, and so on.) This program, far from being any kind of deprivation, is a gift we give ourselves.

A lot of people find that their palates are jaded after so much artificial nonfood, and so much artificially stimulating hard sugar and salty flavor. They are insensitive, at first, to the subtleties of whole, natural foods. If that's you, never fear: As you adjust to eating in this 80–20 ratio, you'll find that your taste buds awaken to the glorious sensations you are treating them to. You'll also leave behind that strange willingness to self-destruct for pleasure I've seen in so many people for whom food is one of life's great entertainments. Some folks live to eat, though it should rightly be the other way around. On this program, food regains its proper perspective—we eat to live—without losing its tremendous sensual appeal. A good meal can still be hugely enjoyable and provide deep satisfaction. It doesn't have to be killing you to do so.

Many of these recipes are not for use during a cleanse (though many of the shakes, juices, and soups are). Many are not for the weeks immediately following a cleanse. And many are meant for use once you've completely rebalanced your system. For as long as you are facing the challenge of symptoms, the simpler, "rawer" choices will be best for you. The majority of them are good just about anytime (though perhaps not on the cleanse), and should always be the bulk of your meals, no matter what stage you're in.

So keep the guidelines you've learned in this book in mind as you select the recipes that are right for you, wherever you are in the program. You can also look for the lists I've included of suggested dishes for different phases to guide you. Take a look, too, at the ideas for breakfasts, healthy snacks, and really quick meals. Once you are familiar with the basics, this program should be not just healthy, but simple and easy—as well as enjoyable and delicious!

RECIPES FOR THE CLEANSE

Alfalfa Sprout Salad**
Alkalizing/Energizing Cucumber Salad**
All-Vegetable Cocktail
Fresh Silky Almond Milk
Anticancer Soup
AsparaZincado Soup
AvoRado Kid Greens Shake
AvoRadoColado Shake
Basic Green Drink*
Basic Green Vegetable Juice
Bean Sprout Salad**
Blood Builder (juice)
Broccoli Salad**
Broccoli/Cauliflower Soup
Cauliflower Toss**
Celery Soup
Celery/Cauliflower Soup
Colorful Cabbage (take carrot out if juicing)**
Creamy or Crunchy Broccoli Soup
Creamy Vegetable Soup
Garden Green Drink
Gazpacho

GRASSoup

Green Power Cocktail*

Green Raw Soup

Healing Soup

High Vitamin C & E Drink*

Insulin Generator (juice)*

LimeyLove Shake

Madrid Gazpacho

Minty Mock Malt Shake

Mock Split Pea Soup

Popeye Soup

Potassium Salad (take carrot out if juicing)**

Potassium Special (juice)*

Rainbow Salad (take out beet, carrot, jicama if juicing)**

Skin Cleanse (juice)*

Spinach Salad**

Spring Green Drink*

Sprouted Lentil Salad**

Sweet Pepper Consommé

Vegetable Minestrone

Vegetable/Grass Drink*

Wheat Sprout Salad (take carrot out if juicing)**

Zucchini Toss**

*Omit carrot and beet during the cleanse. See chapter 7 for more information on using juices.
**Put in a blender and eat as soup during a cleanse. Or put ingredients through a juicer and make into a fresh juice—leaving out any carrots or beets called for when you are on a cleanse.

Breakfast Ideas

• **Shakes.** Green shakes are just as easy to make as fruit smoothies, but without all the acidic sugars, dairy, and fillers. Just throw the alkalizing ingredients of your choice into a blender (I use a Vita-Mix) and whip it up! In the summer, I particularly love the intense wake-me-up flavor of a LimeyLove shake. When we want a more stick-to-your-ribs shake, I add more green powder, or soy sprouts powder, to pump up the protein and calorie content. If you like a creamier shake, experiment with adding avocado, coconut meat, or nut and seed milks or butters. Yum!

• **Soup.** I love to warm up with soup for breakfast on a chilly morning. On warm days, I choose cool soups! AsparaZincado Soup (page 272), Popeye Soup (page 273), and Creamy or Crunchy Broccoli Soup (page 270) are particularly satisfying starts to the day. Hearty soups and stews course through the body creating a good glow that lasts for hours.

• **Vegetable juice.** A fresh glass of juice is a perfect light—but incredibly nutritious—eye opener. Sometimes we mix our fresh veggie juices half and half with Fresh Silky Almond Milk (on page 269) for a creamier green drink in the morning.

• **Zippy Breakfast.** This is, hands down, the favorite around our house. It is a hearty choice. I usually don't feel hungry again until midafternoon after a Zippy Breakfast! It is basically any healthy warm whole grain (we like steamed buckwheat the best) topped with avocado and tomato plus any other veggie garnishes you like, drizzled with good oil, lemon or lime juice, and pure whole salts, then sprinkled with the Zip (Spice Hunter brand) or other zesty seasoning (see Zippy Breakfast on page 358).

• **Pâtés.** Pâtés are hearty, soft-form dips made by putting your recipe ingredients through a juicer that makes nut and seed butters. (I use the SoloStar Juicer.) All the ingredients are pulverized and mixed up together, which leaves lots of license for different types of seasonings. Start with a protein-rich base of soaked sunflower seeds, fresh raw nuts, or edamame (soybeans from the pod) and some sort of healthy fat like coconut meat, nut or seed cheese, or a good oil.

You can dish up your pâté with an ice cream scoop to mold a beautiful mound shape; place it either in the middle of a salad or next to a nice bowl of soup. Or spread it onto a sprouted tortilla for a great breakfast sandwich. Pâtés make perfect baby food, too.

• **Salad.** Especially when the weather's hot, a salad makes a refreshing and crunchy breakfast. Use lots of sprouts, garnished with lemon, pure whole mineral salts, and your choice of oil. (My favorites are hemp seed, olive, or Udo's oil.) Use dehydrated nuts, seeds, and veggies instead of traditional croutons for a crispy crunch.

• **Buckwheat cereal with almond milk** is quick and filling on a cold morning. Buckwheat groats, cracked buckwheat, and cream of buckwheat are available in most health food stores. Or make steamed buckwheat with extra water to create an oatmeal consistency.

• **Sprouted cereal** (page 326).

• **Wraps.** A bunch of fresh or steamed vegetables, soaked seeds or nuts, and a few sun-dried tomatoes with some avocado in a sprouted wheat tortilla (or just about any other combination you dream up) is as portable as it is quick and delicious. This is our usual choice when we're up and out early.

• **Casserole de Cauliflower.** This dish is good anytime (page 368), but particularly satisfying at breakfast.

• **Steamed broccoli.** Steam florets lightly for five minutes. Add chopped onion and/or another green vegetable, stir in some Basic Salad Dressing (page 295), and top with soaked almonds or hazelnuts.

• **Steamed edamame** (green soy beans) with toasted sesame oil and garlic salt will start you off with plenty of protein—and deliciousness!

Quick Meal Ideas

- **Salad.** Keep clean, dried greens, and a few salad dressings, in your refrigerator, so all you have to do is throw on a couple of handfuls of whatever chopped-up goodies catch your fancy that day, and you're ready to eat.
- **Wraps.** Start with a burrito-size sprouted wheat tortilla, spread with pâté, hummus, or another of your favorite spreads. Add some sprouts, beans, avocado, tomato, and/or any other veggies you have on hand or are in the mood for. Top with pure whole salts and/or fresh salsa or pesto. That's a wrap!
- **Soup.** Pick a quick recipe, such as Madrid Gazpacho (page 281), to whip up when you are ready. Or make a big batch over the weekend to see you through the week. With raw soups served chilled, you don't even have to take the time to warm them!

Anytime Recipes

These recipes require no cooking (they are raw) and are 90 to 100 percent alkalizing. They can be used anytime, including the early weeks of the program, immediately following a cleanse, or when you are dealing with any specific imbalances or serious symptoms. Once you are in balance, these are all perfect for that 70 to 80 percent of your meal that is alkaline.

Alfalfa Sprout Salad
Alkalizing/Energizing Cucumber Salad

AvoRado AvoCado Topping
AvoRado Kid Greens Shake
AvoRadoColada Shake
Almond Cheese Mayo
Bean Sprout Salad
Broccoli Salad
Cauliflower Toss
Colorful Cabbage
Edamame Pâté
Fresh Silky Almond Milk
GRASSoup Drink
LimeyLove Shake
Minty Mock Malt Shake
Potassium Salad
Pumpkin Pecan Pâté
Rainbow Salad
Raw Kale Salad
Rawsome Redford Pizza
Spinach Salad
Sprouted Lentil Salad
Tuna-pHishless Pâté
Wheat Sprout Salad
Zucchini Toss

Maintenance Recipes

Once you feel balanced and are no longer dealing with symptoms, you'll have a larger group of recipes to explore while maintaining that 70–30 or 80–20 split to your meals—with these being in that 20 to 30 percent. For example, you might have a big salad with a side of baked Tofu Italian Mock Meatballs.

These choices add more texture and all-important variety to your repertoire. Some of these recipes are warmed, processed, or cooked, and so require more time to digest. These are not good choices in the early weeks after a cleanse, or when experiencing an acute illness or imbalance in the body.

These meals are also good choices for someone who is transitioning slowly into an alkaline way of eating, eliminating acid foods such as meat, dairy, sugar, and fruit gradually.

Alexandra's Favorite Pasta
Almond/Carrot/Ginger-Stuffed Zucchini
Autumn Curry Crêpes with Curried Veggie Filling
Baked Falafel Fritters
Blackened Herbed Fillets
Cabbage-Stuffed Vegetables
Cajun-Style Red Beans and Brown Rice
Casserole de Cauliflower
Cold Tofu Pockets
Doc Broc Casserole
Edamame Patties
Ginger-Almond Paste Topping
Green Chili Tofu Pita
Hearty Harvest Casserole
Maren's Tortilla Pockets
Millet/Buckwheat Oven Cakes
Millet Yam Hash Browns
Nepal Vegetable Curry
Nutty Mock Meat Loaf
Sautéed Edamame Vegetable Soup
Seed Pancakes with Coconut Whipped Topping
Shelley Beans
Shelley's Super Tortillas
Shelley's Super Wraps
Sprouted Bean Casserole
Stuffed Acorn Squash
Stuffed Cabbage Rolls
Sunrise Asian Salad
Three-Bean Salad
Tofu Italian Mock Meatballs
Tofu Patties
Tofu Spinach Quiche
Tofu Stew
Wild Yam Soba Noodles with Kale and Spicy Pine Nuts
Vegetable Steam-Fry
Very Veggie Barley Burgers
Zippy Breakfast

80 or 20?

These recipes fit into either side of that 80–20 or 70–30 split, depending on whether they are raw or cooked. When they are cooked, they move from the 80 to the 20 (or the 70 to the 30).

    Anticancer Soup
    AsparaZincado Soup
    Broccoli/Cauliflower Soup
    Celery Soup
    Celery/Cauliflower Soup
    Chunky Veggie Soup
    Creamy or Crunchy Broccoli Soup
    Creamy Vegetable Soup
    Curried Squash Dhal
    Fresh Silky Almond Milk
    Gazpacho
    Green Raw Soup
    Healing Soup
    Mock Split Pea Soup
    Popeye Soup
    Raw Kale Salad
    Roasted Butternut/Celery Soup with Caramelized Onions
    Special Carrot Soup
    Sweet Pepper Consommé
    Thick Puree of White Bean Soup
    Vegetable Minestrone
    Veggie Borscht

Healthy Snacks

These healthy snacks satisfy the need for crunch and munch that kids of all ages have, and they are perfect when you just need a quick bite or are on the go. Or maybe you have one of those kids in your house who seem to live on snacks? These are also useful in transitioning, and some help during sugar cravings. Some of these travel really well, so you can make sure to continually nourish yourself no matter where you are or what you are doing.

Of course, you can always grab a simple snack like raw almond butter or any of the pâtés on a brown rice cake or a sprouted wheat tortilla. But if you're feeling creative, or just want something different, or are in the mood for a treat, try:

All-Vegetable Cocktail
Almond Pâté
Ashley's Vegetable Nori Roll-Ups
Avocado/Tomato Snack
Camper's Bread
Chilled Cucumber Refresher
Crispy Buckwheat Groats
Crispy Radish Filling
Curried Veggie Filling
Dehydrated Flax Chips
Dried veggies and nuts for crunch and munch
Edamame Pâté
Essene Bread
Fresh Cucumber Dills
Fresh Spinach Filling
Garbanzo Spread
Garden Variety Filling
Great Olé Guacamole
Hearty Nut Filling
Kale with Egyptian Garlic Sauce
Leprechaun Surprise Dip
Mexicali Rice
Mock Pumpkin Pie
Nori Crisps
Okra and Tomatoes Creole
Raw Pecan Pâté
Pumpkin Pecan Pâté
Rawsome Redford Pizza
Refried Beans
Spiced Green Beans
Spiced Winter Squash
Spicy Pecan Croutons
Sprouted Cereal
Sprouted Wheat Bread
Steam-Fried Sprouts
Tofu Salad Spread
Tuna-pHishless Pâté
Veggie Crunch Stix and Crackers
Yummus Hummus
Zippy Garbanzo Spread
Zucchini Italian-Style

RECIPE INDEX

JUICES, SHAKES, AND MILKS

Juices
Basic Green Vegetable Juice 261
Vegetable/Grass Drink 261
Wheat-Beet Juice 262
Basic Green Drink 262
Garden Green Drink 262
Green Power Cocktail 262
Spring Green Drink 263
Potassium Special 263
Insulin Generator 263
High Vitamin C & E Drink 263
Blood Builder 264
Skin Cleanse 264
All-Vegetable Cocktail 264

Shakes
AvoRado Kid Greens Shake 265
AvoRadoColada Shake 266
Minty Mock Malt Shake 266
LimeyLove Shake 267
Salty Shake 267

Nut and Seed Milks
Almond Milk 268
Quick Tahini Milk 268
Fresh Silky Almond Milk 269

SOUPS

GRASSoup   270
Creamy or Crunchy Broccoli Soup   270
Green Raw Soup   271
AsparaZincado Soup   272
Sautéed Edamame Vegetable Soup   272
Popeye Soup   273
Healing Soup   274
Broccoli/Cauliflower Soup   275
Celery/Cauliflower Soup   276
Chunky Veggie Soup   276
Broccoli Creamed Soup   277
Anticancer Soup   277
Mock Split Pea Soup   278
Vegetable Minestrone   278
Celery Soup   279
Special Carrot Soup   279
Creamy Vegetable Soup   280
Gazpacho   281
Madrid Gazpacho   281
Roasted Butternut/Celery Soup with Caramelized Onions   282
Veggie Borscht   282
Sweet Pepper Consommé   283
Thick Puree of White Bean Soup   283
Chilled Cucumber Refresher   284

SALADS

Alkalizing/Energizing Cucumber Salad   285
Rainbow Salad   286
Sprouted Lentil Salad   287
Spinach Salad I   288
Spinach Salad II   288
Bean Sprout Salad   288
Three-Bean Salad   289
Potassium Salad   290
Alfalfa Sprout Salad   290
Wheat Sprout Salad   291
Broccoli Salad   291
Colorful Cabbage   292
Zucchini Toss   292

Cauliflower Toss   293
Fresh Cucumber Dills   293
Raw Kale Salad   294

DRESSINGS, DIPS, PÂTÉS, SPREADS, TOPPINGS, FILLINGS, AND SAUCES

Salad Dressings
Basic Salad Dressing   295
Parsley Dressing   296
Essential Dressing   296
Garlic French Dressing   296
K&L Thousand Island Dressing   297
K&L Ranch Dressing   297
Wowie Zowie Almond Butter Dressing   298
Ginger/Almond Dressing   298
Lemon Basil Dressing   299
Sesame Soy Dressing   299
Pepita Seed Dressing   300
Soy Cucumber Dressing   300
Herbed Salad Dressing   300
Spicy Asian Dressing   301
Curried Carrot Almond Dressing   302
Tahini Dip/Dressing   302
Esther's All-Purpose Dressing   303

Dips
Guacamole   303
Great Olé Guacamole   304
Guacamole Green Mayonnaise Variation   304
Yummus Hummus   305
Tofu/Avocado Dip   305
Zippy Cilantro Dip   306
Leprechaun Surprise Dip   306

Pâtés
Raw Pecan Pâté   307
Almond Pâté   307
Tofu Pâté   308
Edamame Pâté   308
Tuna-pHishless Pâté   309
Pumpkin Pecan Pâté   309

Spreads
Herbed Alkalarian "Butter"   310
Mock Mayo   311
Mock Almond Mayonnaise   311
Esther's Creamy Mayo   312
Green Mayonnaise   312
Garbanzo Spread   313
Zippy Garbanzo Spread   313
Tahini (Sesame Seed Butter)   314
Sweet Carrot Butter   314

Toppings
AvoRado AvoCado Topping   315
Ginger-Almond Paste Topping   316
Basic Seasoning   316
Herb Oil   316
Green Pepper Relish   317
Dehydrated Red Bell Pepper Powder   317

Fillings
Fresh Spinach Filling   318
Crispy Radish Filling   318
Garden Variety Filling   319
Hearty Nut Filling   319

Sauces
Tahini Tofu Sauce   320
Lime Ginger Sauce   321
Rich Raw Tomato Sauce   321
Spring's Pesto   322
Maren's Salsa   322
Tomato Gravy   323
Tomato Sauce   323
Italian Tomato Sauce   324
Sauce Sampler Platter   324

ENTRÉES

Very Veggie Barley Burgers 325
Sprouted Cereal 326
Blackened Herbed Fillets 326
Tofu Salad Spread 327
Tofu Patties 327
Broc & Brussels 328
Sprouted Bean Casserole 329
Tofu Stew 329
Doc Broc Casserole 330
Ashley's Vegetable Nori Roll-Ups 331
Stuffed Cabbage Rolls 332
Curried Squash Dhal 332
Baked Falafel Fritters 334
Shelley's Super Wraps 335
Nepal Vegetable Curry 336
Tofu Italian Mock Meatballs 337
Roasted Pepper Macadamia Sauce 338
Cabbage Stuffed with Vegetables 338
Cajun-Style Red Beans and Brown Rice 339
Beans and Rice 340
Stuffed Acorn Squash 340
Autumn Curry Crêpes with Curried Veggie Filling 341
Curried Veggie Filling 342
Cold Tofu Pockets 343
Vegetable Stir-Fry 343
20-Minute Alkaline Stir-Fry 344
Vegetable Steam-Fry 345
Maren's Tortilla Pockets 346
Sunrise Asian Salad 347
Tofu Spinach Quiche 348
Nutty Mock Meat Loaf 349
Alexandra's Favorite Pasta 350
Rawsome Redford Pizza 350
Pasta with Creamy Pesto Sauce 353
Almond/Carrot/Ginger-Stuffed Zucchini 354
Edamame Patties 354
Hearty Harvest Casserole 356
Seed Pancakes with Coconut Whipped Topping 356
Spiced Winter Squash 357
Fresh Spinach/Zucchini Bake 358

Zippy Breakfast   358
Green Chili Tofu Pita   359

SIDE DISHES

Mexicali Rice   360
Millet Yam Hash Browns   361
Wild Yam Soba Noodles with Kale and Spicy Pine Nuts   362
Millet/Buckwheat Oven Cakes   363
Kale with Egyptian Garlic Sauce   364
Shelley Beans   365
Zucchini Italian-Style   366
Okra and Tomatoes Creole   366
Steam-Fried Sprouts   367
Refried Beans   367
Spiced Green Beans   367
Casserole de Cauliflower   368
Ginger Beans and Carrots   369
Camper's Bread   369
Essene Bread   369
Sprouted Wheat Bread   370
Shelley's Super Tortillas   370

SNACKS

Avocado/Tomato Snack   371
Nori Flower Krisps   371
Veggie Crunch Stix and Crackers   372
Spicy Pecan Croutons   374
Crispy Buckwheat Groats   374
Dehydrated Flax Chips   375
Tortilla Chips   376
Ice Pops   376

DESSERTS

Shelley's Soy Pudding   377
Mock Pumpkin Pie   378

JUICES, SHAKES, and MILKS

JUICES

For all the juicing recipes below, simply combine the ingredients in a juicer (I use Green Power and SoloStar Juicers) and process.

Basic Green Vegetable Juice

SERVES 1

This is a power-packed green drink. Go easy on the parsley, as it has a very strong flavor. Instead of this you can drink 1 teaspoon concentrated green powder in 8 ounces pure water.

2–3 celery stalks
1 cucumber
2–3 large kale leaves
4–5 large lettuce leaves
2 cups spinach
¼–½ cup parsley

Vegetable/Grass Drink

SERVES 1

1–3 oz. carrot juice (3 carrots or fewer; try to keep the drink at least 80 percent green)
3 oz. celery juice (2 large stalks)
½ oz. parsley juice (5 sprigs)
1½ oz. wheatgrass juice

Wheat-Beet Juice

SERVES 1

1½ oz. wheatgrass juice
1 oz. beet juice
6 oz. cucumber juice

Basic Green Drink

SERVES 2

4 cups alfalfa and/or other sprouts
4 cups sunflower and buckwheat greens
½ cup carrots
½ cup sweet red peppers
¼ cup parsley
1 cup cucumber
Add 1 bunch wheatgrass (about ¾ inch thick), if desired

Garden Green Drink

SERVES 2

4 cups sprouts
4 cups green tops
2 cups kale or collard greens
1 cup celery

Green Power Cocktail

SERVES 2

4 cups sprouts
4 cups green tops
1 cup kale
1 cup beets
½ cup wheatgrass

Spring Green Drink

SERVES 2

4 cups sprouts
4 cups greens
½ cup dandelion greens
¼ cup scallion
1 cup carrots

Potassium Special

SERVES 2

3 oz. carrot
4 oz. celery
2 oz. parsley
3 oz. spinach

Insulin Generator

SERVES 2

3 oz. brussels sprouts
3–6 oz. carrots
3 oz. string beans
4 oz. lettuce

High Vitamin C & E Drink

SERVES 2

6 oz. spinach
2 oz. lettuce
2 oz. watercress
4 oz. carrots
2 oz. green peppers

Blood Builder

SERVES 2

8 oz. celery
3 oz. cucumber
2 oz. parsley
3 oz. spinach

Skin Cleanse

SERVES 2

4 oz. potato
4 oz. celery
3–6 oz. carrot
2 oz. watercress

All-Vegetable Cocktail

SERVES 2

1 pt. fresh tomatoes
½ tsp. garlic
1 cucumber, sliced
1 green pepper
Sprigs of fresh parsley
¼ onion, sliced
2–3 lettuce leaves
½ tsp. ginger

Blend all ingredients in a blender on low speed.

SHAKES

AvoRado Kid Greens Shake

SERVES 1

This is by far our favorite cool green shake. We enjoy it for breakfast, lunch, dinner, or as a great anytime snack. (It's good during a cleanse, too.) Rob always has two shakes at a time! This shake gives you the concentrated nutrition of green powders and soy sprout powders and the benefits of avocado all in one. The cucumber and lime act as coolants to the body, and the essential fats in the avocado and the soy sprouts mean this is one really substantial shake that will keep you fueled up for many hours. This is a fantastic way to get greens and chlorophyll into your kids. In the summer, try turning it into pops (page 376) for a really cool treat.

1 avocado
½ English cucumber (organic and wrapped in plastic, if possible)
1 tomatillo (optional)
1 lime (peeled)
2 cups fresh spinach
2 scoops soy powder
1 scoop green powder
½–1 tsp. raw green stevia to taste
6–8 ice cubes

Place all ingredients in a blender; blend on high speed to a thick, smooth consistency. Serve immediately.

Variations:

The shakes that follow are really variations on this one. Here are some other ideas for changing it up :

- Substitute grapefruit or lemon for the lime.
- Add coconut milk or fresh almond milk for a creamier taste.
- Add 1 tsp. almond butter for a nutty flavor.

- Sweeten up your shake by replacing some or all of the ice cubes with fresh coconut water frozen in ice cube trays.
- Use some of the new Frontier flavorings (bottled in oil, not alcohol).

AvoRadoColada Shake

SERVES 1

1 avocado
½ English cucumber (organic and wrapped in plastic, if possible)
1 ruby-red grapefruit (peeled)
2 cups fresh spinach
2 scoops soy powder
1 scoop green powder
½–1 tsp. raw green stevia, to taste
Coconut milk and/or meat, as desired
6–8 ice cubes

Place all ingredients in a blender; blend on high speed to a thick, smooth consistency. Serve immediately.

Minty Mock Malt Shake

SERVES 1

1 avocado
½ English cucumber (organic and wrapped in plastic, if possible)
1 tomatillo (optional)
1 lime (peeled)
2 cups fresh spinach
2 scoops soy powder
1 scoop green powder
½–1 tsp. raw green stevia, to taste
6–8 ice cubes

Place all ingredients in a blender; blend on high speed to a thick, smooth consistency. Serve immediately.

LimeyLove Shake

SERVES 1

This is my favorite when it is hot outside! It's somewhere between a slush and a shake.

½ avocado
½ English cucumber (organic and wrapped in plastic, if possible)
3–4 whole limes (peeled)
2 cups fresh spinach
1 tsp. raw green stevia, to taste
12–16 ice cubes

Place all ingredients in a blender; blend on high speed to a thick, smooth consistency. Serve immediately.

Salty Shake

SERVES 1

This is best during a cleanse, though anyone who prefers an unsweet shake will enjoy it.

1 avocado
½ English cucumber (organic and wrapped in plastic, if possible)
1 tomatillo (optional)
1 lime (peeled)
2 cups fresh spinach
1 tsp. hemp oil
⅓ tsp. whole pure salts
2 scoops soy powder
1 scoop green powder
½–1 tsp. raw green stevia, to taste
6–8 ice cubes

Place all ingredients in a blender; blend on high speed to a thick, smooth consistency. Serve immediately.

NUT AND SEED MILKS

Almond Milk

SERVES 2

½ cup almonds
½ cup pine nuts
1 cup spring- or filtered water

Soak the almonds and pine nuts for 12 hours. Put in a blender and pulverize. Add the water gradually, while continuing to blend on high. Strain through a fine strainer or cheesecloth (you can use the almond pulp as a body scrub). This milk will keep for 3 to 4 days. It is great on hot grains such as quinoa, buckwheat groats, millet, or amaranth. We like to add some soaked almonds to our grains for "crunch." You can thin with more water if desired.

Quick Tahini Milk

SERVES 1–2

Tahini is a butter made from hulled sesame seeds, usually used as a spread. It also makes a very nutritious milk that's high in calcium and protein.

2–4 Tbs. tahini (raw)
1 cup water

In a blender, combine 2 Tbs. of the tahini with the water. Blend thoroughly and taste. Add additional tahini and blend again for a richer milk. This milk will keep for 3 to 4 days.

Fresh Silky Almond Milk

MAKES APPROXIMATELY 1 QUART

This is a quick way to make a rich, creamy nut milk that can be used in any recipe calling for dairy. We mix it half and half with raw green veggie juice for a refreshing breakfast drink. It's also a great way to make a soup, shake, or pudding creamy.

4 cups fresh raw almonds
Water
Stevia, to taste (optional)

Soak the almonds overnight in a bowl of water to cover. Drain and place into a blender until it is one-third full (about 2 cups), then add water to fill the blender. (If you want a thicker almond cream, don't use as much water.) Blend on high speed until the mixture is white and creamy looking. Pour through a fine-mesh strainer (I use a clean white nylon knee-high) into a bowl or pan. Squeeze with your hands to get all the liquid out. Add a bit of stevia to sweeten, if desired, or drink/use as is. Almond milk will stay fresh for about 3 days in the refrigerator. It will separate a bit, but all you need to do is stir or shake it up before serving.

SOUPS

GRASSoup

SERVES 4

I developed this raw recipe for people on a cleanse, but I've found we enjoy it any-time. This silky soup is refreshing on a hot day. It's a gorgeous pastel green, and named for the dill floating on the top, which looks like grass clippings. Sprinkle dehydrated red bell pepper powder (page 317) on top for an instant splash of warm color and sweetness.

2–3 English cucumbers, juiced (no pulp)
1–2 cups Fresh Silky Almond Milk (p. 269)
Water from 1–2 young Thai coconuts (reserve coconut meat for another use; water should be clear and sweet)
1 Tbs. fresh dill (tear or cut leaves off stalk so when added to soup, they float on top and look like grass clippings)
Dehydrated red bell pepper powder (page 317) (optional)

Stir together the first three ingredients. Sprinkle with the dill and red bell pepper powder (if using) just before serving.

Creamy or Crunchy Broccoli Soup

SERVES 4–6

This high-protein soup is a must for broccoli lovers! And it takes just 15 minutes to prepare.

2 cups vegetable stock or water
3–4 cups chopped broccoli
1 red bell pepper, chopped
2 red or yellow onions, chopped
1 avocado

1–2 celery stalks, cut in large pieces
Whole pure salts, to taste
Cumin and ginger, to taste (experiment with different spices!)

In an electric skillet, warm the water or stock, keeping the temperature at or below 118 degrees (finger test). Add the chopped broccoli and warm for 5 minutes.

In a blender, puree the warmed broccoli, bell pepper, onions, avocado, and celery, thinning with additional water if necessary to achieve the desired consistency. If desired, save the broccoli stalks, peeling off the tough outer skin; process them in a food processor until they are small chunks, and add to the soup just before serving to add crunch!

Serve warm, flavoring with whole pure salts, fresh ginger, cumin, or any other spices you like. Add a slice of lemon on top to garnish.

Green Raw Soup

Serves 4–6

This is a wonderfully alkalizing soup that I prefer served cold in the summer months and warmed in the winter months. It's energizing and easy to digest.

1–2 avocados
1–2 cucumbers, peeled and seeded
1 jalapeño pepper, seeded
Juice of ½ lemon
1–2 cups light vegetable stock or water
3 cloves roasted garlic
1 Tbs. fresh cilantro
1 Tbs. fresh parsley
½ yellow onion, diced
1 carrot, finely diced

Puree all ingredients (except the onion and carrot) in a food processor or Vita-Mix. Use more or less water for your desired consistency. Add the onion and raw crunchy carrot bits at the end for a garnish. Yum!

AsparaZincado Soup

SERVES 3–5

This great soup is loaded with zinc and has a rich tomato flavor—and takes only 15 minutes to prepare.

12 medium stalks asparagus (or 17 thin stalks)
5–6 large tomatoes
1 cup fresh parsley
3–5 sun-dried tomatoes (bottled in olive oil)
1–2 tsp. Herbes de Provence (Spice Hunter)
2 tsp. Deliciously Dill (Spice Hunter)
4 cloves fresh garlic
¼ cup dried onion
1 red bell pepper
1 avocado
2 lemons or limes, cut in thin slices

Trim and dice the tips from the asparagus and set aside for garnish. In a food processor or Vita-Mix, blend the asparagus and red tomatoes, parsley, dried tomatoes, spices, garlic, onion, and red bell pepper. Then blend in the avocado until the soup is smooth and creamy. Warm in an electric skillet and garnish with lemon or lime slices on top. Season with whole pure salts to taste or serve cold in the summertime. Sprinkle diced asparagus tips on top of the soup just before serving. Yummy!

Sautéed Edamame Vegetable Soup

SERVES 6–8

This soup gets its wonderful silky broth from straining it after you puree it—an extra step, but well worth it. If you sauté the veggies until they are brown, you will notice a wonderful roasted flavor in this soup. The edamame beans add sweetness.

1 Tbs. grape seed oil
3 large tomatoes, cored and quartered
1 large onion, sliced

1 large red pepper, cut into ½-inch strips
1 carrot, sliced
1 clove garlic, chopped
2 quarts veggie broth (I use Pacific Foods of Oregon brand)
3 large sprigs parsley
¾ tsp. dried thyme
Whole pure salts, to taste
1 (10-oz.) pkg. edamame beans (found in frozen section of grocery store)

Heat the oil in the bottom of a soup pot over high heat. Add the tomatoes, onion, red pepper, carrot, and garlic. Sauté until the vegetables are a deep golden brown, about 15 minutes. Then take about half of those veggies out of the pan, chop fine, and set aside.

Add the veggie broth, parsley, and thyme to the remaining vegetables, heat to a boil, cover, turn the heat down, and simmer for about 10 more minutes. Remove from the heat and cool slightly.

Working in batches, place the soup into a Vita-Mix or any blender and puree. Transfer to a strainer set over a bowl. Pour the puree through the strainer, coaxing the liquid into the bowl. Discard the solids left in the strainer and return the silky broth and the remaining chopped vegetables to the soup pot. This broth should be a beautiful orange color. Add salt to taste at this point. I add a teaspoon. Add the edamame beans and simmer until heated through, about 5 minutes longer.

Popeye Soup

SERVES 4–6

This is a wonderful alkalizing soup because of the cucumbers and greens. It is ready in just 10 minutes. Serve warm with a fresh tortilla for dipping.

1 avocado
1 cup water or vegetable stock (Pacific Foods of Oregon brand is yeast-free)
2 cucumbers, unwaxed
1 cup fresh raw spinach
2 green onions
1 clove garlic
⅓ red bell pepper

Whole pure salt, to taste
Middle Eastern spices (Spice Hunter's Garam Masala, ½–1 tsp., Curry
     Seasoning, ½–1 tsp., and Zip, ½ tsp.)
Fresh lime juice, to taste
4 spearmint leaves, for garnish

In a Vita-Mix or blender, add the avocado and half the water or stock.
Puree, then add the rest of the ingredients (except the spearmint leaves)
one at a time, blending to your desired thickness and thinning with the
remaining water if desired. Add salt to taste, and flavor with spices and lime
juice as desired. You might add a couple of minced sun-dried tomatoes, too.
Experiment! Also, this soup is good while on the liquid cleanse.

Warming options: This soup can be served warm or cold. If you're blending in a Vita-Mix, the longer you blend, the warmer the soup will get. If you
do not have a Vita-Mix, you can carefully warm the soup (not cook it) in an
electric or stovetop skillet over low heat. Warm the soup only until you can
hold your finger in it without having to pull it out. This will keep the food
at about 118 degrees, which will keep the food warm but uncooked. Serve
with spearmint leaves on top. Enjoy!

Healing Soup

SERVES 6–8

*This soup is good anytime, even when you are on the cleanse. It is soothing when
you are tired or stressed, or if you have a cold or flu, and is very antifungal.*

2–3 whole cloves garlic
1 large whole onion
2–3 quarts water
3 Tbs. yeast-free instant vegetable broth
1 cucumber
1–2 carrots (optional)
1 small head cabbage or broccoli (optional)
3 celery stalks (optional)
2 Tbs. fresh cilantro
Whole pure salt, to taste

Crush the garlic cloves and lightly steam-fry. Set aside. Put the whole onion in the water in a deep pan, and simmer until it's transparent (approximately 1 hour). Add the garlic and vegetable broth. Slice the cucumber and any of the optional veggies you are using, and add to the soup. Simmer for 10 to 15 minutes. Add the ginger, cilantro, and salt, adjusting according to taste.

Variation I: You could also bring the water to a boil, then take the soup off the burner and drop assorted finely chopped veggies into the water. This would just warm, but not cook the vegetables.

Variation II: You can grate, juice, or food process the ingredients into a wet paste, and then add them to hot water.

Broccoli/Cauliflower Soup

SERVES 4

½ cup soaked almonds
1 cup cucumber juice or veggie broth (Pacific Foods of Oregon brand)
1 clove garlic, minced
1–2 cups chopped broccoli
1–2 cups chopped cauliflower
¼ tsp. cumin
¼ tsp. curry powder
1 Tbs. lemon or lime juice
1 Tbs. Liquid pHlavor Salt
½ tsp. Real Salt

In a food processor or blender, combine the almonds with the cucumber juice or broth and the garlic. Blend well. With the machine still running, add the broccoli and cauliflower and blend until smooth. Finally, blend in the seasonings, lemon or lime juice, and salts. Add more broth or water to reach your desired consistency.

Variation: Use an avocado instead of the almonds and use this recipe for a salad dressing.

Celery/Cauliflower Soup

SERVES 6–8

1 onion, peeled and chopped
1 Tbs. oil (olive or Udo's)
1 whole head celery, trimmed and chopped (save some celery leaves for
   garnish)
1 head cauliflower, trimmed and chopped
1–2 qts. vegetable stock
½–1 qts. almond milk
Salt, pepper, and seasonings of choice, to taste

Steam-fry the onion in a little water and oil in a large soup pot for about
5 minutes without browning. Pulse-chop the celery and cauliflower in the
food processor until finely chopped.

Add the celery and cauliflower mix to the pot and warm until tender.
Add the vegetable stock and almond milk and simmer for about 15 to 30
minutes—or you can leave this raw and not cook it at all.

Puree the soup mixture in a blender or food processor until a smooth
texture is achieved. Season with salt and other seasonings of choice. Serve
warm or cold.

Chunky Veggie Soup

SERVES 4

2½ cups fresh carrot juice
1 avocado
6–8 celery stalks
1 summer squash
2 carrots
Small bunch arugula
Spice options: parsley, basil, or coriander
Whole pure salts, to taste

For the broth, blend the carrot juice, avocado, and 3 to 4 stalks of the celery.
Grate the squash, carrots, and remaining celery, adding the finely chopped

arugula and other fresh green spices last. Serve in a bowl or cup, decorated with fresh herbs. Add salt to taste.

Broccoli Creamed Soup

SERVES 6

½ cup chopped celery
1 chopped onion
2 Tbs. oil
½ qt. vegetable broth
2 cups pure water, divided
4 cups chopped broccoli
1 medium to large turnip, cut
1 heaping tsp. lecithin powder
Dash of white pepper
½ tsp. Real Salt

Carefully sauté the celery and onion in the oil. Add the broth, 1 cup of the water, and the broccoli. Cook over medium heat until the broccoli is tender-crisp. Meanwhile, steam the turnip until it's hot but not very soft. Let it cool slightly and puree it with enough water to get a thick, smooth consistency. Add the lecithin to the blender and continue mixing for a few seconds. Add the puree to the soup and season. Cook for a few minutes to thicken.

Anticancer Soup

SERVES 2

2 Tbs. caraway seeds
2 broccoli stalks
2 slices each purple and green cabbage
2 carrots
2 green onions, cut
2 cups hot water
Whole pure salts, to taste
3 Tbs. fresh dill weed
1 red pepper, sliced

Soak the caraway seeds in pure water for 24 hours before use, then pour off the liquid. Put finely cut broccoli florets and thinly sliced, peeled stems in a pot with a cover. Grate the cabbage and carrots over the broccoli and add the caraway. Blend the onions into the hot water and pour over the veggies. Cover, steam for 5 minutes, season, and serve, garnishing with dill and sliced red pepper (20 minutes to prepare).

Mock Split Pea Soup

SERVES 4

2 carrots, shaved
2 celery stalks, cut as desired
6 sprigs parsley
1 onion
2 cups crisp steamed green beans
1½ cups crisp steamed asparagus
4 cups water or vegetable stock
1 bay leaf
Dash of mace
½ tsp. whole pure salts, or to taste
½ tsp. cumin, dill, or Spice Hunter's Herbes de Provence (optional)

Chop all the vegetable ingredients in a food processor and add to the water or vegetable stock and bay leaf in a soup pot. Lightly simmer until the vegetables are just softened, about 10 minutes. Remove the bay leaf, then put the contents into a blender and thoroughly puree until a thick, creamy texture is achieved. Add the seasonings. Serve warm.

Vegetable Minestrone

SERVES 4

1 small cabbage
1 red bell pepper
1 onion
2 carrots
2 celery stalks

1 zucchini
1 yellow summer squash
Flax seed oil, to taste
Liquid pHlavor Salt, to taste
Cayenne pepper, to taste

Cut the vegetables as preferred. Cover the carrots and celery with water or vegetable broth in a soup pot. Cook gently until they just begin to "give," then add the remaining vegetables. Do not overcook. Serve hot with flax seed oil, liquid pHlavor salt, and cayenne pepper to taste.

Celery Soup

SERVES 2

4–5 celery stalks (including leaves, if fresh)
1 tsp. coconut oil
3 cups pure water
2 Tbs. yeast-free instant vegetable broth
Flax seed oil, to taste
Whole pure salts, to taste
Cayenne pepper, to taste

Cook the celery in coconut oil until tender. Add the remaining water and broth mix. Pour everything into a blender. Blend for 15 to 20 seconds. Reheat and serve, adding flax seed oil, whole pure salts, and cayenne pepper to taste.

Special Carrot Soup

SERVES 4

1 small onion, chopped
4 large carrots, sliced
1 clove garlic, minced
1 Tbs. coconut oil
¼ tsp. mustard seeds
¼ tsp. turmeric

¼ tsp. ginger
¼ tsp. cumin
Pinch of ground cinnamon
Pinch of cayenne pepper
¼ tsp. Real Salt
7 cups water, divided
⅓ cup kuzu root
1 tsp. lecithin liquid or powder

In a saucepan, steam-fry the onion in oil. Add the carrots, garlic, mustard seeds, spices, and salt. Cook for 2 to 3 minutes, stirring constantly. Add ½ cup of the water, cover, and simmer until the carrots begin to soften. Let cool.

In a large saucepan, bring 5 cups of the water to a near boil and reduce the heat to medium. Stir the kuzu root into 1 cup of cool water. Slowly pour into the heated water and cook until thick.

Place the cooled carrot mixture in a blender and puree on low speed until smooth, adding a bit of water if needed. Add the puree to the thickened water and cook for 5 minutes, stirring as needed. Add the lecithin and stir for a minute. Adjust the thickness if desired.

Creamy Vegetable Soup

SERVES 8

This rich soup gets its creaminess from tofu. Be sure to blend it thoroughly (I think the blender is best) so you get a rich, even, smooth, creamy texture.

1 cup chopped onions
2 cloves garlic, minced
2 cups shredded green cabbage
3 celery stalks, chopped
½ lb. asparagus, cut small
2 large leeks, chopped
4 cups vegetable broth
2 Tbs. chopped fresh parsley
2 tsp. dried dill
2 tsp. dried basil
1 tsp. dried oregano
Real Salt and pepper, to taste
1 pkg. soft tofu

In a skillet, steam-fry the onions and garlic for a few minutes. Add the cabbage, celery, and asparagus. Transfer to a large pot and add the leeks and vegetable broth. Stir in the parsley, dill, basil, oregano, salt, and pepper. Simmer just to brighten the veggies. Let cool a bit, then puree in a blender or food processor 2 cups at a time with some of the tofu, and return to another pot. Heat the soup no higher than 118 degrees, and serve.

Gazpacho

SERVES 6 (¾-CUP SERVINGS)

4 cups tomato juice (you make)
½ cup chopped cucumber
¼ cup chopped green bell pepper
¼ cup finely chopped celery
1 Tbs. olive oil
½ tsp. pepper
1 tsp. basil
½ tsp. minced garlic

Combine all ingredients. Cover and chill overnight.

Madrid Gazpacho

SERVES 6–8

3 large tomatoes
2 cucumbers
1 red bell pepper
1 small jalapeño pepper
1 qt. pure water
3 Tbs. olive oil
2 lemons, juiced
1 tsp. cumin
2 tsp. Real Salt
Garlic, to taste

Blend the vegetables, then add the water, oil, juice, and spices. Blend again (in batches if necessary). Serve chilled, garnished with chopped tomatoes, celery, green onions, cucumbers, red peppers, and avocados.

Roasted Butternut/Celery Soup with Caramelized Onions

Serves 6–8

This is a satisfying soup for chilly autumn and winter days. It is also delicious made with pumpkin and makes a great breakfast, lunch, dinner, or snack.

2 butternut squash
2 Tbs. olive or Udo's oil
3 celery stalks, cut in big chunks
1 onion, peeled and chopped in big chunks
3–4 cups veggie stock (I use Pacific Foods of Oregon brand), divided
Cinnamon and nutmeg or salt and pepper, to taste
1 onion, peeled and sliced into thin rings, for garnish

Preheat the oven to 400 degrees. Cut the squash in half and remove the seeds. Lightly oil the cut side of the squash and chunks of celery and onion. Place the squash (cut-side down) and the celery and onion chunks on an oiled cookie sheet. Roast for about 45 minutes or until tender and lightly browned. Scoop out the soft squash from the skins.

Puree the roasted vegetables in a blender or food processor with some of the stock. If you'd like a smoother texture, pass the soup through a strainer into a clean pot. Add the rest of the stock, season to taste, and keep warm.

To make the onion ring garnish, fry the onion in oil for 10 minutes until brown and somewhat crisp. Top the soup and serve immediately.

Veggie Borscht

Serves 8

6 cups veggie broth
1 cup shredded carrots
1 cup roughly chopped beets
1 cup thinly sliced onions

1½ cups shredded cabbage
1 red pepper, shredded
Vegetized or Real Salt, to taste
Pepper, to taste

Combine the broth, carrots, beets, and onions in a large saucepan. Cook gently until the vegetables are tender. Add the cabbage, red pepper, and salt and pepper to taste; cook for 5 minutes more. The soup will have a richer flavor if you let it cool completely before serving time and then reheat it.

Sweet Pepper Consommé

SERVES 6

3 medium red peppers
2 tomatoes
1 medium onion
¾ tsp. Real Salt
1 whole clove garlic
2 qt. boiling water

Cut the peppers in quarters and remove the seeds. Quarter the tomatoes and onion. Put all the ingredients in boiling water. Simmer, covered, for 1½ hours. Strain and taste for seasoning. A delicate and delicious broth, which may be served hot or cold.

Thick Puree of White Bean Soup

SERVES 8

2 lb. dried white beans, washed and picked over
2 onions, chopped
3 large cloves garlic, minced, divided
7 cups water
1 bay leaf
2 sprigs parsley
1 whole Swiss chard leaf, sliced crosswise

Whole pure salts, to taste
Black pepper, freshly ground, to taste

Soak the beans for 24 hours, in three times their volume of pure water, and
drain. Steam-fry the onions and 1 garlic clove until the onions are tender.
Put in a large pot with 7 cups of water; add the drained beans, remaining
garlic, bay leaf, parsley, and chard, and bring to a boil. Reduce the heat,
cover, and simmer for 1 hour. Add the salt and pepper and continue to simmer until the beans are tender. Remove the bay leaf and parsley. Puree the
soup in batches in a blender. Return to the pot and adjust the seasonings.
This can be frozen.

Chilled Cucumber Refresher

Serves 6

4 cups yeast-free vegetable broth
1 cup shredded cucumber
Dill weed

Combine the broth and cucumber; chill. Sprinkle each serving with dill
weed.

SALADS

Salads are my favorite meal. I'll often have one for breakfast—actually, almost every time I sit down to eat. Traditionally, a salad has been a token gesture compared with the "real" meal, but we need to rethink this. Salads are a main course. Other vegan dishes, including grains, soups, tortillas, pâtés, and other warmed and cooked foods, should be the complement to the salad, rather than the other way around.

Fortunately, making a great salad couldn't be easier. Even complete kitchen novices can shine here, from day one. And the variety is limited only by availability of ingredients and your imagination. True, it may take a bit longer than pushing a few buttons on the microwave to zap a meal. But then a big salad, stored airtight in the fridge, will stay fresh for about three days. (Use a salad spinner to remove excess water and thoroughly dry your greens so they will stay crisp.) Keep clean, dry, dark, leafy lettuces and spinach in your refrigerator in a covered container with a paper towel in the bottom.

Get creative with salads. Showcase the simplicity of vegetables with just a few ingredients, or show off the complex interplay of a whole bunch of additions. Serve them with small piles of each ingredient on its own turf, or tossed all together hodgepodge. Mix up how you prepare the veggies—minced, diced, sliced, shredded, chopped, and so on—or keep all the textures similar. Make them monochromatic (green being a popular color scheme) or brightly jeweled rainbows. Keep them light, or make them extra hearty by adding tofu cubes (or baked or marinated tofu cubes), pine nuts, soaked almonds, sprouts, dehydrated grains (such as Crispy Buckwheat Groats, page 374), or pieces of baked warm falafel. Have fun, explore the salad horizons—and eat well.

Alkalizing/Energizing Cucumber Salad

SERVES 3

Cucumber is one of the most alkalizing and energizing foods that you can eat. It is considered to have a purifying effect on the digestive system and is very beneficial to the hair and skin. For a refreshing lift, lie down with a cucumber slice over each eye for a few minutes or rub a slice over your face after cleansing to tone and purify your skin.

2 cups chopped cucumbers
2 Tbs. chopped parsley
1 Tbs. lemon juice
1 Tbs. flax seed oil or olive oil
⅓ cup finely chopped peppermint
Whole pure salts or Liquid pHlavor Salt, to taste

In a small serving bowl, combine the cucumbers, parsley, lemon juice, oil, mint, and salt. Toss together. Chill for several hours or overnight. Toss again before serving.

Rainbow Salad

SERVES 8–12

I love the colors of vegetables! Presentation of a beautifully arranged alkalizing meal can be an art. Besides, eating a rainbow of colored foods supports the balance of the energy of the body. This is my basic salad recipe, which I make every week. The grating of the vegetables exposes their natural sweetness.

1–2 heads green-leaf lettuce, washed, dried, and ripped into bite-size
    pieces
1–2 heads red-leaf lettuce, washed, dried, and ripped into bite-size pieces
1 pkg. prewashed baby leaf organic spinach
1 head green cabbage, shredded
½–1 head red cabbage, grated
3–4 beets, grated
4–5 carrots, grated
2–3 summer (yellow) squash or zucchini, grated, or ¼ butternut squash,
    grated
⅓–½ large jicama, grated
1 each red, yellow, and orange bell peppers, sliced
1–2 cucumbers, sliced
1–2 pkgs. (approximately 8 oz.) sunflower seed sprouts, or a mix of
    sprouts, or the sprouts of your choice

1 lb. fresh green peas from the pod
1–2 Tbs. per serving salad dressing of your choice

Fill a large salad bowl with lettuces. (You can substitute a packaged salad mix: Get it as fresh as possible, and choose an organic one.) Arrange grated vegetables on top of the greens, starting with the deeper, darker colors on the outside and working into the lighter colors on the inside to create a rainbow effect. Place sliced peppers and cucumbers on top. Sprinkle with sprouts and peas. Top with dressing, or pass it at the table. Choose a dressing from any of the recipes in this book, or any you buy that fits on this program. Or just sprinkle with a healthy oil, whole pure salts, fresh lemon juice, and spices to taste. I hope that once you've tried this, you'll feel free to improvise your own ingredients, proportions, and arrangement.

Sprouted Lentil Salad

SERVES 4

This salad is hearty and also works well as a filling for halved bell peppers.

1 tsp. flax seed oil, Udo's Choice oil, or Omega Nutrition/Essential
    Balance oil
1 Tbs. lemon juice
1 tsp. Liquid pHlavor Salt
1 clove garlic, minced
Pinch of Zip (Spice Hunter)
1 tsp. Curry Seasoning (Spice Hunter)
2 cups sprouted lentils
½ cup chopped onions

In a small bowl, mix the oil, lemon juice, salt, garlic, Zip, and curry powder. In a separate mixing bowl, combine the lentils and onions and toss.

Optional: Add some sprouted garbanzo beans, too!

Spinach Salad I

SERVES 2–3

1 head spinach
½ cup cauliflower, cut in small pieces
2 celery stalks, chopped
6 radishes, chopped

In a large bowl, combine the ingredients and toss well. Top with Essential Dressing (page 296).

Spinach Salad II

SERVES 2–3

1 head spinach
½ cup cauliflower, cut in small pieces
2 celery stalks, chopped
6 radishes, chopped
2 shallots, chopped (or 1 small red onion)
½ cup chopped basil
2 red peppers, chopped
¼ cup pine nuts

In a large bowl, combine all the ingredients and toss well. Top with Essential Dressing (page 296).

Bean Sprout Salad

SERVES 4

¼ cup flax seed oil
2 tsp. fresh lemon juice
2 Tbs. Liquid pHlavor Salt
½ tsp. freshly ground pepper
1 crushed clove garlic
2 Tbs. sesame seeds (soaked overnight)

2 cups fresh bean sprouts
¼ cup finely chopped pimiento
¼ cup finely chopped green onion

For the dressing, combine the oil, lemon juice, salt, pepper, garlic, and sesame seeds in a blender, and puree.

Rinse the bean sprouts in cold water and drain. In a bowl, combine the bean sprouts, pimiento, and onion. Toss lightly in the pureed dressing.

Three-Bean Salad

SERVES 2

Salad

6 oz. steamed fresh green beans
6 oz. steamed fresh wax beans
6 oz. cooked red kidney beans, drained
½ cup chopped green onion
¼ cup snipped fresh parsley

Dressing

¼ cup flax seed oil, Udo's oil, Omega Nutrition/Essential Balance oil, or oil of choice
2 Tbs. Liquid pHlavor Salt
2 cloves garlic, crushed
½ tsp. Italian Seasoning (Spice Hunter)

Mix the salad ingredients in a large bowl. Pour the dressing over the bean mixture and refrigerate for 2 hours. Just before serving, remove the bean mixture with a slotted spoon onto a lettuce bed.

Potassium Salad

Salad

1 head cabbage (green or white), shredded or finely chopped
¾ cup chopped parsley
3 grated carrots
1 avocado, sliced into bite-size pieces (optional—it adds even more potassium)

Dressing

⅔ cup flax seed oil, olive oil, Udo's oil, hemp seed oil, or oil of choice
¼ cup Liquid pHlavor Salt
Dulse, garlic powder, and onion powder, to taste

Combine the vegetables in a large bowl. Mix well. Toss with dressing to taste.

Alfalfa Sprout Salad

Salad

3 cups alfalfa sprouts
3 cups chopped summer squash
2 red peppers, diced
2 chopped green onions
¼ cup chopped red onion

Dressing

1 cup flax seed oil, olive oil, Udo's oil, hemp seed oil, or oil of choice
Juice of 1 fresh lemon or lime
1 tsp. Real Salt or Liquid pHlavor Salt
1–2 tsp. seasoning blends (optional), such as Italian or Mexican (I use
    Spice Hunter brand)

Combine the vegetables in a large bowl. Toss with dressing to taste.

Wheat Sprout Salad

SERVES 6

3 cups fresh sprouts
1 cup grated carrots
¾ cup minced onion
3 Tbs. flax seed oil, Udo's oil, Omega Nutrition/Essential Balance oil or oil of choice
1½ Tbs. fresh lemon juice
Paprika

Mix all the ingredients except the paprika. Sprinkle with paprika. Serve on a bed of lettuce, adding whole pure salts to taste.

Broccoli Salad

SERVES 2

1 head broccoli
1 cup diced celery
4 chopped scallions
1 large chopped red onion
⅓ cup Parsley Dressing (page 296) or Herbed Salad Dressing (page 300)

Cut the raw broccoli into bite-size pieces. Mix all the ingredients and chill for 1 hour.

Colorful Cabbage

Cabbage is considered one of the most powerful therapeutic foods in the world. Many studies have linked eating cabbage with a reduction of cancer, especially colon cancer. Also, cabbage juice has been proven to help heal stomach ulcers and prevent stomach cancer.

2 cups thinly sliced red cabbage
2 cups thinly sliced green cabbage
1 carrot, grated
1 red pepper, slivered
1 yellow pepper, slivered
1 green pepper, slivered
1 orange pepper, slivered
¼ cup chopped scallions
¼ cup minced parsley
¼ cup lemon juice
3 Tbs. water
1 Tbs. oil (extra-virgin olive, flax seed, Udo's Choice, hemp seed oil, or oil
    of choice)
1–2 tsp. dried red chili pepper
Dash of whole pure salts

In a bowl, combine all ingredients. Toss thoroughly and let the flavors mix for at least half an hour before serving.

Zucchini Toss

Salad

1 medium head red-leaf lettuce
1 small head romaine lettuce
2 medium zucchini, thinly sliced
1 cup sliced radishes
3 green onions, sliced

Dressing

¼ cup flax seed oil
2 Tbs. Real Salt
Garlic clove(s) to taste, crushed
¼ tsp. dried tarragon leaves

Combine all the vegetables in a large bowl. Toss with the dressing.

Cauliflower Toss

SERVES 4

Salad

½ medium bunch romaine lettuce, torn
½ small head cauliflower (broken into florets—2 cups)
¼ cup sliced radishes

Dressing

¼ cup flax seed oil
1 green onion, sliced
¼ Tbs. dried dill weed
Vegetized or sea salt
Freshly ground pepper

Layer half of the lettuce and cauliflower in a salad bowl. Top with the radishes and the remaining lettuce and cauliflower. Combine the dressing ingredients, mix, and pour over the salad.

Fresh Cucumber Dills

SERVES 6

2 large cucumbers, peeled and thinly sliced
2 Tbs. fresh dill weed
1 Tbs. fresh lemon juice

3 Tbs. distilled water
½ tsp. Real Salt
Dash of cayenne pepper

Drain the cucumbers well. Stir the remaining ingredients together and add
to the cucumbers; mix well. Cover and chill overnight.

Raw Kale Salad

SERVES 4–6

This chewy, hearty salad is one of our mainstays.

2 heads or bunches green kale (organic if possible)
1 red onion, diced
⅓ cup olive oil
Whole pure salts, to taste
Sun-dried tomatoes (optional)
Pine nuts or nuts of choice (optional)
Dehydrated Veggie Blend Mix (optional)

Wash the kale by submerging it in a large bowl (or clean sink) filled with
water, with salt added. (We use Real Salt or Liquid pHlavor Salt.) Swish
the kale around to completely wash the curly-edged leaves. Rinse, and shake
off the extra water.

Carefully cut the leaves away from the core stems and cut or gently tear
into bite-size pieces. (Save the stems for use in a soup.) Dry the kale pieces
in a salad spinner.

Combine the kale and diced red onion in a bowl with a resealable lid (I
use Tupperware) and stir in the olive oil, adding salts to taste. Make sure all
the kale gets coated with the oil, so it's shiny. Use more oil if necessary. Stir
in any of the optional ingredients you like (or wait until just before serving
to maintain crunch).

Seal the bowl with a lid and place in the refrigerator overnight to marinate and soften the kale.

DRESSINGS, DIPS, PÂTÉS, SPREADS, TOPPINGS, FILLINGS, AND SAUCES

Try thinning the spread recipes with veggie juice, water, or oil and using them as salad dressings.

SALAD DRESSINGS

You can thicken dressings to your liking with ground flax seeds, ground psyllium seed powder, agar agar, or kuzu root, all of which you can find at your local health food store.

Basic Salad Dressing

SERVES 6

⅓ cup fresh lemon or lime juice
1 cup cold-pressed extra-virgin olive oil, or any other preferred oil, such as
    Essential Balance
½ tsp. ground oregano
½ tsp. ground cumin
½ tsp. garlic powder
½ tsp. Zip (Spice Hunter) or a dash of cayenne pepper
1 Tbs. Liquid pHlavor Salt

Put all ingredients in a blender or food processor and blend until smooth.

Parsley Dressing

SERVES 4

1¾ cups water
2 celery stalks
⅓ cup preferred oil (virgin olive, Essential Balance, flax seed, hemp seed, etc.)
1–3 cloves garlic
¼ cup parsley
Salt, Liquid pHlavor Salt, or other seasonings of choice (optional)

Blend all ingredients. Use on salads and veggies.

Essential Dressing

SERVES 4–6

1 cup preferred oil (Udo's, Essential Balance, hemp seed, olive, flax seed,
    grape seed, or oil of choice)
¼ cup Liquid pHlavor Salt or 1 tsp. Real Salt (adjust to taste)
Juice of 1 fresh lemon
½–1 tsp. of any seasoning you prefer, such as Italian, Mexican (Spice
    Hunter), pesto, garlic powder, onion powder, parsley, basil, or oregano

Combine all ingredients in a food processor and mix well, or simply place
them in a salad dressing jar and shake to mix well. Chill and serve.

Garlic French Dressing

MAKES 2–3 CUPS

½ cup sun-dried tomatoes
Juice of 1 lemon
3 cloves garlic
1 tsp. whole pure salts
1 tsp. paprika
½ tsp. cayenne
1–2 packets stevia
2 cups pure water

Blend all ingredients in blender until smooth and creamy. Add water (up to ¼ cup more) to reach your desired consistency.

K&L Thousand Island Dressing

MAKES ¾ CUP

½ cup unsweetened soy milk (I like WestSoy)
¼ tsp. dry mustard
1 Tbs. lemon juice
½ tsp. salt
1¼ tsp. paprika
6 Tbs. olive oil, mild flavor
$\frac{1}{16}$ tsp. stevia, or to taste
2 sun-dried tomatoes, packed in olive oil
1 Tbs. chopped onion
1 Tbs. chopped green bell pepper
1 Tbs. chopped celery

Combine all ingredients in a blender and blend until smooth.

K&L Ranch Dressing

MAKES ¾ CUP

½ cup unsweetened soy milk (I like WestSoy)
6 Tbsp. olive oil, mild flavor
2 Tbsp. lemon juice
3 Tbsp. chopped green onion
1 Tbsp. chopped parsley
¼ tsp. dry mustard
1 tsp. onion powder
¼ tsp. paprika
¼ tsp. Real Salt
⅛ tsp. red pepper
$\frac{1}{16}$ tsp. white stevia

Combine all ingredients in a blender, and blend until smooth.

Wowie Zowie Almond Butter Dressing

Serves 6

This is a rich, sweet dressing that tastes great on salads, over rice, or on top of any steamed veggies. Children will especially like this dressing because of its creamy nut butter taste. Add additional water to thin if desired.

1 cup raw almond butter (I use MaraNatha brand)
½–1 cup water
Juice of 1 lemon
1 Tbs. Liquid pHlavor Salt or 1 tsp. Real Salt
2 tsp. chicory root powder (a sweetener) or raw green stevia
1 heaping Tbs. dried onion
2 cloves garlic
1 Tbs. grated fresh gingerroot
1 Tbs. sesame oil
½ tsp. Zip (Spice Hunter)

In a blender or food processor, combine the almond butter, water, lemon juice, salt, and chicory root or stevia. After this is well blended, leave the blender on and add the onion, garlic, ginger, oil, and Zip. Blend well, adding additional water if required for a thinner consistency. Serve warmed or cool.

Ginger/Almond Dressing

Serves 4

3 scallions (white part only)
3-inch piece peeled fresh ginger
2 cloves garlic
¼ cup almond butter
1 tsp. flax seed oil
Whole pure salts, to taste
1 cup water (add more if desired)
1–2 sun-dried tomatoes packed in olive oil (optional)

In a food processor, process the scallions, ginger, garlic and tomatoes (if using) until smooth. Add the almond butter, oil, and whole pure salts and process until the mixture is blended. Slowly add the water to your desired consistency, and continue processing until well blended. Serve on non-starchy veggies, salads, and so on.

Lemon Basil Dressing

Makes 1½ cups

1 lemon, juiced, then rind grated finely
3 Tbs. finely minced fresh basil
Dash of stevia
1 block soft tofu
1 cup olive oil

Mix the first three ingredients until blended. Puree with the tofu. Whisk in the oil.

Sesame Soy Dressing

Makes 1¼ cup

1 Tbs. toasted sesame seeds, divided
1 tsp. toasted sesame seed oil
1 clove garlic
1 tsp. whole pure salts
1 cup olive oil

Put 2 tsp. of the sesame seeds in a blender, add the sesame oil, garlic, salts, and olive oil, and blend until combined and smooth. Stir in the remaining sesame seeds.

Pepita Seed Dressing

MAKES 1½ CUPS

¾ cup olive oil
¼ cup fresh lemon juice
Whole pure salts, to taste
Zip (Spice Hunter), to taste
1 cup green raw pepita seeds

Combine the oil and lemon juice in a blender, and add salts and Zip to taste. (This is a basic lemon vinaigrette.) Toast the seeds lightly in the oven on a dry pan. Reserve 1 Tbs. seeds for garnish. Blend the remaining seeds with the rest of the dressing.

Soy Cucumber Dressing

SERVES 4

A subtle, refreshing dressing.

2–3 tsp. carrot juice
1 large cucumber (I prefer peeled and seeded)
½ red bell pepper
½ small onion
1 cup soy milk
1 tsp. dried basil (or 2 tsp. fresh)
1 Tbs. Real Salt, to taste

Blend all the ingredients in a food processor or blender until smooth.

Herbed Salad Dressing

SERVES 2

1 tsp. dry mustard
1 tsp. fresh parsley
1 tsp. dill weed

½ tsp. Real Salt
¼ tsp. tarragon
¼ tsp. ground black pepper
⅛ tsp. thyme
⅓ cup preferred oil (virgin olive, grape seed, Udo's, flax seed, Essential Balance, or oil of choice)
Pinch of oregano

Combine all the ingredients.

Spicy Asian Dressing

Serves 4–6

This dressing is easily whipped up in the food processor and gives your salads a wonderful Asian zing. If you tend not to like too much spice, then use half the amounts of spices listed.

⅓ cup plus 1 Tbs. sesame tahini
½ cup water (plus more to thin, as needed)
½ cup Liquid pHlavor Salt
2 tsp. dried onions
6 Tbs. flax seed oil
½–1 tsp. chicory root powder (sweetener)
3 Tbs. grated gingerroot
½ tsp. Chinese Five-spice seasoning
⅛–¼ tsp. cayenne pepper or Hot Zip (Spice Hunter)
½ tsp. cumin

Place all the ingredients in a food processor and process until smooth and well mixed. This dressing will last several days in the refrigerator.

Curried Carrot Almond Dressing

SERVES 4

This dressing is simple, fast, and full of great flavor. I have found that it's best if you first blanch the soaked almonds to remove their skins. Since this dressing has fresh carrot juice in it, it is highly perishable; make only enough to use up in a day or two.

½ cup almonds, soaked and blanched with skins removed (a rubber garlic cylinder roller takes the skins off fast)
1 cup fresh carrot juice
⅓–½ tsp. curry powder
½ tsp. dried onion
Whole pure salts, to taste
Dash of lemon or lime juice, to taste
1 clove fresh or 2 cloves roasted garlic (optional)

Put all ingredients in a blender and blend at high speed until smooth. If you want this for more of a dip, then use more almonds and less carrot juice and process to your desired thickness.

Tahini Dip/Dressing

SERVES 4

1 cup raw tahini
1 tsp. dried parsley or ½ cup fresh parsley
1 Tbs. dried onion or 1 small onion, chopped
2–3 sun-dried tomatoes
½ cucumber, peeled and chopped
1 fresh tomato, chopped
2 Tbs. lemon or lime juice (I use more)
1 tsp. finely chopped fresh cilantro
½ tsp. cumin
1–3 cloves garlic or 4–6 cloves roasted garlic
Whole pure salts, to taste
1 tsp. Real Salt
Pinch of cayenne or Zip (Spice Hunter)

Put all ingredients in a food processor and blend until smooth. Thin with water or oil for a dressing, or let the mixture set up in the fridge for a dip.

Esther's All-Purpose Dressing

MAKES 1 QUART

This is great as sauce on quinoa, rice, buckwheat, or veggie burgers (page 325). It makes a great salad dressing, too!

1 bunch green onions or ¼ cup white onions
1 cup water and 1 tsp. Real Salt
Pinch of cayenne pepper, or to taste
½ cup lemon juice
¼-½ packet stevia, to taste
3 Tbs. raw tahini or raw hemp butter
1 tsp. gingerroot
2 cups olive oil

Combine all ingredients in a blender and blend on high until creamy.

DIPS

Guacamole

SERVES 2

1 large ripe avocado
1 tomato, finely chopped
1/4 tsp. Real Salt
⅛ cup lime or lemon juice
Chili powder, to taste

Mash the avocado and mix with the remaining ingredients. Use as a salad dressing or serve as a dip for raw bell peppers, celery, eggplant, cucumber, or summer squash.

Great Olé Guacamole

SERVES 6–8

Spice Hunter's Mexican Seasoning and Zip really give this guacamole a kick! Use this as a dip for fresh veggies. Cut veggies like bell peppers and cabbage with small cookie cutters for children.

Juice of 1 lemon or lime (or use both)
1 large tomato
3 avocados
1 tsp. Mexican Seasoning (Spice Hunter)
¼ tsp. cumin
½ tsp. Zip (Spice Hunter)
1 tsp. Real Salt or to taste

In a food processor fitted with an S-blade, blend the lemon juice with half the tomato and half the avocado until smooth. Finely dice the remaining half tomato. Mash the remaining avocado, leaving the pulp chunky. Combine both mixtures, seasoning with the Mexican Seasoning, cumin, Zip, salt, and additional lemon juice to taste, if desired. Olé!

Guacamole Green Mayonnaise Variation

SERVES 4

1 tomato, chopped, peeled
½ onion, chopped
2–3 seeded green chili peppers

Blend all the ingredients in a processor until you reach mayonnaise consistency.

To make Guacamole from the Green Mayonnaise recipe, add the ingredients listed for this recipe to the ingredients for Green Mayonnaise (page 312).

Variation: Add parsley, chives, tarragon, or other spices of choice.

Yummus Hummus

SERVES 6–8

2–3 Tbs. olive oil
Juice of 1 lemon
1–2 cloves garlic, minced
1/8–1/4 cup tahini (raw)
1 (17-oz.) jar garbanzo beans, drained (save water)
Whole pure salts, to taste
1/2–1 tsp. Garlic Herb Bread Seasoning (Spice Hunter)
1/2–1 tsp. cumin
Zip (Spice Hunter), to taste

In a food processor, process the oil, lemon juice, garlic, and tahini until smooth. Add the beans and seasonings and process until creamy. You may need to thin with extra water (from the beans) to your desired consistency. Serve on wraps, with raw veggies, or in pita sandwiches.

Great variations: Add an avocado to this recipe to make the hummus green and creamier, or add 1 or 2 red or orange bell peppers to make the hummus sweeter and a more vibrant orange. Add a few sun-dried tomatoes for a more flavorful and deeper-colored hummus. Experiment and enjoy!

Tofu/Avocado Dip

SERVES 6

1 pkg. soft fresh tofu, drained
1 1/2 tsp. lemon juice
1 tsp. garlic powder
1 Tbs. diced onion
2 Tbs. chopped fresh cilantro
1/2 tsp. chili powder
1 small tomato, diced (optional), or 2–3 sun-dried tomatoes
1 medium avocado, mashed
1/2–1 tsp. Real Salt

In a blender or food processor, combine the tofu, lemon juice, garlic powder, onion, cilantro, and chili powder; process until well blended. Put the mixture in a bowl, add the tomato, avocado, and salt, and mix well. Chill and serve with chips or fresh veggies. You can also put all the ingredients in the food processor again; process until smooth and serve chilled.

Zippy Cilantro Dip

SERVES 6–8

½ cup chopped fresh cilantro
1 or 2 hot chili peppers
2 cups frozen petite peas, thawed
1 pkg. fresh tofu, drained
1 Tbs. lemon juice
1 tsp. ground cumin
¼ tsp. freshly ground pepper
Whole pure salts, to taste
1 medium cucumber

Combine one-quarter of the cilantro with all the remaining ingredients except the cucumber in a food processor and process until smooth, approximately 30 seconds on high. Refrigerate for 1 hour. Lay out overlapping thin cucumber slices and rim with the remaining cilantro. Serve with the dip.

Leprechaun Surprise Dip

SERVES 6–8

2 cups very finely chopped spinach
2 cups very finely chopped parsley
1 cup very finely chopped green onions
½ cup Mock Mayo (page 311)

Mix well. Serve with fresh vegetables.

PÂTÉS

Raw Pecan Pâté

SERVES 8

This pâté spreads well on tortillas and celery. The fresh raw pecans and shredded veggies make it a sweet pâté that's great for children!

2 cups fresh raw pecans
¼–½ red onion
1–2 tsp. poultry spice (e.g., Spice Hunter)
4–6 fresh basil leaves
¼ cup finely grated carrots, beets, and/or raw squash
¼ cup finely minced parsley (optional)

In a food processor fitted with an S-blade, blend the pecans, onion, poultry spice, and basil leaves. Thin with enough water (optional) to reach your desired consistency—like pâté. Add the grated veggies and keep blending until well mixed and moist. Stir in the minced parsley and mix well. You can even make this into patties and warm them in a food dehydrator to the desired warmth and crispness (4 to 8 hours) if you wish. If you are in a hurry, you could warm the pâté lightly in an electric skillet right before you serve it. Other spices can be added to the pâté, too, such as Spice Hunter's Garlic Herb Bread Seasoning or Cowboy BBQ Rub. Experiment!

Almond Pâté

SERVES 8–10

3 cups soaked almonds
1 cup lemon juice
¼ cup Liquid pHlavor Salt
½–1 clove garlic (you could use roasted garlic, too)

In a food processor, process the almonds, lemon juice, salt, and garlic until smooth. Store in an airtight container in the fridge.

Variations: This is a basic pâté spread recipe. You can vary it by using pine nuts, sesame seeds, or other nuts, such as soaked hazelnuts or pecans. You can cream it up more by adding tahini. Also, try seasoning it differently with various Spice Hunter spices. Fresh herbs or dehydrated veggies can color and flavor it up. Be daring and creative! Use it to stuff peppers or celery. Spread it on crackers or wraps.

Tofu Pâté

SERVES 6–8

1 lb. firm fresh tofu, drained
1 Tbs. Liquid pHlavor Salt
1 Tbs. sesame tahini
1 Tbs. flax seed oil
2 Tbs. yeast-free vegetable broth
1 Tbs. minced chives
1 Tbs. minced fresh basil

Place all ingredients in a mixing bowl and mix thoroughly until smooth. Press the mixture into a mold and refrigerate for 2 hours.

Slice or scoop out and serve with nonstarchy vegetables.

Edamame Pâté

SERVES 6

This is a beautiful bright green pâté with an Asian flair.

1 fresh Thai coconut
1 (10 oz.) bag frozen edamame (green soy beans), not in the pod
1 tsp. Real Garlic Salt or any garlic salt
1 Tbs. toasted sesame seed oil

Drain the coconut water and reserve for another use. It's a very refreshing drink all by itself. Or it can be used in the GRASSoup recipe (page 270). Open the coconut and, using a spoon, dig out the white flesh meat. Put the coconut meat and edamame through a juicer that does nut butters and pâtés

(I use a Samson Juice Extractor), catching into a container. Add the seasonings and mix well. Spread on crackers, use as a dip with chips, or mound with an ice cream scoop on top or on the side of a salad or soup.

Tuna-pHishless Pâté

SERVES 6 (APPROXIMATELY 2 CUPS)

This will remind you of the tuna salad you used to take in your lunch box, complete with dill seasoning (instead of pickles) and chopped celery for crunchy texture. Use it as a dip or spread.

1 cup soaked raw sunflower seeds
1 cup coconut meat from a young Thai coconut
1–2 celery stalks, finely chopped
1 tsp. Deliciously Dill (Spice Hunter)
½–1 tsp. Herbamare seasoning
Dehydrated Red Bell Pepper Powder (page 317) (optional)

Place the sunflower seeds and coconut meat through a juicer that does nut butters and pâtés (I use a Samson Juice Extractor), and put into a bowl or other container. Add the celery and seasonings and mix well. Garnish with red bell pepper powder if desired. Chill in the fridge.

Pumpkin Pecan Pâté

SERVES 6

1 cup raw, soaked, blanched almonds
1 cup coconut meat from a young Thai coconut
⅓ cup raw pecans (no need to soak)
1 tsp. pumpkin pie spice (Spice Hunter makes a good one), or more to
  taste
Raw green stevia, to taste (optional)

Place all the ingredients through a juicer that does nut butters and pâtés (I use a Samson Juice Extractor).

SPREADS

Herbed Alkalarian "Butter"

APPROXIMATELY 2 CUPS

Dr. Johanna Budwig, a great advocate of the healing properties of flax seed oil, gave me the inspiration for this alkalarian answer to butter. The combination of healthy oils makes a solid butter-type spread that melts beautifully once it hits something warm, spreading a mix of herbs, seasonings, and healthy omega and lauric oils over your dish. The coconut oil keeps it solid in the fridge, and the flax oil gives it a rich golden appearance. You can experiment with different herbs, spices, and flavorings. Try adding lemon juice, or fresh or dried mint, or diced pecans or almonds, or Frontier Herbs flavorings (bottled without alcohol).

Whatever combination you come up with, just put a pat or two on steamed veggies or warmed grains such as quinoa, buckwheat, or millet, or use it as a spread on a wrap.

1 cup coconut oil (organic extra-virgin cold-pressed; I use Wilderness
    Family Naturals), divided
1 yellow onion
8 large cloves garlic
½–1 tsp. whole pure salt
2 tsp. Italian seasonings (Spice Hunter or your choice)
1 tsp. minced fresh rosemary
2 tsp. minced sun-dried tomatoes (optional)
½ cup Barlean's Flax Oil (in the refrigerated section of your health food store)

In a nonstick pan, heat 3 Tbs. of the coconut oil. Sauté the diced onion and garlic until the onion is clear, stirring constantly. If desired, slightly brown the onion and garlic for a more roasted flavor. Add the remaining coconut oil, letting it melt until clear. Stir to mix. Take off the burner; do not cook. Strain the mixture through a strainer to take out the pieces of onion and garlic if desired—or leave them in for a stronger taste. Add the salt, spices, and seasonings of choice, along with the Barlean's Flax Oil. Stir well, pour into small tubs, and place in the refrigerator to set.

Do not cook or fry with this Herbed Alkalarian Butter—the heat will cause trans-fatty acids to form. Keep the mixture raw and use only after you have cooked or warmed your food. Great on the Zippy Breakfast (page 358)!

Mock Mayo

SERVES 4

1 cup steamed cauliflower
Water
Flax seed oil
¼ tsp. Real Salt
¼ tsp. dry mustard
¼ tsp. paprika
½ tsp. powdered lecithin (optional)
½–1 tsp. Udo's oil, to emulsify (optional)
Cayenne pepper, to taste

Whip the cauliflower with a little water and flax seed oil, and add the remaining ingredients or process in a food processor until creamy and smooth.

Mock Almond Mayonnaise

SERVES 4

1 cup soaked almonds
½ cup water or veggie broth
1 Tbs. dried onion or 3 Tbs. chopped onion
3 Tbs. chopped red pepper
1 clove garlic
1 lemon, peeled and chopped
1 Tbs. oil (Udo's Choice or flax seed oil)
1 tsp. dried oregano or 1 Tbs. fresh
2 tsp. dulse flakes
2 tsp. Liquid pHlavor Salt
Pinch each of cumin, curry, and Zip (Spice Hunter)

In a food processor or blender, combine the almonds with the water or broth and process until smooth. Add the onion, red pepper, garlic, lemon, oil, oregano, dulse flakes, salt, and spices. Blend until smooth, using additional water if necessary to achieve your desired consistency. This can be a great dressing for salad or a dip with dehydrated veggies added. Enjoy!

Esther's Creamy Mayo

MAKES 1¼ CUPS

2 fresh young coconuts (meat only)
2 Tbsp. lemon juice
½ tsp. whole unprocessed salt
¼ tsp. mild mustard powder
½ tsp. garlic powder
¾ cup olive oil

Combine all ingredients except the olive oil in a blender and blend. Slowly drizzle the oil into the mixture while you continue to blend. Store in the refrigerator with an airtight lid.

Note: Use only the meat of the coconut; you can save the water for another purpose. Try pouring it into ice cube trays, freezing it, and using it instead of plain ice cubes in a shake. It will slightly sweeten your shake.

Green Mayonnaise

SERVES 6–8

1 lb. tofu, drained
2 avocados
½ Tbs. curry powder
3 Tbs. lemon juice
Salt, to taste
Zip (Spice Hunter), to taste

Place all ingredients in a food processor and process until smooth and creamy.

Garbanzo Spread

SERVES 6–8 (3 CUPS)

2 cups sprouted or canned garbanzo beans (chickpeas)
1 chopped medium onion
2 Tbs. dried parsley
1 tsp. Real Salt
1 tsp. coriander
Dash of cayenne or chili powder
¼ cup water

Blend all ingredients in a blender until smooth. Spread on sprouted whole wheat tortillas and top with alfalfa sprouts, or use with veggies.

Zippy Garbanzo Spread

SERVES 6–8 (3 CUPS)

4 cups sprouted, cooked garbanzo beans (chickpeas)
3 Tbs. tahini
3 lemons or limes
5–6 cloves garlic, pressed
1 medium onion, chopped
2 Tbs. dried parsley
Dash of cumin
1 tsp. Real Salt
1 tsp. coriander
Dash of cayenne, chili powder, or Spice Hunter's Zip
¼ cup water

Blend all ingredients in a blender until smooth. Spread on sprouted whole wheat tortillas, topped with alfalfa sprouts, or eat with veggies.

Tahini (Sesame Seed Butter)

SERVES 6

1 cup sesame seeds
2 tsp. flax seed oil (or preferred oil)

Combine the ingredients in a food processor or blender. Blend into a smooth paste. This is a protein food, for use with nonstarchy vegetables. Use it up quickly. Keep refrigerated, tightly covered.

Sweet Carrot Butter

SERVES 8–10

This is a sweet, creamy spread that is wonderful on wraps or used as a dip for raw veggies. It's especially nice when something sweet is called for. Kids like this one, too.

2 cups raw macadamias
2–3 shredded organic carrots
Vanilla or stevia, to taste
Olive oil and water, to thin

In a food processor, mix the nuts and carrots and process until smooth and creamy. Add a few drops of vanilla or a couple of drops of stevia while processing if desired. While the processor is running, add olive oil and/or water to reach your desired consistency.

TOPPINGS

AvoRado AvoCado Topping

SERVES 6

This is a great topping that is all raw and will work well with various seasonings of your choice. It is great as a veggie dip or wonderful when spooned on top of Millet/Buckwheat Oven Cakes (page 363).

1 cup raw almonds
½ cup oil (I use olive)
¼ cup water
1 avocado
2 Tbs. lemon or lime juice (I use both)
½–1 tsp. Real Salt
½–1 tsp. Spice Hunter spices (I use Mexican Seasoning or Zip)
⅓ cup chopped red pepper
⅓ cup chopped red onion
1 carrot

Place the almonds in a Vita-Mix and grind to a powder, then add the oil, water, avocado, lemon or lime juice, salt, and seasonings of choice. Mix well in a blender, coaxing the batter down the sides with a spatula. Take out of the blender and put in a bowl.

In a food processor, finely chop the red pepper and red onion, then put the shredding blade on and shred the carrot into the red pepper and onion mixture. Stir everything together and then spoon into the avocado mixture in the bowl. Stir until well combined and chill before serving.

Ginger-Almond Paste Topping

SERVES 2–3

This recipe is similar to the Wowie Zowie Almond Butter Dressing (page 298), but much thicker. Try it on Millet Yam Hash Browns (page 361) hot out of the oven.

½ cup almonds (I've used ½ cup almond butter in a pinch, or you could use other nuts, such as macadamias or pecans)
¼–½ tsp. Real Salt (to taste)
Juice of 1 lemon
1 Tbs. minced fresh ginger
½ tsp. dried onion
1 clove garlic, minced (could be roasted for a nice flavor difference)

Put all ingredients into a food processor and let it fly! Add water to thin if desired.

Basic Seasoning

SERVES 6–8

1½ oz. onion powder
½ oz. garlic powder
2 oz. comfrey leaf or celery leaf powder, or a mix
½ tsp. red cayenne pepper
½ tsp. whole pure salts
½ oz. gingerroot powder

Mix all ingredients together. Store in a tightly capped jar and use as a vegetable seasoning.

Herb Oil

SERVES 4 (¾ CUP)

½ cup flax seed, olive, Essential Balance, or Udo's oil
2 Tbs. lemon juice
½ tsp. Real Salt

⅛ tsp. freshly ground black pepper
¼ cup finely chopped fresh parsley
½ tsp. dried tarragon leaves
Dash of cayenne pepper

Mix all ingredients well. Store in a jar in the refrigerator. Great on salads and steamed veggies.

Green Pepper Relish

MAKES 5 CUPS

6 large green peppers
2 small fresh hot chili peppers
Flax seed oil
Whole pure salts, to taste
Cumin, to taste

In preheated 450-degree oven, place the green peppers and chili peppers in a shallow baking dish. Bake for 20 minutes, turning once. Put the peppers in a pan of cold water, skin them, and remove the seeds. Chop the peppers very fine. Add enough flax seed oil to create a spreading consistency. Season with whole pure salts and cumin to taste. For sweeter relish, use red peppers instead of green. Store in a jar with a tight lid in the refrigerator.

Dehydrated Red Bell Pepper Powder

MAKES ABOUT ½ CUP

This is a very concentrated flavorful seasoning powder made simply from red bell peppers. Sprinkle over anything where you want color plus a deep, rich, sweet flavor. I use it on salads, in soups and wraps, and over nut milks and puddings. We also snack on dehydrated red bell pepper strips as if they were red licorice, and sometimes eat the powder by the spoonful for a treat.

10 large red bell peppers, stemmed, cored, and cut into ½-inch slices.

Place the red pepper slices on dehydrator trays and dry until snap-crisp (usually about 24 hours, or at least overnight). Transfer into a blender (I use a Vita-Mix) and grind into a fine powder. Store in an airtight container.

FILLINGS

Fresh Spinach Filling

SERVES 6

1¼ cups finely chopped fresh spinach
3 Tbs. Mock Mayo (page 311)
1 Tbs. chopped pimiento
¼ tsp. onion powder

Combine all ingredients and mix well. Season to taste. Delicious in sprouted wheat tortillas.

Crispy Radish Filling

SERVES 6

¾ cup finely chopped celery
½ cup finely chopped radishes
¼ cup Mock Mayo (page 311)
1 Tbs. chopped chives
¼ tsp. Real Salt
Few grains of pepper

Combine all ingredients and mix well. Great for stuffing celery, on sprouted wheat bread, or on sprouted wheat tortilla roll-ups.

Garden Variety Filling

SERVES 6

¾ cup grated carrot
½ cup finely chopped celery
2 Tbs. grated jalapeño soy cheese
3 Tbs. Mock Mayo (page 311)
1 Tbs. finely chopped green pepper
1 Tbs. Liquid pHlavor Salt
¼ tsp. Real Salt
¼ tsp. cayenne pepper
Few grains of black pepper

Combine all ingredients and mix well. Excellent for stuffing celery sticks or to eat with vegetables.

Hearty Nut Filling

SERVES 6

½ cup almond butter
¼ cup finely chopped green pepper
¼ cup grated carrot
1 tsp. minced onion
¼ cup Mock Mayo (page 311)
1½ tsp. salt
½ medium red onion, finely chopped

Mix all ingredients; you can put them in a food processor if desired. Excellent for stuffing celery sticks or with vegetables.

SAUCES

Tahini Tofu Sauce

SERVES 2 (⅔ CUP)

Serve this creamy, cool sauce with Baked Falafel Fritters (page 334), or use as a dip for fresh veggie stix or on top of steamed veggies. It can also be used as a main spread in a wrap!

1 garlic clove, finely chopped
2 Tbs. (or more) fresh lemon or lime juice
¼ cup tahini
½–1 tsp. salt (or 1½ tsp. Liquid pHlavor Salt)
1 Tbs. olive oil
⅓ cup soft silken tofu (Nori brand)
Sesame seeds, raw or toasted, for garnish

In the food processor, put the garlic, lemon juice, tahini, and salt. Process until combined. With the machine running, slowly add the olive oil through the feed tube, then add the soft tofu and pulse until smooth. Garnish with sesame seeds. This sauce can be stored in the refrigerator in an airtight container for a day or two.

To dry-toast sesame seeds, heat a heavy skillet over medium-low heat. Add the sesame seeds and shake the skillet gently to move the seeds around so that they toast evenly and do not burn. Toast the seeds until they are aromatic and barely take on color. Allow them to cool slightly before serving.

Lime Ginger Sauce

SERVES 4–6

This makes a wonderful sauce, dressing, or marinade.

¼ cup lime juice
¼ cup oil (flax seed, olive, or Udo's Choice)
1 Tbs. Liquid pHlavor Salt
¼ cup water
1 Tbs. fresh mint
1 Tbs. fresh cilantro
1 tsp. minced gingerroot
¼ tsp. dried red chili pepper
2–3 tsp. fresh jicama or carrot juice
1 tsp. Real Salt, to taste
Dash of Zip (Spice Hunter)

In a processor or blender, combine all ingredients and blend well.

Rich Raw Tomato Sauce

SERVES 4–6

This is a wonderfully fresh-tasting raw tomato sauce that goes great over pasta. I use it over raw yellow crookneck squash angel hair, which I make with a gadget called the Saladacco. It also is a wonderful dipping sauce, and can be served cold or warmed but not cooked.

3–5 sun-dried tomatoes (I use Melissa's brand packed in olive oil)
4 fresh, firm tomatoes, chopped
½ cup fresh basil, chopped
1 tsp. dried onion
1 tsp. roasted garlic
1 tsp. Real Salt

Put all the ingredients in a food processor and blend to your desired consistency. Store in an airtight container in the refrigerator for up to 3 days.

Variation: Instead of the fresh basil and roasted garlic, just use ¼–⅓ cup Garlic Galore brand pesto. This is a lovely dairy-less pesto that is also great on wraps. It is found in most large health food stores.

Spring's Pesto

SERVES 4

6 cloves garlic
4 cups fresh basil or 1 cup dried basil
1 cup fresh parsley
6 Tbs. raw nuts (pine, almond, hazelnut, pumpkin—I use a combination
    and soak them overnight)
1 cup or more olive oil
½ tsp. Real Salt
½ tsp. pepper
2 Tbs. sun-dried tomatoes

Combine all ingredients in a food processor (with an S-blade) or in a blender. Blend until smooth.

Maren's Salsa

SERVES 6–8

6 cloves minced garlic
1 yellow onion, finely chopped
½ cup finely chopped fresh cilantro
½ cup finely chopped fresh parsley
7 ripe tomatoes, finely chopped
1 green pepper, finely chopped
1 red pepper, finely chopped
Juice of 1 lemon and 1 lime (about 10 Tbs.)
Real Salt, to taste
Mexican Seasoning (Spice Hunter), to taste
Cajun Seasoning (Tone's), to taste
Cayenne pepper, to taste
Cumin, to taste

Blend together and refrigerate.

Tomato Gravy

SERVES 6–8

1 qt. peeled tomatoes, pureed
1 small eggplant, diced
6 Tbs. finely chopped green pepper
3 Tbs. olive oil
Real Salt, to taste

Cook the pureed tomatoes in a saucepan over medium heat. After 15 minutes of cooking the puree, stir in the eggplant and pepper and shut off the heat. When the mixture has cooled slightly, add the remaining ingredients and blend. Serve warm on raw or steamed zucchini.

Tomato Sauce

SERVES 4–6 (ABOUT 3½ CUPS)

½ cup chopped onion
½ cup vegetable stock
3 cups coarsely chopped tomatoes
½ tsp. oregano
½ tsp. thyme
½ tsp. basil
1 tsp. garlic powder
Freshly ground pepper

Cook the onion in the stock until soft. Add the tomatoes, then other herbs and spices as desired. Bring to a boil, cover, and simmer for 30 to 45 minutes. Store in a glass jar and refrigerate until ready to use. For good food combination, eat with celery, bell peppers, cucumbers, eggplant, okra, or summer squash.

Italian Tomato Sauce

SERVES 14 (½-CUP SERVINGS)

2 (28-oz.) cans Italian tomatoes (crushed)
1 tsp. basil
½ tsp. oregano
1 (6-oz.) can tomato paste
1 bay leaf
5 tsp. minced garlic
½ tsp. cayenne pepper

Mix all the ingredients; simmer on the stove for 2 hours. Use in your favorite Italian recipe or serve over spaghetti.

Sauce Sampler Platter

SERVES 8–12

This is a great way to serve a variety of tastes and textures. It makes a great appetizer or can be used as a main meal for anytime. It's wonderful for parties, too!

Roasted Pepper Macadamia Sauce (page 338)
Sweet Carrot Butter (page 314)
Spring's Pesto (page 322)
Yummus Hummus (page 305)
Maren's Salsa (page 322)
Raw veggies of your choice (for example, carrot sticks, bell pepper strips,
    broccoli and cauliflower florets, raw yam slices, cucumbers, jicama
    sticks)
Baked tortilla chips
Crackers

On a plate, scoop a big mound of each of the sauces, and serve with veggies, crackers, and chips for dipping.

Entrées

Very Veggie Barley Burgers

SERVES 6–8

These hearty burgers have a great meat-like texture. Barley is higher in protein than rice or other grains, and is a great source of fiber. Try different seasonings to give these burgers the flavor you like.

2 cups steamed pearled barley (cook as you do rice)
1 cup veggie broth
⅓ cup flax seeds, ground
1 cup any raw shelled nuts: almonds, pine nuts, walnuts, pecans, macadamias, or sunflower seeds
2 zucchini, chopped (or shredded in food processor)
3 onions, peeled and chopped (or shredded in food processor)
2 tomatoes, chopped (or shredded in food processor)
4 carrots, peeled and chopped (or shredded in food processor)
2 cloves garlic, peeled and chopped (or shredded in food processor)
2 cups sprouted wheat tortilla crumbs (dry and grind in blender or food processor into flour)
2 Tbs. dried herbs of choice (Spice Hunter has several good blends) *or* 3 Tbs. fresh herbs of choice
1 tsp. whole unprocessed salt, or more to taste

Preheat the oven to 375 degrees. Stir together the barley, veggie broth, and ground flax seeds in a bowl. Combine with the remaining ingredients; mix well. Divide the mixture into even portions, form into patties, and arrange on an oiled cookie sheet. Bake until golden brown, approximately 15 minutes on each side. Serve hot, or cool and crumble over a salad.

Sprouted Cereal

SERVES 2

2 cups wheat or rye grains (organic, unstored)
½–1 tsp. cinnamon

Soak the grain overnight in distilled water. Drain and set the jar on its side
to sprout. Rinse the sprouts morning and evening, and let them sprout for
2 days.

Add enough water to the sprouts to blend in a blender. Pour into a saucepan and cook until toasty warm. May be served in a bowl with soy milk.

Blackened Herbed Fillets

SERVES 4–6

*This is a somewhat spicy coating that could be used for red snapper, trout, salmon,
or even extra-firm tofu that has been sliced thin (¼ to ⅓ inch). I usually double or
triple this recipe, because I like a heavy coating on the fillets.*

3 Tbs. paprika
2½ tsp. dried onions
½ tsp. Zip (Spice Hunter) or cayenne pepper (start with ¼ tsp; you can
    always add more)
1½ tsp. dried thyme
1½ tsp. dried oregano
1½ tsp. dried basil
¾ tsp. ground cumin
1 tsp. Real Salt
½ cup grape seed oil
4–6 fresh fish or tofu fillets (4–6 oz.)
¼ cup mint leaves (fresh), minced for garnish
Lemon and lime wedges

Combine all the dry seasonings except the mint in a shallow bowl and mix
well. Put the oil into another shallow bowl. Set the bowls side by side. Heat
an electric fry pan or large skillet-type pan on a burner over high heat. Dip
the fillets in the oil and coat well, then dip into the herb mixture and coat

both sides. Cook in the hot pan on one side until the herbs turn dark but not burned (1 to 3 minutes), then flip over and cook on the other side.

Sprinkle minced mint on top of the fillets and garnish with lemon and lime wedges before serving.

Note: To cook fish more thoroughly, I sometimes fry it first, over medium heat, for a while until it's cooked through. Then I dip it in the oil and coat and fry on the outside for a crisper finish.

Tofu Salad Spread

SERVES 4 (3½ CUPS)

8 oz. fresh tofu, well drained
¾ cup chopped green onion
1 cup finely chopped celery
¾ cup finely chopped carrot
6 Tbs. Mock Mayo (page 311)
1 Tbs. dried parsley
¼ tsp. basil
¼ tsp. sage
¼ tsp. thyme
1½ tsp. vegetable salt or Real Salt
½ tsp. garlic powder
⅛ tsp. cayenne pepper

Mix all the ingredients. Serve on a bed of greens.

Tofu Patties

SERVES 6

1 carton fresh tofu, drained
3 Tbs. chopped onion
½ Tbs. vegetable broth mix
1 cup grated zucchini
³⁄₈ tsp. Real Salt
Egg replacer equal to 2 eggs

Slice the tofu and steam for 5 to 10 minutes. Chop and drain well. Steam-fry the onion. Add the vegetable broth mix and zucchini and stir well. Add the salt, tofu, and egg replacer and combine. Make into patties. Put on sprayed baking sheets and flatten slightly. Bake lightly at 350 degrees. Turn the patties when the bottoms are barely brown. Finish baking—do not overbake.

Broc & Brussels

Serves 6–8

This is a hearty green dish that is great anytime, even breakfast.

1 lb. brussels sprouts, washed and ends trimmed
Grape seed or coconut oil
1 tsp. Herbamare and/or garlic salt
3 cups broccoli, cut into individual florets
2-4 Tbs. sun-dried tomatoes (preferably organic)
¼ tsp. whole unprocessed salt
2 Tbs. Manitoba Hemp Seed Oil
⅓ cup olive oil
3 Tbs. pine nuts

Preheat the oven to 350 degrees. Cut the brussels sprouts in half, rinse them thoroughly in salt water, and drain. Lay out on a cookie sheet. Drizzle with grape seed or coconut oil and sprinkle liberally with Herbamare and/or garlic salt. Roast for 30 minutes. Meanwhile, steam the broccoli for 10 to 15 minutes, then rinse in cold water to avoid overcooking. Chop the sun-dried tomatoes with some oil from the jar in a food processor, using the S-blade, until it forms a chunky paste. Cut the roasted brussels sprouts and steamed broccoli into smaller bite-size pieces, if desired, and stir together with 1 to 2 Tbs. of the sun-dried tomato paste, the hemp and olive oils, the unprocessed salt, and the pine nuts.

Sprouted Bean Casserole

SERVES 6

1 large onion, chopped
1 clove garlic, finely chopped
3 cups chopped leeks
3 Tbs. Liquid pHlavor Salt
Freshly ground pepper, to taste
1 large red or green pepper, finely chopped
1 cup mung beans, sprouted
1 cup baby lima beans, sprouted
1 cup pinto beans, sprouted

Steam-fry the onion and garlic. Add the leeks, salt, and pepper. Simmer for 15 minutes. Add the chopped pepper and simmer for 5 minutes. Pour over the sprouted beans in a casserole dish. Stir gently. Bake at 350 degrees for 15 minutes.

Tofu Stew

SERVES 8

2 medium onions, sliced
3 cups water
1 bay leaf
3 kale leaves, torn into bite-size pieces
1½ cups fresh green beans
2 leeks, cut into bite-size pieces
3 large onions, quartered
1 pkg. fresh tofu, firmness of choice

In a 3-quart pan with a lid, steam-fry the sliced onions. Add the water, bay leaf, and kale. Cover and simmer until the kale begins to soften. Remove the bay leaf. Add the green beans, leeks, and quartered onions and continue to simmer until the beans are tender.

Meanwhile, drain and slice the tofu and add it to the pan to warm, or steam separately in a steamer. Season if desired. Arrange tofu on top of the stew to serve.

Doc Broc Casserole

SERVES 6

This is a great casserole guaranteed to fool your kids into thinking they are eating hamburger. Little kids and big kids alike will love the herbed potato chips sprinkled on top.

Florets from 2 large bunches broccoli (save leaves and stalks; peel and clean stalks)
1 cup soft tofu
1 tsp. ground mustard seed (I use hot)
1 small bunch fresh basil or fresh tarragon, stemmed and minced
Whole pure salts and pepper, to taste (could use Spice Hunter's Zip)
2/3 cup olive oil
1 pkg. Lightlife Smart Ground (a soy protein substitute that resembles ground beef)
1 pkg. Terra Red Bliss Potato Chips (I use the olive oil and fine herbs flavor)

Steam the broccoli with a little water in a covered pan for about 4 to 5 minutes, until it's bright green and just crisp-tender.

Mince the broccoli leaves and peeled stalks in a food processor until very fine (scrape down the sides if necessary).

Add the soft tofu, mustard, basil or tarragon, salt, and pepper into the food processor with the fine broccoli mixture and process. While the machine is running, slowly add the olive oil until well emulsified and let the processor run until the mix is creamy and mixed well.

In a large electric fry pan, heat a small amount of oil, add the Smart Ground, crumble it up, and fry it for a couple of minutes, then add the steamed broccoli and pour the sauce (from the food processor) over the top. Stir in, mixing well.

With a rolling pin, mash the Terra Potato Chips while they're still in the bag until they are crumbs. Then sprinkle over the top of the broccoli mixture and serve.

Ashley's Vegetable Nori Roll-Ups

Serves 4–6 (2–3 rolls)

Juice of 1 lemon
2 Tbs. Liquid pHlavor Salt
1 tsp. extra-virgin olive oil or flax seed oil
Dash of cinnamon or cayenne pepper
2 carrots, slivered
3 scallions, slivered
1 avocado, slivered
1 zucchini, slivered
1 cucumber, slivered
2 cups cooked rice (basmati or brown)
1 pkg. nori sheets
Alfalfa sprouts
Buckwheat or sunflower seed sprouts

In a small bowl, combine the lemon juice, salt, oil, and cinnamon or cayenne. Place the vegetables in a shallow pan and pour the lemon juice mixture over them. Set aside.

Drain the vegetables thoroughly by tossing them in a colander or blotting them with paper towels.

Spread a thin layer of rice over each nori sheet, leaving about a ⅓-inch nori border at the end. Arrange the marinated vegetables on the sheets, top them with a lot of sprouts, and roll them up (I use a sushi mat for this). Let them sit until they will hold their form and cut into bite-size pieces with a sharp knife.

Variations: Use any vegetables and sprouts you like. You can also serve with dips or sauces on top.

Stuffed Cabbage Rolls

SERVES 4

1 medium head cabbage
1 bay leaf
1 clove garlic
1 cup finely chopped onion
1 pkg. drained fresh tofu (break into fine pieces)
⅛ tsp. black pepper
½ tsp. Real Salt or vegetized salt
1 tsp. Liquid pHlavor Salt
3 cups vegetable broth, cold
½ cup vegetable broth mix

Grease a shallow, 2-quart range-top casserole with a tight-fitting lid. Remove and discard any wilted outer leaves from the cabbage. Rinse it and cut in half through the core. Remove eight large leaves. Shred enough remaining cabbage to yield 2 cups and spread it into the casserole dish. Add the bay leaf and garlic clove; set the casserole aside.

Pour boiling water into a large pan to the 1-inch level. Add the eight leaves of cabbage and the Real salt. Cover and simmer for 2 to 3 minutes.

Meanwhile, steam-fry the chopped onion, tofu, pepper, and liquid salt. Place ¼ cup of this mixture into the center of each of the eight cabbage leaves and roll up each leaf, tucking the ends in. Secure with wooden picks and place on the shredded cabbage in a casserole dish.

Stir the veggie broth mix into the cold veggie broth and pour over the cabbage rolls with a few grains of pepper. Cover and simmer over low heat for 30 minutes. Remove the bay leaf and picks and serve.

Curried Squash Dhal

SERVES 8

You can use any kind of squash for this wonderfully warm dish. This can be made thick as a stew and served over rice or thinned down as a soup that's great to start the day on a wintry morning!

1 medium yellow onion, quartered
½ can unsweetened coconut or almond milk

3 cloves garlic, sliced
2 serrano or Thai chili peppers, seeded and diced
1 Tbs. minced fresh gingerroot
2 tsp. garam masala
2–4 sun-dried tomatoes, minced
1 tsp. ground cumin
½ tsp. cinnamon
1 tsp. Real Salt
¼ tsp. turmeric
¼ tsp. ground coriander
2 cups vegetable stock or water, divided
1 Tbs. Udo's Choice oil or olive oil
2 cups fresh tomatoes, diced
4 cups peeled and diced butternut squash
2 cups cooked black-eyed beans or lentils
1 cup green peas
2 cups chopped spinach or kale
3 Tbs. minced mint

Combine the onion, almond milk, garlic, chili peppers, gingerroot, garam masala, sun-dried tomatoes, cumin, cinnamon, salt, turmeric, coriander, and 3 Tbs. of the stock or water in a blender. Puree the mixture to a paste, scraping down the sides of the blender a few times.

Heat the oil in a large saucepan, then add the spice paste and cook, stirring often, for 10 minutes. Add the remaining stock, tomatoes, and butternut squash. Cook over medium heat, stirring often, until the squash is just tender, about 20 minutes.

Mix in the black-eyed beans, green peas, and spinach. Continue to cook, stirring often, until the spinach is tender, about 10 more minutes. Remove from the heat. Taste and adjust the seasonings. Stir in the mint just before serving. Yum!

Baked Falafel Fritters

Serves 8 (2½ dozen)

This recipe is wonderfully fast to whip up in your food processor. Fresh cilantro and the red hot chili pepper add fun color. (The red hot chili pepper is not that hot, but remember to take the ribs and seeds out of the middle first.) I serve these warm in cabbage leaves or butter lettuce leaves, rolled up as hors d'oeuvres, but they would also make a great side dish to a big salad or could even be thrown into a wrap or pita sandwich! These are very hearty because they have both chickpeas and beans, making them high in calcium and protein. I use different kinds of beans to change the flavor and color of the fritters. The other plus is that they are baked instead of deep-fried like most falafel.

Serve with Tahini Tofu Sauce (page 320).

¼ cup coarsely chopped fresh parsley
¼ cup coarsely chopped fresh cilantro
1½ cups canned chickpeas, rinsed and drained (15-oz. can)
8 oz. (1 cup) beans, soaked overnight (drain well and cook in boiling water
    for about 10 minutes, or you could use canned in a pinch. I use black-
    eyed beans, cranberry beans, or lima beans)
1 clove garlic, minced
1 tsp. cumin
1 tsp. turmeric
1 tsp. salt
¼ cup chopped red onion
1 red hot chili pepper, seeds and ribs removed, minced
1 Tbs. fresh lime juice
3 Tbs. flour (spelt, millet, or whole wheat)
2 heads butter lettuce or savoy cabbage, leaves separated; tear big ones in
    half
6 cherry tomatoes, quartered, or 1 small tomato, finely chopped
Tahini Tofu Sauce (page 320)
1 Tbs. toasted or raw sesame seeds

In the bowl of a food processor, process the parsley and the cilantro until fine. Add the chickpeas, beans, garlic, cumin, turmeric, salt, red onion, chili pepper, and lime juice. Pulse until the mixture forms a very thick paste that is fairly smooth (this will involve scraping the sides down and processing a few times). Add the flour and pulse to combine. Transfer the mixture to a bowl and set aside. This mixture can be made one day ahead and refrigerated in an airtight container.

On a nonstick cookie sheet, drop the falafel mixture 1 Tbs. at a time and bake at 350 degrees for 10 to 12 minutes. You can also brush these with olive oil and bake until golden brown if you like.

Serve each fritter warm on a piece of lettuce or cabbage cup. Garnish with the tomatoes, a dollop of Tahini Tofu Sauce, and a sprinkling of sesame seeds. Wrap the cabbage around the fritter and eat like a finger food hors d'oeuvre, or serve by a salad for a great meal!

Shelley's Super Wraps

Serves 4

Wraps are today's answer to healthy fast food. If you stock your refrigerator with some basics, you can make a wrap in just a few minutes. They travel well, and if you include your favorite spices, they can be to-die-for delicious!

4 tortillas (see notes)
1 cup Yummus Hummus (page 305) or other hummus
1 jar pesto (I use Garlic Galore brand) or Spring's Pesto recipe (page 322)
1 head romaine lettuce or any other preferred lettuce or greens (most of the time, I just dig into our Rainbow Salad, page 286, for the greens to fill in these wraps)
½ cup soaked almonds
8 sun-dried tomatoes (bottled in olive oil)
½ red, yellow, orange, or green pepper, sliced thin
2 carrots, chopped or shredded
1 cup chopped broccoli
1 cup chopped cauliflower
½ red onion, sliced
4–8 cloves roasted garlic
1 pkg. sunflower seed sprouts
1 (8-oz.) pkg. raw pine nuts
Juice of 1 lemon or lime
Favorite spices, to taste

Lay each tortilla flat and spread with hummus or nondairy pesto (I always use both!), or any spread you like. The Roasted Pepper Macadamia Sauce (page 338) and even the Raw Pecan Pâté (page 307) also work well. Then lay several leaves of romaine lettuce down the center. You could also use any other lettuce or even mixed green salad. On top of the green lettuce, place any of the ingredient items. Then roll up the wrap and secure tightly in plastic wrap (a couple of layers). Repeat with the remaining tortillas. Eat immediately, or at least on the same day, as the tortilla can become soggy. Enjoy!

Notes: You can start with tortillas made from the Shelley's Super Tortillas recipe (page 370) or sprouted wheat tortillas from the health food store; sometimes you can get a "wraps" café or restaurant to sell you its tortillas, and can keep them in the freezer or fridge. Look for hummus and nondairy pesto at your local health food store.

Nepal Vegetable Curry

SERVES 4–6

1 onion, chopped
1 bay leaf, broken
1 green chili, chopped
1 clove garlic, minced
1-inch piece ginger, grated
¼ tsp. turmeric
Whole pure salts or vegetized salt to taste
1 lb. carrots, cubed
½ cauliflower, broken into florets
1 cup green peas
1 tsp. each coriander and cumin
1 cup hot water

Lightly steam-fry the onion. Add the bay leaf, chili, garlic, ginger, turmeric, and salt. Stir in the carrots and sauté lightly. Add the remaining ingredients. Cook gently over medium heat until the vegetables are tender.

Tofu Italian Mock Meatballs

SERVES 8–10 (TEN 2-INCH OR FORTY 1-INCH BALLS)

This is a great transitional food when you're phasing off meat. If wild rice is used, a sweet nutty flavor will result. The meatballs can be served warm for a main course, and also make a great cool snack right out of the fridge. (I always double this recipe, because everyone loves them!)

8–10 sprouted wheat tortillas
2 celery stalks with leaves, finely chopped
1 medium red onion, finely chopped
2 cloves garlic, minced
2 lbs. firm tofu (Nigari), crumbled
1 cup vegetable stock (Pacific Foods of Oregon brand)
¼ cup whole rolled oats
3 Tbs. Liquid pHlavor Salt
2 cups finely chopped fresh basil
1 cup parsley
¼ tsp. black pepper, freshly ground
2 tsp. Zip (Spice Hunter) or pinch of cayenne pepper
½ cup cooked brown rice
½ cup cooked wild rice
1 Tbs. olive oil
Herbes de Provence, to taste (about 1 tsp.)

Leave the tortillas out to dry on a counter, or quick-dry them in a low-heat oven. Break them into small pieces and blend in a Vita-Mix or food processor until they are finely ground into crumbs. Set aside in a bowl.

In an electric skillet, steam-fry the celery, onion, and garlic, cooking until softened, about 6 minutes. Transfer to a large bowl. Put the tofu, vegetable stock, oats, and salt in a blender and blend until smooth. Add the basil, parsley, black pepper, Zip, and Herbes de Provence; pulse until well blended. Add to the onion mixture.

Add the cooked brown and wild rice to the onion mixture, along with the tortilla crumbs to create a mixture that's slightly sticky but forms into balls easily.

Preheat the oven to 400 degrees. Lightly oil a baking dish or cookie sheet. Shape the mixture into balls and roll each ball into the remaining tortilla crumbs to coat. Bake until lightly browned, 20 to 30 minutes. Serve with Roasted Pepper Macadamia Sauce (below) to dip the balls in. Enjoy!

Roasted Pepper Macadamia Sauce

SERVES 6–8

This is a rich, beautifully colored sauce that can be made thick for dipping with grilled tofu slices or the Tofu Italian Mock Meatballs. Or it can be thinned and used as a wow salad dressing.

4–5 big pieces of roasted red peppers (you can roast them or buy bottled)
6 cloves roasted garlic
3 large fresh basil leaves
½–1 cup olive oil, divided
1 lb. macadamia nuts (raw is best; roasted will give a different flavor)
Whole pure salts and pepper, to taste

Put the roasted bell peppers, garlic, basil leaves, and a third of the oil in a food processor and process until well blended. With the machine still running, add the macadamias down through the top and continue blending until well emulsified. Finally, add the rest of the oil with the machine still running; add water to thin, if desired.

Cabbage Stuffed with Vegetables

SERVES 6

8 cabbage leaves
1 cup French-style green beans
1 Tbs. dehydrated onion flakes moistened with tomato juice or veggie
    broth
2 celery stalks
½ cup bean sprouts
½ green bell pepper
1 tsp. chopped parsley
2 cups vegetable broth
Liquid pHlavor Salt, to taste

Flax seed oil, to taste
Cayenne pepper, to taste

Scald the cabbage leaves with boiling water and leave them covered in the pot for 30 minutes. Chop all the vegetables fine, add the parsley, and mix. Spoon the vegetable mixture onto each cabbage leaf. Roll tight and tuck in the ends. Fasten with toothpicks and simmer in the vegetable broth for 1 hour. Serve, seasoning with salt, flax seed oil, and cayenne pepper.

Cajun-Style Red Beans and Brown Rice

Serves 8

1 lb. dried pinto beans
2 cups chopped yellow onion
1 cup chopped green onion
1 cup chopped green bell pepper
½ tsp. minced garlic
¼ tsp. red cayenne pepper
¾ tsp. black pepper
½ tsp. Real Salt
¼ tsp. oregano
¼ tsp. garlic powder
1 oz. Liquid pHlavor Salt
6 oz. tomato paste
¼ tsp. thyme
1 tsp. celery flakes
6 cups cooked brown rice

Wash the beans and then soak them for 12 hours. Drain the water. Fill a large pot with the beans, adding water to ½ inch above them. Add the remaining ingredients except the rice, and cook over low heat 2 to 2½ hours, covered. Serve over cooked brown rice.

Beans and Rice

SERVES 4–6

2 cups dried beans such as kidney, pinto, or garbanzo, soaked and cooked
    according to package directions, drained
½ tsp. cumin
½ tsp. chili powder
1 tsp. Real Salt
1–2 cloves minced garlic, to taste
2 cups vegetable broth
¼ cup chopped fresh parsley
½ onion, chopped
1 red bell pepper, chopped
2 carrots, grated
Whole pure salts
2–3 tomatoes, chopped
Basmati or brown rice

Season the beans with the cumin, chili powder, salt, and garlic. Add enough
of the vegetable broth to just cover the bean mixture. Stir in the parsley,
onion, pepper, and carrots, and simmer until the onion is soft. Add whole
pure salts to taste. Mix in the tomatoes just before serving with a scoop of
basmati or brown rice. In a pinch, you could also use canned beans. For
a more raw and energizing dish, use sprouted beans such as garbanzo or
lentils.

Stuffed Acorn Squash

SERVES 4

Nonstick vegetable spray
2 small acorn squash, halved and seeded
¼ cup water
½ cup diced onion
½ cup diced carrot
½ cup diced red bell pepper
½ cup thickly sliced zucchini
½ tsp. minced garlic

Preheat the oven to 350 degrees. Spray a large baking dish with cooking spray. Steam the acorn squash halves by placing the cut sides down in a pan on the stovetop with ¼ cup water for 10 to 15 minutes. Lightly steam-fry remaining ingredients, a few minutes only, stirring frequently. Spoon the vegetables into the squash halves. Bake for 20 to 25 minutes or until the squash is tender.

Autumn Curry Crêpes with Curried Veggie Filling

Serves 6

This wonderfully colorful Thai-tasting dish can be served as an hors d'oeuvre, snack, or side dish to your main course. Serve the crêpes fresh from the grill as you make them, or save them in the fridge and fill them the next morning for a really spicy warm breakfast!

1 cup almond milk (I use Pacific Foods of Oregon brand)
3 Tbs. unsweetened coconut milk
1½ tsp. egg replacer or 1½ Tbs. agar agar flakes (seaweed gel, found in your health food store)
⅓ cup water
1 Tbs. olive oil
½ tsp. turmeric
¼ tsp. curry powder
Dash of cinnamon
1 cup all-purpose flour (or spelt, millet, or whole wheat flour)
½ tsp. salt (optional)

In a bowl, whisk together the almond milk, coconut milk, egg replacer or agar agar flakes, water, oil, turmeric, cinnamon, and curry. Then whisk in the flour and salt until there are no lumps left in the batter. If you are using agar agar, put the mixture in a food processor and process until smooth. Put plastic wrap over the bowl and refrigerate for at least 30 minutes or up to 1 day.

Heat a small nonstick crêpe pan or skillet (I use my electric fry pan) over medium-low heat. If the batter has begun to separate, gently stir it to blend again. Once the pan is hot, drop 2 Tbs. of crêpe batter into the skillet and swirl the pan to coat the bottom evenly with the batter. If the batter does not swirl easily, add a little water to thin it down a bit. Cook the crêpe until the top appears dry, about a minute or two. Using a spatula, gently flip the crêpe and cook until the bottom appears lightly browned and the crêpe slides easily in the pan, about a minute or two more. Transfer the crêpe to a paper towel or plate. The crêpes may be made in advance and refrigerated or frozen.

Curried Veggie Filling

SERVES 6

This filling is spicy and colorful! You can substitute veggies of your choice—it always comes out tasty! This dish is especially good in the autumn or winter because of its warming spices and grounding effect from being cooked.

¼ cup olive oil
10–12 thin stalks asparagus, cut into 3-inch segments
½ cup snow peas
1 yellow onion, thinly sliced
4 cloves minced garlic
2 medium red bell peppers, seeds and ribs removed, cut into matchsticks
2 medium orange or yellow bell peppers, seeds and ribs removed, cut into matchsticks
1 Tbs. grated fresh ginger
1½ tsp. ground cumin
1 Tbs. curry powder
½ tsp. cinnamon
½–1 tsp. ground mustard seeds
1 tsp. whole pure salts, to taste
½ cup pine nuts
⅓ cup coconut milk (unsweetened)

Heat the olive oil in a large skillet or electric fry pan over medium-high heat. Add the asparagus and snow peas and cook, stirring constantly, until they barely begin to brighten and soften. Add the onion and garlic and reduce the heat to medium. Continue to cook until the onion softens a bit. Add the bell peppers and steam-fry with a little water if necessary to barely soften the peppers.

Add the ginger, cumin, curry, cinnamon, and mustard seeds, and a little more olive oil, and continue to stir-mix and cook. Add the salts, pine nuts, and coconut milk, and cook until the mixture reaches your desired softness. I keep my veggies medium-crisp. Serve warm with the Autumn Curry Crêpes (page 341), or serve over rice or any other cooked grain you prefer.

Cold Tofu Pockets

SERVES 2

1 tsp. sesame seeds
1 pkg. firm or extra-firm fresh tofu
3 scallions
¼ cup chopped fresh coriander
¼ red bell pepper
1 cup Liquid pHlavor Salt

Soak the sesame seeds overnight. Drain the tofu. Cut in half on the diagonal to form two triangles, then cut a pocket in each triangle. Finely chop the scallions, coriander, and pepper. Combine with the sesame seeds. Stuff half the scallion mixture into each piece of tofu. Pour Liquid pHlavor Salt over the tofu pockets and marinate in the refrigerator for 10 minutes before serving.

Vegetable Stir-Fry

SERVES 4

1 Tbs. oil
⅛-inch slice fresh ginger, pared
¼ tsp. Real Salt
1 small clove garlic, crushed
½ cup chopped broccoli (cut small)
½ cup cauliflower slices
½ cup red pepper strips
½ cup onion slices
1 cup pea pods
½ cup sliced celery
Whole pure salts, to taste

Preferred oil, to taste
Cayenne pepper, to taste

Put the oil, ginger, salt, and garlic into a wok or large skillet. Cook, uncovered, over heat that will not burn the oil, stirring constantly for 2 minutes. Add the broccoli, cauliflower, peppers, onions, pea pods, and celery, stirring constantly for 3 minutes. Shut off the heat, cover, and let set for 5 minutes. Serve, flavoring with whole pure salts, your preferred oil, and cayenne to taste. If the broccoli is not cooked sufficiently for your taste, try slightly steaming before adding.

20-Minute Alkaline Stir-Fry

SERVES 4

1 pkg. buckwheat soba noodles
½ package extra-firm tofu, cubed
Whole pure salts, to taste
Vegetable broth, as needed
1 red bell pepper, chopped
1 onion, chopped
1 head broccoli, cut into florets, and/or 1 bunch asparagus, cut into 1-inch
    lengths
Olive oil
Raw, unhulled sesame seeds
Garlic
Stir-fry spice combination and/or ginger

Break the noodles into fourths, prepare according to package directions, and drain. While the noodles are cooking, sauté the tofu, in a large pan, in a little whole pure salts and vegetable broth for about 5 minutes. Remove from the pan and set aside. Sauté the veggies for about 5 minutes in more whole pure salts and broth. Add the tofu and noodles. Sprinkle with olive oil, sesame seeds, garlic, and spices, and stir gently.

Vegetable Steam-Fry

Serves 4

1–2 tsp. grated fresh ginger (use a hand grater)
2–3 cloves garlic, crushed
½ cup chopped broccoli (cut small)
½ cup cauliflower slices
½ cup red pepper strips
½ cup onion slices
½ cup yellow squash
1 cup pea pods
Other veggies as desired, cut julienne
1 cup fried tofu (or use marinated tofu from the health food store)
¼ tsp. Real Salt

Steam-Fry Sauce

⅓ cup water or veggie stock
1 tsp. any Asian stir-fry spice containing ginger
Juice of ½ lemon or lime
Whole pure salts, to taste

Heat an electric fry pan. Add a small amount of water and steam-fry the ginger and garlic for a couple of minutes. Add the veggies, tofu, and salt, and steam-fry until the veggies are very bright and slightly softened. Pour the steam-fry sauce mixture over the top and steam for 1 or 2 more minutes. Serve immediately!

Variation: Sometimes I add pine nuts or pecans to enrich this dish!

Maren's Tortilla Pockets

SERVES 2–4

This makes two sealed-pocket sandwiches (four sections), and they are delicious! Serve with soup or salad. These little sealed sandwiches are a great way to hide the insides, too! Children especially love them. They would also make great appetizers.

2 large sprouted wheat tortillas or other tortillas
Filling of your choice, such as:
- ½ cup hummus, ½ cup rice, ¼ cup salsa
- ¼ cup pesto, ¾ cup steamed veggies, 1 tsp. almond butter
- ¼ cup salsa, ½ cup black beans, ½ cup cooked millet or buckwheat
- ½ cup avocado, ⅓ cup salsa, ½ cup grilled tofu cubes
- ¾ cup grated veggies, ¼ cup sun-dried tomatoes, ¼ cup soaked almonds, chopped
- 1 cup stir-fried veggies
- 1 cup Casserole de Cauliflower (page 368)

Preferred oil
Whole pure salts
Spices (optional), such as Mexican, Italian, barbecue (I use Spice Hunter brand)

Set up a sandwich press or grill, brush with oil. Make a cardboard pattern the size of your sandwich press. Set the heat on the appliance to medium to medium high and leave it open. Stack your tortillas. Place the pattern in the middle and, with a sharp knife, cut out tortillas. (Use extra pieces to make chips by baking on a cookie sheet at 325 degrees for 10 minutes.) Place one shaped tortilla on the bottom half of the appliance. Place fillings into center of each section of the press with a spoon, keeping it away from the edges, and season with salt and spices to taste. Place the second tortilla on top and close and lock the lid for about 3 minutes, or until lightly golden.

Serve with soup or salad or use as a healthy snack. You can make these ahead of time; they travel well. Experiment and come up with your own favorite combinations for fillings!

Sunrise Asian Salad

SERVES 4

This is a hearty, chewy salad with the addition of beans and wild rice.

½ cup adzuki beans
½ cup black beans
½ cup black-eyed peas
½ cup brown rice
½ cup wild rice
⅓ cup fresh lemon juice
1 Tbs. Liquid pHlavor Salt or 1 tsp. Real Salt
1 tsp. curry powder
1 clove fresh garlic, minced
1 tsp. Zip (Spice Hunter) or 2 tsp. black pepper
1-inch cube fresh ginger, grated
⅔ cup olive oil
½ medium red onion, sliced thin
1 carrot, julienned (use mandolin)
½ cup snow peas, trimmed and sliced
1 cup bean sprouts or 1 cup sprouts, any kind (I use Pro-Vita-Mix sprouts
   from Life Sprouts)

Place the beans and rice into a large bowl.

In a small food processor, place the lemon juice, salt, curry powder, garlic, pepper, and ginger. Gradually add the olive oil and process until well emulsified.

Pour the dressing over the beans-and-rice mixture. Add the remaining vegetables. Toss well and chill for 2 hours before serving.

Tofu Spinach Quiche

SERVES 6–8

Pastry

4 cups whole wheat flour
6 Tbs. preferred oil
Pinch of whole pure salts
A little cold water

Filling

2 onions (diced)
¾ cup vegetable oil
2 Tbs. chopped parsley
2 Tbs. dill weed
2 cups fresh spinach (chopped and cooked) *or* 2 (10-oz.) pkgs. frozen
    spinach, defrosted
Whole pure salts, to taste
2 cups tofu
¼ cup soy milk (if necessary)

Pastry

Combine the ingredients and knead the dough into a cohesive ball. Roll out
the pastry on a floured board, then press it into an oiled pie dish.

Filling

Sauté the onions in the oil until they are transparent. Add the parsley, dill
weed, spinach, and salts; mix them in well.

Blend the tofu in a processor, adding the soy milk if it is difficult to blend
on its own. (You might also put the parsley into the blender to chop it up
more easily.) Pour this over the vegetable mixture and mix thoroughly.

Place the filling in the pastry shell and bake it at 375 degrees for about
30 minutes.

Nutty Mock Meat Loaf

Serves 6

1 cup almonds, raw
⅔ cup sunflower seeds, raw
½ cup Brazil nuts, raw
¼ cup flax seeds, ground
2 small onions, diced
½ cup parsley, fresh
½ tsp. Real Salt
½ tsp. sweet basil
½ tsp. sage
⅓ tsp. thyme
½ cup water

Sauce

½ cup almonds, ground
2 cups water
1 tsp. seasoning, your choice
2 Tbs. arrowroot flour
Dash of cayenne pepper
2 Tbs. olive oil
¼ tsp. Real Salt

Preheat the oven to 350 degrees. Grind the nuts and seeds in a processor, blender, or grinder. Combine with the onions and seasonings; mix well. Add the water and mix again. Place in a well-oiled loaf pan and bake for 25 minutes.

To make the sauce, combine all the ingredients, bring to a low boil, and stir constantly. Turn the heat down and simmer over low until thick. Pour over the top of the baked nut loaf. Serve with tossed salad or steamed vegetables.

This is a good snack and freezes well. As an alternative to the listed spices, I use Spice Hunter's Cowboy BBQ Rub and 3 sun-dried tomatoes.

Alexandra's Favorite Pasta

SERVES 6

1 (28-oz.) can plum tomatoes, undrained
2 cloves garlic, minced
2 tsp. olive oil
1 lb. spaghetti or fettuccine, uncooked
8 oz. raw, store-bought almond cheese
1/8 tsp. red pepper flakes

Cube the tomatoes and heat them with their juices over medium heat with the garlic and olive oil for 20 minutes.

Meanwhile, cook the pasta, drain, and place in a serving bowl. Add the tomatoes, cheese, and red pepper flakes; toss. Cover the bowl for 5 minutes to allow the cheese to melt. Toss again before serving.

Rawsome Redford Pizza

SERVES 6

This 100 percent raw pizza is wonderfully filling and packed with calcium, magnesium, lycopene, protein, vitamins, and minerals—and replaces an acidic meal with an alkaline one. Perfect!

You can make the crust, almond cheese, and Rich Tomato Topping ahead of time, and if you do your pizza will take hardly any time at all to assemble.

Crust

I use the Excalibur dehydrator to make perfect crusts that can also double as great crackers or tostada flatties.

1/2 cup ground flax seeds
Water to cover ground flax seeds, approximately 1 cup
1 cup soaked raw almonds
2 cups soaked raw sunflower seeds
1 cup raw ground buckwheat
1/2 cup ground Deluxe Vegetable Blend (Jaffe Bros. blend of dehydrated cubed carrots, onions, tomatoes, celery, parsley, green peas, and green bell peppers)

Juice of 1 lemon
1 clove garlic
¼ cup olive oil
1 Tbs. whole pure salt (or to taste)
2 Tbs. Italian Seasoning (Spice Hunter)
1 Tbs. Spice Hunter Garlic Herb Bread Seasoning
¼–½ cup water

Grind the flax seeds into powder and place in a bowl with enough water to cover. Stir the ground flax seeds into the water and set aside to thicken. Rinse and drain the soaked seeds (soak for 15 to 20 minutes) and nuts and add them to your food processor with all the remaining ingredients. Mix well until you have a smooth, thick paste consistency. You may have to stop and stir a few times to get this mix well blended. Adjust with water at the end until the dough has a good consistency and can be rolled out with a rolling pin or pressed in a tortilla press between two pieces of thick plastic. (I use the plastic bags that my Jaffe products come packaged in.) Make pizza crust rounds the desired size. I usually do 5 to 7 inches across, for individual pizzas. Once you get them pressed between your plastic sheets, carefully peel off the top plastic layer to expose the top side of the crust, then flip it over onto the dehydrator sheet and carefully peel off the remaining plastic sheet. (For the dehydrator, you can use a Teflex sheet, but I usually prefer the screened sheet with small holes in it to allow the crust to dehydrate on both sides evenly.) Dehydrate overnight. Will keep for up to 2 weeks if kept dry and cool.

Almond Cheese

This fluffy, creamy spread is concentrated and rich. Use it in wraps, or to stuff celery stalks, or wherever you would use mayonnaise.

2 cups soaked almonds
1 lemon, juiced
¼ cup olive oil (or oil of choice: coconut, Udo's, grape seed)
½ cup water
½–1 tsp. whole unprocessed salt (to taste)
¼ tsp. ground mustard
¼ tsp. Spice Hunter Cafe Solé (mix of lemon, pepper, onion, and sea salt)

Blanch the almonds in boiling water for 30 seconds. When they're cool, pinch off their skins and discard. Place lemon juice, oil, and water into a food processor and begin blending. With the food processor running, drop almonds through the top opening and blend well until emulsified to a thick fluffy consistency. Add the spices. Scrape the sides and stir as needed; adjust the consistency with water. Store in the refrigerator in an airtight container for up to 3 to 5 days.

Tomato Sauce

2 pints cherry or grape tomatoes (or 4 regular tomatoes)
1 Tbs. dried oregano (or fresh if desired)
½ cup sun-dried tomatoes
⅓ cup fresh basil
½ tsp. whole unprocessed salt
1 clove garlic (remove middle section of clove to quiet odors)
1–3 tsp. psyllium seed husk (the more you use, the thicker your sauce will
   be)

Place all the ingredients into a food processor and pulse-chop to a chunky consistency. Set aside. This sauce will keep in the fridge for 3 to 5 days.

Toppings

Choose any of the following to sprinkle over the top of your pizza: chopped, sliced, shredded, or julienned zucchini, carrots, jicama, cabbage, romaine lettuce, beets, spinach, or bell peppers.

Pizza Assembly

Place a finished crust on the counter and spread with a thick layer of Almond Cheese, then a thick layer of Tomato Sauce. Sprinkle with toppings. Serve immediately.

Pasta with Creamy Pesto Sauce

Serves 4–6

This is a colorful, wonderful way to veggie up your pasta. Even better, you can just eat the veggies and sauce without the pasta. I serve the sauce raw and the dish cold in the summer, and warm it all up in the winter.

3 cups shaved small yellow squash (zucchini would work also)
2 red bell peppers, cleaned and sliced into long thin strips
1 red onion, sliced in thin rings (marinated in Liquid pHlavor Salt and/or some Real Salt)
1 cup chopped tomato
½ cup sun-dried tomatoes, chopped fine in food processor
½ cup chopped fresh basil (or 1 Tbs. dried basil)
2 Tbs. chopped fresh oregano (or 1 tsp. dried oregano)
1 Tbs. destemmed and chopped fresh rosemary (or ½ tsp. dried rosemary)
½ tsp. Zip (Spice Hunter)
1 tsp. minced garlic (or ½ tsp. garlic powder)
1 tsp. minced ginger (or ¼–½ tsp. powdered ginger)
⅓ cup fresh lemon juice
1 lb. vegetable pasta made without eggs
1 recipe Spring's Pesto (page 322) or 1 bottle Garlic Galore pesto with sun-dried tomatoes
1 can coconut milk
Whole pure salts to taste
Soy Parmesan (optional)

With a vegetable peeler, shave the yellow squash (or zucchini) lengthwise into long, thin strips, cutting any remaining parts with seeds into long strips with a knife; or you can put the squash through a Saladacco machine, which cuts it into angel-hair pasta. In a bowl, combine with all the ingredients up through the lemon juice; mix well and set aside. Prepare the pasta according to package directions. Drain and toss with a small amount of olive oil to prevent sticking. Keep warm. Put the pesto and coconut milk into a food processor and process until creamy. While the processor is still running, add water to your desired consistency. Add salt to taste. To serve, arrange the pasta on a plate, topping with veggie mix and then creamy pesto sauce. Sprinkle with a soy Parmesan if desired.

Almond/Carrot/Ginger-Stuffed Zucchini

SERVES 4

1 large onion, peeled and chopped
2 Tbs. olive oil
4 medium zucchini
1 clove garlic, minced
4 medium carrots, scraped and finely diced
1 tsp. grated fresh ginger
2/3 cup soaked almonds, chopped, or raw unsoaked macadamia nuts,
    chopped
Whole pure salts, to taste
Zip (Spice Hunter) or pepper, to taste

Preheat the oven to 375 degrees.

Sauté the onion in the oil in a medium saucepan for 5 minutes. Halve the zucchini lengthwise and scoop out the soft centers to make good cavities for stuffing.

Chop the scooped-out centers of the zucchini and add to the onion, along with the garlic, carrots, and ginger. Cover and sauté gently for about 10 minutes, until the veggies are slightly soft.

Remove from the heat and add the chopped almonds or macadamias and seasonings to taste.

Place the zucchini skins in an oiled shallow casserole and fill them with the carrot mixture. Cover and bake for about 30 to 40 minutes. Serve immediately.

Edamame Patties

SERVES 4

These are hardy little veggie burgers that can be pan-fried if you're in a hurry, or dehydrated for 4 to 6 hours to make a more crusty outside. They are made with a base of edamame (soybeans from pods) that you can find in your health food store in the frozen section.

3 Tbs. flax seeds
6 Tbs. water

1 carrot, grated fine or processed to fine pulp

2 cloves garlic

1 tsp. dried onion

2 sun-dried tomatoes (packed in olive oil)

½ cup parsley

½ tsp. dried mustard

½ tsp. turmeric

1 tsp. Mexican Seasoning (Spice Hunter)

⅓ tsp. Deliciously Dill (Spice Hunter)

1 tsp. Real Salt

1 (10-oz.) pkg. vegetable soybeans (Sno Pac carries a brand already depodded; or you can get them in the pod and slip the beans out yourself)

Grind flax seeds to powder using a blender or coffee grinder and put in a bowl. Add the water and stir to mix well. Set aside to gel up.

Put the flax mixture, carrot, garlic, dried onion, sun-dried tomatoes, and all the seasonings into a food processor and process to your desired consistency. (I do this quite smooth.) Then add the edamame beans and process until well mixed. You can make this coarse and more chunky with the beans showing, or smoother and more mixed if you like. Also, you can use more edamame beans if the mixture seems to be too moist. You should be able to form this into patties easily. Then make into small patties and put into a dehydrator for 4 to 6 hours, or use a little grape seed oil, dip the patties in some sprouted wheat tortilla crumbs, and fry on both sides. Serve with the Rich Raw Tomato Sauce (page 321) on top for a real treat!

Optional: You can use all sorts of different spices for these. Sometimes I use Italian Seasoning or Garlic Herb Bread Seasoning by Spice Hunter. Also you could add some garbanzo or other beans of choice to stretch the recipe or add more bean flavors. Experiment! Enjoy!

Hearty Harvest Casserole

SERVES 12

2 large onions, cut and separated into rings ¾ inch thick
1 each medium green and red pepper, cut into 1-inch strips
1 cup sprouted barley, partially cooked (reserve 1 cup water)
¼ cup vegetable broth mix
3 medium carrots, cut into chunks
2 large tomatoes, peeled and quartered
2 medium zucchini, cut into 1½-inch chunks
1 lb. green beans, snapped in half
½ head cauliflower florets
2 cloves garlic, crushed
1 Tbs. Real Salt
¼ tsp. black pepper
1 tsp. paprika
¼ cup chopped parsley

Steam-fry the onions and bell peppers. Combine all the ingredients in a casserole dish. Cover. Bake at 350 degrees for 1 hour. The barley should be tender.

Seed Pancakes with Coconut Whipped Topping

Serves 6–8

This combination of seeds guarantees a good intake and ratio of essential fats. Make sure you start with very fresh organic raw seeds and nuts. One good source is Jaffe Bros.

¼ cup raw pumpkin seeds
¼ cup raw sunflower seeds
¼ cup raw sesame seeds
½ cup raw flax seeds
1 cup millet or spelt flours, or a combination of other flours (quinoa, amaranth, buckwheat, bean)
1½ tsp. baking soda
1 tsp. Real Salt
1/16 tsp. stevia (optional)
Unsweetened soy milk or water, as needed

Mix the seeds together. Place ⅓ cup of this seed mixture at a time into a coffee grinder and grind into a flour. (Or you can grind it all at once in a Vita-Mix blender.) Measure out 1 cup and put in a bowl. (Store the rest in fridge or freezer.) Add the remaining dry ingredients and stir. Then add soy milk or water until you reach your desired consistency. The batter will thicken after sitting a couple of minutes. Heat some olive, coconut, or grape seed oil in a frying pan, spoon in the batter, and brown the pancakes on both sides.

Buckwheat Pancakes: Use 2 cups buckwheat (made from raw buckwheat kernels) instead of the flour.

Whipped Topping

½ carton soft tofu
⅓ cup Thai coconut milk
½ tsp. Frontier non-alcohol vanilla
⅛ tsp. white stevia powder
1 Tbs. fresh lemon juice

Whip all the ingredients in a blender and serve over Seed Pancakes. Store in the fridge.

Spiced Winter Squash

SERVES 2

2 cups grated butternut squash
1 cup grated acorn or banana squash
2 Tbs. olive oil
2 tsp. Garam Masala or Curry (Spice Hunter)
Pinch of cinnamon
1 Tbs. lemon or lime juice, or both
1 Tbs. Liquid pHlavor Salt
2 Tbs. minced onion

Combine the squash, oil, spices, juice, salt, and onion. Mix well and toss. Then turn into an electric fry pan and gently warm this dish right before serving.

Fresh Spinach/Zucchini Bake

SERVES 6

2½ Tbs. oil, divided
2 cloves garlic, 1 chopped
20 oz. fresh spinach
¾ cup chopped onion
1 Tbs. basil leaves
2 cups diced zucchini
Egg replacer equal to 6 eggs
¼ cup sprouted wheat bread crumbs
¾ tsp. vegetized or Real Salt

In a large, warm saucepan, put 1 Tbs. of the oil with the whole garlic clove and washed spinach. Cover and cook for 4 minutes, wilting the spinach leaves. Remove the garlic and drain the spinach. Heat the oven to 350 degrees. Reheat the pot, adding 1½ Tbs. oil with the chopped garlic, onion, basil, salt, pepper and zucchini. Cook until the onion is soft. Mix in the spinach. Oil a baking dish. Spread the spinach-zucchini mixture over the bottom of the dish. Pour egg substitute over the vegetables, tilting to evenly distribute the mixture. Sprinkle with crumbs. Bake 10–14 minutes or until egg substitute is set.

Zippy Breakfast

SERVES 1

This would make a delicious meal anytime, but we love it to start our day.

1–2 cups cooked rice or grain of your choice (I use basmati, brown, or wild
    rice, millet, quinoa, or buckwheat)
1 avocado, sliced
1 firm tomato, chopped
1–2 tsp. oil (flax, Udo's, olive)
1–2 tsp. Liquid pHlavor Salt
Juice of 1 lemon or lime (or both)
Zip (Spice Hunter), to taste

Start with the warm rice in a bowl. Arrange the sliced avocado and tomato on top. Then drizzle the oil, salt, and lemon juice over the top. Sprinkle with Zip to taste.

Variation: Sometimes I throw some chopped red bell pepper, sunflower seed sprouts, and soaked almonds over the top for extra crunch! Enjoy!

Green Chili Tofu Pita

SERVES 6

These are great little Mexican triangles stuffed with a fresh tofu-cilantro filling. Great for a snack or appetizer or as a main course beside a big salad.

1 pkg. pita bread or tortillas
3 cloves garlic, minced
1 small can green chilies (chopped)
1 tsp. Mexican Seasoning (Spice Hunter)
2 tsp. dried onion, or ¼ cup minced fresh onion
¼ cup soy Parmesan cheese substitute
1 Tbs. fresh cilantro
½ tsp. Real Salt
1 pkg. extra-firm tofu (Nigari)
1 jar or can enchilada sauce
Avocado slices, for garnish
3–4 sun-dried tomatoes, for garnish

Cut each pita like a pie into eight triangular pieces, then open each one up so you can put the filling in. In a food processor, mince the garlic, then add all other ingredients except the tofu, the enchilada sauce, and the garnishes; process until finely chopped. Put the grater attachment on the processor and grate the tofu into the mix. Process for a few seconds more to mix.

Spoon the filling into the pita triangles and place into a pie pan. Spoon enchilada sauce over each pita and inside over the filling mixture. Bake at 350 degrees for 10 to 15 minutes. Arrange avocado slices and sun-dried tomatoes on top as a garnish just before serving warm.

SIDE DISHES

Mexicali Rice

Serves 6–8

This is a salsa rice that is a great complement to a Mexican dinner. Serve with Great Olé Guacamole (page 304) and Green Chili Tofu Pita hors d'oeuvres (page 359).

3 Tbs. olive oil, divided
1 onion, chopped
1 clove garlic, minced
½ cup diced celery
2 large tomatoes, coarsely chopped
2 serrano chilies, seeds and stems removed, chopped
2 Tbs. chopped fresh cilantro
1 tsp. fresh lime juice
½ tsp. oregano
1 tsp. Real Salt
3–4 cups cooked rice

Put half the olive oil in a skillet or electric fry pan and sauté the onion and garlic until the onion softens. Then add the rest of the ingredients (I chop them all up in a food processor) except the rice and remaining olive oil and steam-fry until the veggies are bright and still somewhat crisp. Add the cooked rice and the rest of the olive oil. Mix well and serve warm.

Millet Yam Hash Browns

SERVES 4

Millet is a good source of iron, lecithin, and choline, and yams are high in vitamin E. This is a nice recipe to help wean yourself off starchy deep-fried hash browns. I doubled this recipe, and it was gone in two days!

2½ cups water
½ tsp. Real Salt
1 cup millet
1 yam (carrot or sweet potato works, too), peeled and processed in food
    processor to semi-fine/coarse chunks
1 tsp. dried onions
½ tsp. Deliciously Dill (Spice Hunter)
½ tsp. Garlic Herb Bread Seasoning or other favorite spice blend (Spice
    Hunter)
½ tsp. dried garlic powder (could use fresh or roasted)
Grape seed oil, for brushing
Minced fresh cilantro, for garnish

Preheat the oven to 400 degrees. Bring the water and salt to a boil in a medium saucepan. Add the millet, lower the heat, cover, and simmer for 15 minutes.

Open the lid and place the processed yam on top of the millet. Return the lid and continue to simmer for 10 more minutes. Transfer to a large bowl.

Add all remaining spices and toss. Add Real Salt to taste, but don't douse the natural sweetness of the yams. The mixture should be sticky and stiff enough to hold its shape when formed into oval patties.

Using a ¼-cup measuring cup, scoop out the batter and form oval patties about ⅓ to ½ inch thick. Place on an oiled cookie sheet and bake at 400 degrees for 20 minutes or until brown.

Sprinkle the minced fresh cilantro and some Ginger-Almond Paste Topping on top (page 316).

Enjoy. These are incredible right out of the oven. Later we spread hummus on top and have them as a snack!

Wild Yam Soba Noodles with Kale and Spicy Pine Nuts

SERVES 4

This is a nice, filling side dish that warms the body.

1 bunch kale or fresh spinach
2 Tbs. grape seed oil
3 cloves garlic, minced
⅓ cup veggie broth
2 Tbs. Liquid pHlavor Salt
Juice of ½ lemon
½ cup pine nuts, spiced (see Spicy Pecan Croutons recipe on page 374)
1 pkg. Wild Yam Soba Noodles (Eden brand)
2 Tbs. crumbled nori (optional)

Slice the kale (or spinach) stems thinly. Chop the leaves coarsely or put them in a food processor and pulse-chop until coarse.

Heat the oil in a large electric fry pan over medium heat. Sauté the garlic and kale stems for a few minutes, then add the leaves, veggie broth, and salt; continue sautéing until the kale is tender and bright, about 8 minutes. Add the lemon juice and mix well. Take out of the electric fry pan and set aside. Note: At this point you can put the kale/spinach in a food processor and process to a finer smooth pâté if you'd like.

In the same fry pan, prepare the pine nuts according to Spicy Pecan Croutons recipe (page 374) and set aside for garnish.

In a large pot of boiling water, cook the soba noodles until tender, then rinse and drain well. Put the cooked noodles into the electric fry pan and add the kale mixture on top. Mix together well, sprinkling the spicy nuts and the crumbled nori on top.

Millet/Buckwheat Oven Cakes

SERVES 6

These are incredibly hearty, dense pancakes made of ground raw hulled buckwheat and millet. They have an "eggy" consistency and are made from a thick batter. Buckwheat has a binding quality and is gluten-free. It is a seed, not a grain, and thus it is more alkalizing. My family likes these served fresh from the oven, on the side of a big salad, or just as a snack for breakfast, lunch, or dinner. They would also travel well. I use a Vita-Mix to grind the buckwheat and millet into flour. Sometimes it's best to do a cup at a time.

Experiment with this basic recipe and change the vegetables and seasonings to come up with several different versions (there are suggestions below).

1 cup millet
1½–2 cups raw hulled buckwheat
1 small yam, peeled and shredded
1 onion, sliced or chopped
2 cloves garlic
1 Tbs. dried parsley (or ½ cup chopped fresh parsley)
¼ tsp. cinnamon (I use more)
¼ tsp. nutmeg (I use more)
1 tsp. spice blend of your choice
1 tsp. Mexican Seasoning (Spice Hunter)
1 tsp. Real Salt
2 cups water, Rice Dream, almond milk, or soy milk
3 Tbs. grape seed or olive oil, for frying

Grind the millet and buckwheat to flour in a Vita-Mix. Mix well together in a large bowl and set aside.

In the Vita-Mix (or any blender), place the shredded yam, chopped onion, garlic, parsley, spices, salt, and water; blend until smooth. Pour into the dry flour mixture and mix well. The batter should be quite thick and stiff.

In an electric fry pan, heat the oil over medium heat and spoon the batter (about 3 to 4 Tbs. per pancake) into the oiled pan. Cook until golden brown on one side, then flip over to the other side and cook until done. You may need to add more oil as you continue to cook the rest of the pancakes. Serve hot, or serve cold as a snack.

Another baking option is to make square pancakes (my family likes these best): Get a 9-by-13-inch glass pan and oil it well. Pour in the entire batter mixture. Bake in an oven preheated to 375 degrees for 30 minutes covered, then uncover and let bake for 20 to 30 minutes more to slightly brown the top. Let cool and cut into squares. These can be served with any sauce, pesto, or dressing you like on top. The AvoRado AvoCado Topping (page 315) works great!

Substitution suggestions:
- Try adding sesame seeds, sprouted sunflower seeds, or pine nuts for a nuttier texture.
- Instead of yam, substitute a sweet potato, beet, or carrots.
- Instead of parsley, substitute kale, spinach, or grated zucchini.
- Try these other spices as seasonings from Spice Hunter: Deliciously Dill, Garlic Herb Bread Seasoning, Herbes de Provence, and Zip.

Kale with Egyptian Garlic Sauce

SERVES 4

Kale is a tasty green and deserves to be better known. Its ruffled leaves cook to a deep green and are an appealing accompaniment for rice or other whole grains. Kale is delicious with an Egyptian sauce of sautéed garlic and ground coriander. It's not exactly a sauce, but more a seasoning mixture—a way to add a quick burst of flavor to a cooked vegetable. It's also good with okra or baked eggplant, and can be mixed with brown rice and zucchini.

1 lb. kale
4 medium garlic cloves, minced
2 tsp. ground coriander
Real Salt, to taste
Cayenne pepper, to taste

Rinse the kale and remove the stems, including the tough part of the leaf. Pile the leaves and cut into manageable size. Steam the kale until tender-crisp, then transfer to a bowl. Steam-fry the garlic, about 1 minute. Add the coriander, salt, and cayenne and stir over low heat for 15 seconds to blend. Immediately toss with the kale in the pan or bowl. Taste and adjust seasonings. Serve hot.

Shelley Beans

SERVES 4

In Indiana and Ohio, shelley beans are known as cranberry beans. These beans, with their red-striped and cream coloring, are much sweeter and more delicate than pinto beans. When cooked, they lose their marking and become solid in color. This rich recipe includes macadamias, ginger, and lime, which make the beans especially creamy and tasty.

15–20 raw macadamia nuts
2 cloves garlic
⅓–½ inch piece ginger, grated on fine cheese grater
1 cup water, divided
1 tsp. grape seed oil
1 small jalapeño chili, seeded and minced
1 tsp. coriander
½ tsp. cumin
2 cups cooked cranberry beans (soaked overnight then cooked in water
    and 1 tsp. Real Salt until done)
Lime juice, to taste
Sections from 1 lime (skins included), minced in processor
Chopped fresh basil or cilantro, for garnish

Combine the macadamias, garlic, and ginger in a food processor. While processing, add ½ cup of the water and blend to a thick milky sauce.

In a fry pan, heat the oil over medium heat. Add the jalapeño and cook for a few minutes, then add the coriander and cumin. Continue cooking for another minute. Add the cooked beans and continue to stir, warming the beans for another few minutes.

Stir in the nut milk mixture and add more of the water if desired for a thinner consistency. Just before serving, add the lime juice and minced lime sections. Stir and mix well. Serve with the chopped cilantro on top, adding Real Salt to taste. Grapefruit sections make a nice garnish as well.

Zucchini Italian-Style

SERVES 8

8–10 medium zucchini
⅔ cup coarsely chopped onion
2 cloves garlic, minced
1½ cups tomatoes
1 tsp. Real Salt
⅛ tsp. pepper
3 Tbs. olive oil

Wash the zucchini, trim the ends, and slice. In a saucepan, steam-fry the onion, garlic, and sliced zucchini over low heat for 10 minutes, turning and moving the mixture occasionally.

Remove the zucchini mixture from the heat and sieve in the tomatoes with salt and pepper. Blend lightly and thoroughly.

Turn the mixture into a casserole dish, cover, and simmer for 30 minutes. Add the olive oil to the dish before serving.

Okra and Tomatoes Creole

SERVES 6–8

4 cups sliced okra
1 cup chopped onion
⅓ cup chopped green pepper
2 cups chopped tomatoes
½ tsp. Real Salt
⅛ tsp. black pepper
⅛ tsp. curry powder
1 tsp. powdered lecithin
⅛ tsp. thyme

Wash the okra, cut off the stem ends, slice, and set aside. Steam-fry the onion and green pepper in a large skillet to the transparent stage. Add the okra and tomatoes. Stir in a mixture of the salt, pepper, curry powder, lecithin, and thyme. Simmer, covered, for 30 to 40 minutes or until the okra is tender.

Steam-Fried Sprouts

SERVES 4

½ cup finely chopped onion
½ cup finely chopped green or red pepper
2 Tbs. Liquid pHlavor Salt
2 cups fresh bean sprouts, any kind

Steam-fry the onion and pepper in a skillet, with the salt. Add the sprouts and steam gently for 30 seconds. Serve immediately.

Refried Beans

SERVES 6 (3 CUPS)

½ cup chopped onion
1 tsp. minced garlic
3 cups cooked pinto beans
Garlic powder, to taste
Cayenne pepper, to taste
Black pepper, to taste
Real Salt, to taste

Steam-fry the onion and garlic. Puree the pinto beans in a food processor or blender. Pour the pureed beans into the skillet and stir the mixture constantly over low to medium heat until thickened; season while cooking. Serve hot with vegetables.

Spiced Green Beans

SERVES 6

1 lb. green beans
½ tsp. Real Salt
½ cup boiling water
1 cup thinly sliced onion
¼ tsp. black pepper
¼ tsp. nutmeg
1 Tbs. flax seed oil
1 Tbs. parsley

Wash the green beans, break off the ends, then cut them lengthwise into fine strips. Carefully place the beans and salt into a saucepan of boiling water. Cook, loosely covered, until tender-crisp. Meanwhile, steam-fry the onion in a skillet. Drain the beans and add to the skillet with a mixture of salt, pepper, and nutmeg. Sauté for 5 minutes. Add the flax seed oil and parsley. Toss well and serve.

Casserole de Cauliflower

SERVES 4–6

This dish takes 20 minutes to prepare. It's a lot like couscous in texture and makes a great breakfast, lunch, or dinner side dish.

2 tsp. oil (olive, flax, or Udo's Choice)
2–4 tsp. cumin
½ tsp. turmeric
½ yellow or red onion, finely minced
1 cup water
Florets from 1 very large or 2 small cauliflowers
7–8 sun-dried tomatoes (Melissa's brand are packed in olive oil)
1 red bell pepper, finely chopped
¼ cup minced fresh parsley
2 cloves garlic, minced
½ cup raw pine nuts
Whole pure salts, to taste
Lemon or lime juice, to taste

In an electric skillet, warm the oil, cumin, and turmeric. Keeping the temperature on warm or low, add the onion and allow the flavors to blend for 2 to 4 minutes, then add the water and warm.

In a food processor fitted with an S-blade, process the cauliflower into very small pieces (like couscous). Also process the sun-dried tomatoes and red pepper into fine, small pieces.

Add the cauliflower to the skillet and gradually warm, adding the parsley, garlic, sun-dried tomatoes, pepper, and pine nuts. Season with whole pure salts and lemon or lime juice to taste. Enjoy!

Ginger Beans and Carrots

SERVES 4

1 lb. fresh green beans
¼ cup oil
1 tsp. mustard seeds
½–¾ cup chopped onion
4 carrots, thinly sliced
¼ tsp. ground ginger
1 tsp. Real Salt
2 Tbs. fresh lemon juice

Wash and snap the beans. Carefully heat the oil in a skillet. Add the mustard seeds and sauté for 30 to 40 seconds (the seeds will pop). Stir in the onion, carrots, and beans. Cook, stirring, for 5 minutes. Stir in the ginger and salt; lower the heat. Cook for 10 minutes. Stir in lemon juice just before serving.

Camper's Bread

SERVES 2

2 cups sprouted wheat flour
¼ cup nonaluminum baking powder
1 Tbs. Real Salt
2 Tbs. oil (olive, Udo's, or oil of choice)
1 cup pure water

Mix the dry ingredients, cut in the oil, add the water, and mix well. Grease a frying pan; pour in the batter and cook very slowly. Turn.

Essene Bread

SERVES 2

1 qt. sprouted grain
⅔ cup pure water

Add the water to the grain and grind up in a Vita-Mix. Form into a small loaf and bake at 275 degrees for 3 hours or until a crust forms. Very moist.

Sprouted Wheat Bread

SERVES 1–2

2 cups wheat

Sprout 2 cups wheat for 2 days, then grind.

Make a pad ⅛ inch thick from this dough.

Bake on a flat stone in full summer sun from morning until noon on one side, then from noon until evening on the other side. If the weather is bad, bake it in a slow oven (275 degrees) until slightly crisp.

This recipe is adapted from the Dead Sea Scrolls and is the same type of bread Jesus broke at the Last Supper. It's a tasty, hardtack-like bread.

Shelley's Super Tortillas

SERVES 6–8

4 cups flour (use any mix of flours you like, such as whole wheat, unbleached white, or spelt)
2 tsp. Real Salt
4 tsp. seasonings of your choice (I use Spice Hunter's Mexican and California Pizza)
2 Tbs. dried onions
12 sun-dried tomatoes (packed in olive oil)
2 tsp. garlic powder
2–4 leaves fresh basil
1½ cups coconut milk or water
2 Tbs. olive oil

Mix all the ingredients in a food processor with a dough S-blade. Use the pulse-chop action to prevent overheating the motor. When the dough forms into one big ball, turn it out onto a floured flat surface; break off balls and roll them out to about ⅛- to ¼-inch thickness. Transfer to an electric pan that has been lightly oiled and heat on both sides until you see a few air pockets rise. Take off the burner and let cool, then wrap in an airtight bag and keep in the fridge or freezer. Do not overcook, unless you want a crisped tortilla to use with dips or soups. Or you can decrease the milk or water and add fresh vegetable juices instead, such as spinach, parsley, or carrot.

SNACKS

Avocado/Tomato Snack

Serves 2–3

2 avocados
1 small eggplant, diced
1 tsp. curry powder
2 Tbs. lemon juice
2 seeded green chili peppers
Real Salt and seasoning, to taste
2 or 3 tomatoes, thickly sliced

Blend all the ingredients except tomatoes in a blender until smooth. Spoon onto warmed tomato slices.

Nori Flower Krisps

Makes about 10 Krisps

These delicious cracker-type snacks make a great on-the-go treat, but they also work placed elegantly alongside a beautiful salad at the dinner table.

Experiment with any of the pâté recipes (Edamame Pâté, Tuna-pHishless Pâté, and so on) in place of the Brazil nuts. Try using equal parts of any nut and raw coconut meat run through the juicer. Add sun-dried tomatoes, use different types of nuts, like macadamias, and use different seasonings to create unique variations of Nori Flower Krisps every time you make them.

Nori sheets can be found in an Asian grocery or in the macrobiotic section of your health food store.

1 lb. raw Brazil nuts
Juice of 1 lemon
Garlic salt to taste
¼ cup Liquid pHlavor Salt

¾ cup lime juice *or* coconut water
Dehydrated red bell pepper powder (page 317)
1 package nori seaweed sheets

Run the Brazil nuts through a Samson Juice Extractor to make a paste.
Then add the lemon juice and garlic salt (or other seasonings) and mix well.
Set aside. In a spray bottle, combine the liquid salt and lime juice or coconut milk. (Or, place 1 cup vegetable broth in a spray bottle instead.) Lay
4 sheets of nori on top of a dehydrator tray with a mesh underlining and
spray the sheets front and back to soften them. Spread the nut paste in the
middle of the nori sheets, leaving a margin of an inch or two. With cupped
hands, coax the softened nori edges in toward the middle to create a flower
shape. Sprinkle the center nut paste liberally with dehydrated red bell pepper powder and place into a dehydrator. Dehydrate until snap-crisp (usually
overnight). Break or cut into cracker-size pieces—or serve whole and let
everyone break off portions as they eat.

Veggie Crunch Stix and Crackers

SERVES 8–10

*These colorful treats are a great way to wean children and adults from yeast
breads. They are a wonderful grab-snack and also complement and give crunch
to a vegan-based meal such as soup and salad. They work up very fast and travel
well. I use small cookie cutters and make little dinosaur, airplane, and heart crackers. Also, you can season them any way you want by adding a couple of teaspoons
of your favorite spice.*

2 cups flour (all-purpose, millet, whole wheat—I use half all-purpose and
    half whole wheat)
½–1 tsp. salt
1½ tsp. baking powder
3 heaping Tbs. soft tofu (Nori brand is good)
2 Tbs. olive oil
½–¾ cup cold water or fresh vegetable juice, or mix
1–2 tsp. Seasonings of your choice (optional)

In a food processor, pulse the flour, salt, and baking powder to combine.
Add the tofu and olive oil and pulse until the mixture resembles coarse

meal. With the machine running, gradually add between ½ and ¾ cup ice water or fresh veggie juice until the dough comes together in a soft ball (approximately 1 minute).

Turn the dough out onto a lightly floured surface. Form it into a smooth rectangle, about 4 by 6 inches, then roll it out into an 8-by-10-inch sheet, ¼ inch thick. With a sharp knife cut the dough lengthwise into ¼-inch-wide strips.

Using your hands, gently roll each strip into a 16-inch-long stick. For a twisted version, grab each end of the dough strip with your fingers and carefully stretch and twist it in opposite directions. For crackers, use cookie cutters (children love these!). Arrange the stix on two baking sheets, side by side but not touching, and press the ends into the baking sheet to keep the stix straight while they cook. If desired, brush each stick lightly with olive oil and sprinkle with salt or seasonings of your choice. Bake at 350 degrees until firm and cooked through, 14 to 18 minutes.

Transfer the stix or crackers to a wire rack to cool. Store in an airtight container at room temperature for 2 to 3 days.

Variations:

- Beet Stix: Combine 2 Tbs. beet juice (from 1 small beet) with ½ cup cold water.
- Popeye Stix: Combine ½ cup parsley or spinach juice with ¼ cup cold water.
- Bugs Bunny Stix: Combine ¼ cup carrot juice (from about 3 carrots) with ¼ cup cold water.
- Tomato Stix: ¼ cup fresh tomato juice, with 1–2 Tbs. sun-dried tomato pesto. Combine with ⅓ cup cold water.

Or try these spicing options:

- Curry/Turmeric Stix: 1 tsp. curry powder and ½ tsp. ground turmeric.
- Cumin Stix: 2 tsp. ground cumin.
- Garlic Stix: 2 tsp. Garlic Herb Bread Seasoning (Spice Hunter).
- Mexi Stix: 2 tsp. Mexican Seasoning (Spice Hunter).
  Experiment!

Spicy Pecan Croutons

SERVES 4–6

These spicy, toasty pecan croutons will add pizzazz to any salad. That's if they make it into the salad—they usually go down as a pop-in-the-mouth snack around my house. The cayenne pepper adds magnesium and bioflavonoids to enhance circulation.

2 Tbs. grape seed or olive oil
1 cup raw pecans (almonds or pine nuts also work great)
½–1 tsp. cayenne pepper (start with ½ tsp. and work up if you like them
   hotter)
1 tsp. Spice Hunter's Curry or plain ground cumin (Spice Hunter's
   Cowboy BBQ Rub would also work; experiment!)
¾ tsp. Real Salt

In a fry pan, heat the oil over medium-low heat. Add the pecans and all other ingredients and sauté until the nuts are well coated and lightly toasted. Serve warm from the pan over salads. And serve immediately. These croutons are also wonderful sprinkled over stir-fried veggies such as asparagus or green beans. And you can cool and eat for a snack. Enjoy!

Another great serving idea: Make the Blackened Herbed Fillets (page 326) and sauté some asparagus to place on top of the fish when done. Then as a garnish, sprinkle these pecan croutons over the top. Serve with a big helping of Rainbow Salad (page 286). Bon appétit!

Crispy Buckwheat Groats

SERVES 6–8

2 cups hulled buckwheat groats, soaked 6–8 hours
Whole pure salts, to taste
Lemon or lime juice (I use both)
Zip (Spice Hunter) or any seasoning, to taste

Drain the buckwheat groats and put them in a shallow bowl. Add whole pure salts and juice to cover. Add spices to taste. Let the groats soak in this solution for 1 hour, then drain again. Put the groats in a food dehydrator on Teflex liners and dehydrate until dry (2 to 3 hours).

These are great little munchy snacks and can be used as croutons in a salad or wrap.

Dehydrated Flax Chips

SERVES 6–8

1 cup flax seeds
2 cups water
1 tomato
½ red bell pepper
1 clove garlic
1–2 tsp. Spice Hunter's Mexican Seasoning, Italian, Garlic Herb Bread, or any other spice combo you like
½ small red onion or 1 tsp. dried onion flakes
½ beet
Real Salt to taste

Soak the flax seeds in the water for 2 to 4 hours. Process the tomato, bell pepper, garlic, Mexican spices, onion, beet, and Real Salt. Keep it chunky. Add the soaked flax seeds into the blended mixture. Spoon 2-inch rounds onto a Teflex sheet and dehydrate at 105 to 110 degrees for 8 to 12 hours, or to the desired crispness. Turn the crisps over after 4 to 6 hours to ensure even drying.

Optional: Sprinkle sesame or soaked pumpkin seeds on top before dehydrating.

Tortilla Chips

SERVES 4–8

4 large sprouted wheat tortillas, or tortillas of your choice
¼ cup olive oil, grape seed oil, or other preferred oil
Seasonings of choice, such as sesame seeds, garlic, or Spice Hunter's
    Italian, Mexican, Cowboy BBQ, or Herbes de Provence

Lay out the tortillas on two nonstick cookie sheets. With a pastry brush
or napkin, wipe over each tortilla so that the surface is covered with oil.
Sprinkle your seasonings of choice over the top of the tortillas and bake at
350 degrees until golden or just almost crisp, around 10 minutes.

Cool and then break into pieces for eating with dips, soups, or salads.
You can also precut the tortillas with a pizza cutter before you bake them if
you want cleaner-edged crackers.

Ice Pops

MAKES ABOUT 12 ICE POPS, OR 1 ICE CUBE TRAY FULL

1 shake recipe (pages 265–267)

Make the shake recipe, then pour it into ice cube trays or small paper cups
(1- to 2-oz. size), insert toothpicks or Popsicle sticks, and freeze. Or forget
the sticks; instead, thaw the frozen shakes a little, remove from the cups or
trays, and chop into a slushie.

DESSERTS

Shelley's Soy Pudding

SERVES 2

This is a great way to have a delicious treat while staying alkaline. We eat this for breakfast sometimes, and use it in place of one of the soups on a cleanse. It is high in good fats, vitamin E, calcium, and potassium thanks to the almonds and avocados, and high in good proteins from the soy powder.

1 cup Fresh Silky Almond Milk (page 269)
2 avocados
1 lime
2 scoops soy powder
½ tsp. raw green stevia
6–8 ice cubes

Place all the ingredients in a blender and blend on high until the mixture is rich, smooth, and pudding-like.

Variations:

- Add 2 Tbs. nonsweetened dried coconut to the pudding while blending, and sprinkle some more over the top before serving.
- Use lemon instead of lime.
- Replace the lime with the juice from ½ grapefruit.
- Add ½ scoop greens powder or 1 cup fresh baby spinach.
- Add a ½- to 1-inch piece of fresh ginger, grated, and 1 or 2 peeled whole limes
- Add 2 heaping Tbs. raw powdered carob and a capful of Frontier liquid mint seasoning.
- Add a capful of Frontier liquid cinnamon flavoring and sprinkle nutmeg on top.
- Sprinkle the pudding with chopped raw almonds or any desired nut (pecan, macadamia, and so on).

- This recipe makes good ice pops, too. Poor any variation into small paper cups (1- to 2-oz. size) or ice cube trays, add toothpicks, and freeze. Or forget the sticks; instead, thaw the frozen shakes a little, remove from the cups or trays, and chop into a slushie.

Mock Pumpkin Pie

SERVES 6–8

This recipe was the result of trying to come up with something healthy in place of pumpkin pie at Thanksgiving. It is a healthy alternative made out of carrots. Experiment using pumpkin and other squashes.

Piecrust

2 cups raw almonds
2–3 Tbs. soy milk or almond milk
2 Tbs. wheat bran flakes

Pie Filling

1 lb. carrots, peeled and grated
½ tsp. nutmeg
½ tsp. cinnamon
⅛ tsp. clove
1 tsp. vanilla
½ cup slivered or whole almonds, for garnish

To make the crust, place the raw almonds in a food processor and pulse-chop until fine. Add the soy milk and bran 1 Tbs. at a time until the mixture holds together. Press evenly into a pie plate.

To make the filling, steam the carrots until they're soft. Place in a blender or food processor and process until smooth. Add the spices and vanilla. Pour the mixture into the almond crust, garnishing the top with slivered or whole almonds. Chill in the fridge overnight and serve cold.

Recipe Substitutions

You can most certainly rely on many of your old favorite recipes while you are on this program. And with a few creative substitutions, even more of them will fit right in with your new way of eating. Here are the most common substitutions necessary to get you started:

If a Recipe Calls For	Substitute
1 pkg. yeast	1 tsp. nonaluminum baking powder
Whole wheat or white flour	Try spelt, buckwheat, or millet flour, or a combination
Milk	Soy milk, rice milk, almond milk, sesame milk
Vinegar	Lemon or lime juice
Soy sauce or tamari	Liquid pHlavor Salt
Regular cooking oils or salad oil	Good oils such as olive, hemp, coconut, sunflower, flax seed, borage, almond, grape seed, or Udo's Choice
Butter or margarine	Good oils, as above, or (if not cooking) Herbed Alkalarian "Butter" (page 310)
Cheese	Sprouts (obviously, this doesn't work in every instance—for example, when the cheese is to be melted)
Meat	Soy products (make sure they contain no yeast)
Eggs	Egg replacer (as directed on package)

If a Recipe Calls For	Substitute
Salt	Real Salt, Celtic Sea Salt, or salt with dehydrated veggies
Walnuts or cashew nuts	Almonds, hazelnuts, pecans, pine nuts
White rice	Organic brown rice, brown or natural white basmati rice, spelt, buckwheat groats, millet, kamut, quinoa, amaranth
Bread	Unleavened, yeast-free sprouted breads
Pasta	Vegetable, spelt, or artichoke pasta

Resources

Medical

For referrals for live blood analysis and the Mycotoxic/Oxidative Stress Test, (MOST) or for health retreats or consultations, contact the pH Miracle Center at 760-751-8321. This is also the place to call for information about products used in this book that this resource section does not provide.

The pH Miracle Healing Centers
16390 Dia Del Sol
Valley Center, California 92082
760-751-8321
760-751-8324 Fax
www.phmiracleliving.com

For general information, recipes, articles, and testimonials: www.phmiracleliving.com.

For further video education on the New Biology™ and the pH Miracle Lifestyle and diet: www.phmiracleliving.com.

Promotes preventative medicine, encourages higher standards for ethics and effectiveness in research, and advocates broader access to medical services.

Physicians Committee for Responsible Medicine
5100 Wisconsin Ave., NW
Suite 404
Washington, DC 20016

202-686-2210
www.perm.org

Empowers consumers to make informed health choices in the areas of dietary supplements, complementary and alternative medicine, food and water safety.

Citizens for Health
P.O Box 2260
Boulder, CO 80306
800-357-2211
www.citizens.org

The cutting-edge catalogue carries many items in the category of health technology, including pH meters, water systems, and books.

Cutting Edge Catalogue
P.O. Box 5034
Southampton, NY 11969
Orders: 800 497-9516
Information: 516 287-3813
Fax: 516-287-3112
www.cutcat.com
E-mail: cutcat@i-2000.com

Leads tenacious and effective public campaigns against toxic food and water technologies, including food irradiation, pesticides, and GMOs, while stimulating efforts to build safe, sustainable alternatives.

Food and Water Journal and Wild Matters
389 Rt. 215
Walden, VT 05873
800-EAT-SAFE
www.foodandwater.org

Promotes vegetarianism throughout the world by supporting and connecting national and regional groups, and holding International Vegetarian Congress.

International Vegetarian Union
P.O. Box 9710

Washington, DC 20016
202-362-VEGY
www.ivu.org

Dedicated to promoting the vegetarian way of life by sponsoring regional and national conferences and campaigns, distributing educational materials, and publishing *Vegetarian Voice*.

North American Vegetarian Society (NAVS)
P.O. Box 72
Dolgeville, NY 13329
518-568-7970
www.navs-online.org

Dedicated to children with serious health challenges, including obesity, and helping their parents and their child with alternative health education.

InnerLight Biological Health and Education Foundation
16390 Dia Del Sol
Valley Center, CA 92082
760-751-8321
www.phmiracleliving.com

Food

- Organically grown California avocados, picked fresh off the tree and shipped to you next day: 760-751- 8321, www.phmiracleliving.com
- Extra virgin coconut oil: Garden of Life, 800-622-8986, or www .gardenoflifeusa.com
- New Frontier flavorings bottled in oil (without alcohol): www.frontier coop.com
- Pomona's Universal Pectin available at health food or grocery stores, Whole Foods, or from Workstead Industries, P.O. Box 1083, Greenfield, MA 01302, (413) 772-6816
- Heat Wave Seasoning from the Cape Herb and Spice Company, distributed by Profile Products, www.elements-of-spice.com, P.O. Box 140, Maple Valley, WA 98038, 425-432-4300
- Lite House Spice Company, www.litehousefoods.com
- Spice House dehydrated tomato powder and veggie granules, www .thespicehouse.com

- Mauk Family Farms brand raw wheat free crusts, www.Maukfamily-farms.com
- Recommended brands: Sweet Leaf stevia with fiber; Pacific free-range organic chicken broth and yeast-free vegetable broth; Pomi strained tomatoes with no preservatives, additives, or vinegar; White Wave baked seasoned tofu; Veat gourmet, baked seasoned tofu; Garden Burgers; Boca Burgers; Spice Hunter spice combinations; Real Salt
- Real Salt; Redmond Minerals, Inc., 800 367-7258, www.realsalt.com
- For a wonderful, easy-to-get-started program on sprouting, kits in different sizes, instructions on how to sprout, information on nutritional aspects of different seeds, single seeds, and seed mixes: Life Sprouts, P.O. Box 150, Hiram, Utah, 435 245-3891
- There are many organic food distributors, many of which are based in California due to the year-round growing climate. Here's one I like: Diamond Organics, P.O. Box 2159, Freedom, CA 95019, orders by phone: 888-674-2642, fax: 888-888-6777, or email: organics@diamondorganics.com
- Pacific Foods of Oregon, Tualatin, OR 97062, 503-692-9666, www.pacificfoods.com
- Udo's Choice, Flora, Inc., Lyden, WA 98264, 800-446-2110, www.udoerasmus.com, www.florainc.com
- Barlean's Organic Oils, 4936 Lake Terrell Road, Ferndale, Washington 98248, 800-445-FLAX. Look for this cold-pressed oil in the refrigerator case of your local natural foods store.
- Arrowhead Mills (Omega Nutrition/Essential Balance Oil), Vancouver, BC V5L 1P5, 800-661-3529, www.omeganutrition.com
- Image Foods, Inc., 350 Cambridge Ave., Suite 350, Palo Alto, CA 94306, www.imagefoods.com
- For workshops on preparing alkalizing meals: Shelley Young's Academy of Culinary Arts, The pH Miracle Healing Center, Dia Del Sol, Valley Center, CA 92082, 760-751-8321, www.phmiracleliving.com

Books

- *The Omega Diet,* Artemis P. Simopoulos, MD and Jo Robinson
- *The Oil–Protein Diet,* Johanna Budwig, MD
- *Flax: The Super Food,* Barb Bloomfield, Judy Brown, Seigfied Gursche
- *The Trans Fat Solution,* Kim Severson

- *The Healing Miracles of Coconut Oil,* Bruce Fife, ND
- *Fat Wars,* Brad J. King
- *The Miracle of Magnesium,* Carolyn Dean, MD, ND
- *Water and Salt, the Essence of Life,* Barbara Nendel, MD
- *Molecules of Emotion,* Candace B. Pert, PhD
- *Urban Rebounding,* J.B. Berns
- *Taking Charge of Your Weight and Well-Being,* Joyce D. Nash, PhD, and Linda H. Ormiston, PhD
- *The Food Revolution,* John Robbins
- *The Blood and Its Third Anatomical Element* by Antoine Béchamp
- *Soy Smart Health,* Neil Solomon, MD, PhD
- *Understanding Acid-Base,* Benjamin Abelow, MD
- *Fats That Heal and Fats That Kill,* Udo Erasmus
- *Slow Burn,* Stu Mittleman
- *Muscles in Minutes,* Mike Mentzer
- *Static Contraction,* Peter Sisco and John Little
- *The Complete Book of Massage,* Claire Maxwell Hudson
- *The Touch That Heals,* William N. Brown, PhD, ND, DSc
- *Rainbow Green Live-Food Cuisine,* Gabriel Cousens, MD

Websites

- www.phmiracleliving.com

Equipment

- pH strips: http://thephmiracle.us/products.html
- pH meters: Cutting Edge Catalogue, P.O. Box 5034, Southampton, NY 11969; 800-497-9516; www.cutcat.com; e-mail: cutcat@I-2000.com
- pH Miracle Mark I Plasma Activated Alkaline Water Ionizers: www.phmiracleliving.com
- pH Miracle Whole Body Vibrational Exercise Equipment: www.phmiracleliving.com
- Cellerciser mini tramp: The pH Miracle Center, 760-751-8321, for more information or go to www.phmiracleliving.com
- Infrared sauna: www.phmiracleliving.com, or Nova: http://www.novacompanies.com

- pH Miracle Mark I Electro-Magnetic MicroIonization Water Machine: www.phmiracleliving.com
- VitaMix blender with the plunger, 8615 Usher Road, Cleveland, OH 44138-2199, 800-848-2649.
- Green Power, Green Star, Green Life Juicer; Orders: 888-254-7336; Inquiries: 562-940-4240, www.greenpower.com

Supplements

- pH Miracle Living Nutritionals, 16390 Dia Del Sol, Valley Center, CA 92082, www.pHmiracleliving.com or 760-751-8321
- Nordic Naturals, 54 Hangar Way, Watsonville, CA 95076, 800-662-2544, www.nordicnaturals.com
- Source Natural, Inc., 19 Janis Way, Scotts Valley, CA 95066, 800-815-2333, www.sourcenaturals.com
- Solaray, Nutraceutical Corporation, 1400 Kearns Blvd., Second Floor, Park City, UT 84060, 800-669-8877, www.natraceutical.com
- InnerLight, Inc., 867 East 2260 South, Provo, UT 84606, www.innerlightinc.com
- InnerLight Worldwide Inc., 867 E. 2260 S., Provo, UT 84606, e-mail: info@innerlightcorp.com
    - U.S. Headquarters: +1 801 655 0605
    - European Union: +36 1 382 0223
    - Norway: +47 456 18000
- Green Kamut Corporation, 1965 Freeman, Long Beach, CA 90804

References

2004 Physicians' Desk Reference, 58th ed. Stamford: Thomson Health Care, Inc.; 2003.

Adetumbi, M. A., Javor, C. F., and Lau, B. H. S. Anti-Candida activity of garlic—effect on macromolecular synthesis. Presented at the American Society for Microbiology, Loma Linda University, 1985.

Alberts, B., et al., eds. *Molecular Biology of the Cell*, 2d ed. New York: Garland Publishing, Inc., 1989.

Aleksandrowixz, J., and Smyk, B. Mycotoxins and their role in oncogenesis with special reference to blood diseases. *Polish Medical Science Historical Bulletin*, 1971; 24: 25–30.

Alexander, J. G. Allergy in the gastrointestinal tract. *Lancet*, 1975; 2: 1264.

Alpert, M. E., Hutt, M. S. R., Wogan, G. N., and Davidson, C. S. Association between aflatoxin content and hepatoma frequency in Uganda. *Cancer*, 1971; 28: 253.

Anderson, M.E., Luo, J.L. Glutathione therapy: from prodrugs to genes. *Semin Liver Dis.*, 1998; 18:415–424.

Aso, H., et al. Induction of interferon and activation of NK cells and macrophages in mice by oral administration of Ge-132, an organic germanium compound. *Journal of Microbiology and Immunology*, 1985; 29(1): 65–74.

Avdic, E., "Bicarbonate versus acetate hemodialysis: effects on the acid-base status" (Med Arh 2001; 55(4):231–3).

Aw, T.W., Wierzbicka G., Jones D.P. Oral glutathione increases tissue glutathione in vivo. *Chemico-biological Interactions*, 1991; 80:89–97.

Bains, J.S., Shaw, C.A. Neurodegenerative disorders in humans: the role of glutathione in oxidative stress-mediated neuronal death. *Brain Research Reviews*, 1997; 25:335–358.

Bakhir, V. *Electrochemical Activation*, 2 vol. All-Russian Institute for Medical Engineering, Moscow, 1992.

Barker, N. et al. Identification of stem cells in small intestine and colon by marker gene Lgr5. *Nature*, 449, 1003–7 (25 October 2007).

Batmanghelidj, F. *Your Body's Many Cries for Water.* Global Health Solutions, Falls Church, VA, 1992.

Béchamp, Pierre Jacques Antoine. *The Blood and Its Third Anatomical Element* (Montague R. Leverson, translator). London: John Ouseley Limited, 1912.

Becker, Robert O., M.D., and Selden, Gary. *The Body Electric. Electromagnetism and the Foundation of Life.* New York: Quill/William Morrow, 1985.

Bertz, A., et al. Modulation by cytokines of leukocyte endothelial cell interactions. Implications for thrombosis. *Biorheology*, 1990; 27: 455.

Bick, R. L. Disseminated intravascular coagulation. *Hematology/Oncology Clinics of North America*, 1993; 6: 1259.

Bird, Christopher. *Gaston Naessens.* Tiburon, Calif.: H. J. Kramer, Inc., 1991.

———. *The Galileo of the Microscope.* St. Lambert, Quebec, Canada: Les Presses de l'Université de la Personne, Inc., 1990.

———. To Be or Not to Be? A paper presented in an address to L'Orthobiologie Somatidienne Symposium 1991, Sherbrooke, Quebec, hosted by Gaston Naessens.

Blank, F. O., Chin, G., Just, B., et al. Carcinogens from fungi pathogenic for man. *Cancer Research*, 1968; 28: 2276.

Bleker, Dr. Maria. *Blood Examination in Darkfield According to Professor Dr. Günther Enderlein.* Gesamtherstellung, Germany: Semmelweis-Verlag, 1993.

Boeing, H., Schlehofer, B., Blettner, M., Wahrendorf, J. Dietary carcinogens and the risk for glioma and meningioma in Germany. *International Journal of Cancer*, 1993; 53(4): 561–65.

Bohn T, Walczyk S, Leisibach S, Hurrell RF. Chlorophyll-bound magnesium in commonly consumed vegetables and fruits: relevance to magnesium nutrition. *The Journal of Food Science*, 2004; 69(9): S347–S350.

Bolton, S., and Null, G. The medical uses of garlic: Fact and fiction. *American Pharmacy*, August 1982.

Borok Z, Buhl R, Grimes GJ, et al. Effect of glutathione aerosol on oxidant-antioxidant imbalance in ideopathic pulmonary fibrosis. *Lancet.* 1991; 338:215–216.

Bowers W.F. Chlorophyll in wound healing and suppurative disease. *Journal of the American Society of Plastic Surgeons*, 1947;73:37–50.

Bowie, E. J., et al. The clinical pathology of intravascular coagulation. *Bibliotheca Haematologica*, 1983; 49: 217.

Bredbacka, S., et al. Laboratory methods for detecting disseminated intravascular coagulation (DIC): New aspects. *Acta Anaesthesiologica Scandinavica*, 1993; 37: 125.

Breen, F. A., et al. Ethanol gelation: A rapid screening test for intravascular coagulation. *Annals of Internal Medicine*, 1970; 69: 1197.

Breinholt, V., Hendricks, J., Pereira, C., Arbogast, D., Bailey, G. Dietary chlorophyllin is a potent inhibitor of aflatoxin B1 hepatocarcinogenesis in rainbow trout. *Cancer Research*, 1995;55(1):57–62.

Breinholt, V., Schimerlik, M., Dashwood, R., Bailey, G. Mechanisms of chlorophyllin anticarcinogenesis against aflatoxin B1: complex formation with the carcinogen. *Chemical Research in Toxicology*, 1995;8(4):506–514.

Broquist, H.P. Buthionine sulfoximine, an experimental tool to induce glutathionine deficiency: elucidation of glutathionine and ascorbate in their role as antioxidants. *Nutrition Review*, 1992; 50:110–111.

Brown, L.A., Bai, C., Jones, D.P. Glutathione protection in aveolar type II cells from fetal and neonatal rabbits. *American Journal of Physiology*, 1992; 262:L305–L312.

Burkitt, D. Some disease characteristics of modern Western civilization. *British Medical Journal*, 1973; 1: 274.

Carp, H., et al. In vitro suppression of serum elastase-inhibitory capacity by ROTS generated by phagocytosing polymorphonuclear leukocytes. *Journal of Clinical Investigation*, 1979; 63: 793.

Carpenter, E.B. Clinical experiences with chlorophyll preparations. *American Journal of Surgery*, 1949; 77: 167–171.

Cascinu, S., Cordella, L., Del Ferro, E., et al. Neuroprotective effect of reduced glutathione on cisplatin-based chemotherapy in advanced gastric cancer: a randomized double-blind placebo-controlled study. *Journal of Clinical Oncology*, 1995; 13:26–32.

Chandler, W. L., et al. Evaluation of a new dynamic viscometer for measuring the viscosity of whole blood and plasma. *Clinical Chemistry*, 1986; 32: 505.

Chen, F., Cole, P., Mi, Z., Xing, L. Y. Corn and wheat-flour consumption and mortality from esophageal cancer in Shanxi, China. *International Journal of Cancer*, 1993; 4(2): 163–69.

Chernomorsky, S.A., Segelman, A.B. Biological activities of chlorophyll derivatives. *New Jersey Medicine*, 1988; 85(8):669–673.

Cheung, P-Y, Wang, W., Schulz, R. Glutathione protects against ischemia-perfusion injury by detoxifying peroxynitrite. *Journal of Molecular and Cellular Cardiology*, 2000; 32:1669–1678.

Chimploy, K., Diaz, G.D., Li, Q., et al. *International Journal of Cancer,* 2009; in press.

Cho, T. H., et al. Effects of *Escherichia coli* toxin on structure and permeability of myocardial capillaries. *Acta Pathologica Japonica,* 1991; 41: 12.

Christiansen, S.B., Byel, S.R., Stromsted, H., Stenderup, J.K., Eickhoff, J.H. [Can chlorophyll reduce fecal odor in colostomy patients?]. *Ugeskr Laeger,* 1989; 151(27): 1753–1754.

Colucci, M., et al. Cultured human endothelial cells: An in vitro model of vascular injury. *Journal of Clinical Investigation,* 1983; 71: 1893.

Cooper, L. A., and Gadd, G. M. Differentiation and melanin production in hyaline and pigmented strains of *Microdochium bolleyi.* In Constantini, A. V., Weiland, H., Qvick, Lars I. *The Fungal/Mycotoxin Etiology of Human Disease,* Vol. 2. Freiburg, Germany: Johann Friedrich Oberlin Verlag, 1994.

Cope, Freeman W. Evidence from activation energies for superconductive tunneling in biological systems at physiological temperatures. *Physiological Chemistry and Physics,* 1971; 3: 403–10.

Costantini, A. V., Weiland, H., Qvick, Lars I. *The Fungal/Mycotoxin Etiology of Human Disease,* Volumes 1 and 2. Freiburg, Germany: Johann Friedrich Oberlin Verlag, 1994.

Cusumano, V. Aflatoxin in patients with lung cancer. *Oncology,* 1991; 48: 194–95.

Dashwood, R., Yamane S, Larsen R. Study of the forces of stabilizing complexes between chlorophylls and heterocyclic amine mutagens. Environ Mol Mutagen. 1996;27(3): 211–218.

Dashwood, R.H., Breinholt, V., Bailey, G.S. Chemopreventive properties of chlorophyllin: inhibition of aflatoxin B1 (AFB1)-DNA binding in vivo and anti-mutagenic activity against AFB1 and two heterocyclic amines in the Salmonella mutagenicity assay. *Carcinogenesis,* 1991; 12(5):939–942.

Dashwood R.H. The importance of using pure chemicals in (anti) mutagenicity studies: chlorophyllin as a case in point. Mutat Res. 1997; 381(2):283–286.

Dawson-Huges, B. "Treatment with Potassium Bicarbonate Lowers Calcium Excretion and Bone Resorption in Older Men and Women," *The Journal of Clinical Endocrinology & Metabolism,* Vol. 94, No. 1 96–102.

De Mattia, G., Bravi, M.C., Laurenti, O., et al. Influence of reduced glutathione infusion on glucose metabolism in patients with non-insulin-dependent diabetes mellitus. *Metabolism,* 1998; 47:993–997.

Dement'eva, I.I. "Calculation of the dose of sodium bicarbonate in the treatment of metabolic acidosis in surgery with (and) deep hypothermic circulatory arrest" (Anesteziol Reanimatol 1997 Sep–Oct; 5:42–4).

Dickens, L. *Carcinogenesis: A Broad Critique.* Baltimore: Williams & Wilkins, 1967.

Dickens, R., and Jones, H. E. H. Further studies on the carcinogenic action of patulin-induced mammary adenomas and local sarcomas or fibrosarcomas in mice and rats. *British Journal of Cancer,* 1965; 19: 392.

Dingley, K.H., Ubick, E.A., Chiarappa-Zucca, M.L., et al. Effect of dietary constituents with chemopreventive potential on adduct formation of a low dose of the heterocyclic amines PhIP and IQ and phase II hepatic enzymes. *Nutrition and Cancer,* 2003; 46(2): 212–221.

Duke, Don, M. S. Materials rich in monoatomic elements [report on personal research]. Phoenix, Ariz., 1995.

Egner, P.A., Munoz, A., Kensler, T.W. Chemoprevention with chlorophyllin in individuals exposed to dietary aflatoxin. *Mutat Res.* 2003;523–524:209–216.

Egner, P.A., Stansbury, K.H., Snyder, E.P., Rogers, M.E., Hintz, P.A., Kensler, T.W. Identification and characterization of chlorine (4) ethyl ester in sera of individuals participating in the chlorophyllin chemoprevention trial. *Chemical Research in Toxicology,* 2000; 13(9): 900–906.

Egner, P.A., Wang, J.B., Zhu, Y.R., et al. Chlorophyllin intervention reduces aflatoxin-DNA adducts in individuals at high risk for liver cancer. *Proceedings of the National Academy of Sciences,* 2001; 98(25):14601–14606.

El-Osta, Assam et al. "Transient high glucose causes persistent epigenetic changes and altered gene expression during subsequent normoglycemia." *Journal of Experimental Medicine,* Vol. 205, No. 10, 2409–2417.

Encyclopedia of Chemical Technology. New York: John Wiley and Sons, 1983.

Enderlein, Prof. Dr. Günther. *Akmon,* Volume I, Books 1 and 2. Hamburg, Germany: Ibica-Verlag, 1957.

———. *Bakterien Cyclogenie.* Hamburg, Germany: Ibica-Verlag, 1925.

Enomoto, M. Carcinogenicity of mycotoxins. In *Toxicology, Biochemistry and Pathology of Mycotoxins* (Uraguchi, K., and Yamazaki, M., eds.). New York: John Wiley & Son, 1978.

Erickson, B.L. and Wullaert, R.A. Expanding a new scientific view of the functional properties of water.

———. *Proceedings of the Functional Water Symposiums,* (1994–2000), Tokyo, Japan.

Exner, R., Wessner, B., Manhart, N., Roth, E. Therapeutic potential of glutathione. *Wiener Klinische Wochenschrift,* 2000; 112: 610–616.

Favilli, F., Marraccini, P., Iantomasi, T., Vincenzini, M.T. Effect of orally administered glutathione levels in osme organs of rats: role of specific transporters. *British Journal of Nutrition,* 1997; 78: 293–300.

Feriani, M., Randomized long-term evaluation of bicarbonate-buffered CAPD solution. *Kidney International,* 1998; Nov; 54(5):1731–8.

Fernandes, G. Effect of Electrolyzed Water Intake on Lifespan of Autoimmune Disease Prone Mice. *FASEB Journal,* 12 (1998); A794.

Fink-Gemmels, J. The significance of mycotoxin assimilation of meat animals. *Deutsche Tierärztliche Wochenschrift,* 1989; 96(7): 360–63.

Flagg, E.W., Coates, R.J., Eley, J.W., et al. Dietary glutathione intake in humans and the relationship between intake and plasma total glutathionine level. *Nutrition and Cancer,* 1994; 21:33–46.

Franceschi, E. A. Meat, poultry, cooked ham, salami, sausages, cheese, butter and oil-related thyroid cancer. *International Journal of Cancer,* 1993; 53(4): 561–65.

Fungalbionics Convention: The Fungal/Mycotoxin Etiology of Chronic and Degenerative Disease. Metro Toronto Convention Centre, September 30, 1994.

Furukawa, T., Meydani, S.N., Blumberg, J.B. Reversal of age-associated decline in immune responsiveness by dietary glutathione supplementation in mice. *Mechanisms of Ageing and Development,* 1987; 38:107–117.

Gamba, G., Bicarbonate therapy in severe diabetic ketoacidosis. A double blind, randomized, placebo controlled trial. *Revista de Investigacion Clinica,* 1991, Jul-Sep; 43(3):234–8). Miyares Gomez A. in Diabetic ketoacidosis in childhood: the first day of treatment. *Anales de Pediatria,* 1989 Apr; 30(4): 279–83).

Ghadirian, P. Thermal irritation and esophageal cancer in northern Iran. *Cancer,* 1987; 60(8): 1909–14.

Giovannucci, E., Rimm, E. B., Colditz, G. A., Stampfer, M. J., Ascherio, A., Chute, C. C., and Willett, W. C. A prospective study of mycotoxins and risk of prostate cancer. *Journal of the National Cancer Institute,* 1993; 85(19): 1538–40.

Gogel, H.K., Tandberg, D., Strickland, R.G.. Substances that interfere with guaiac card tests: implications for gastric aspirate testing. *American Journal of Emergency Medicine,* 1989;7(5):474–480.

Griffith, O.W. Biologic and pharmacologic regulation of mammalian glutathione synthesis. *Free Radical Biology & Medicine,* 1999; 27:922–935.

Grimstad, I. A., et al. Thromboplastin release, but not content, correlates with spontaneous metastasis of cancer cells. *International Journal of Cancer,* 1988; 41: 427.

Gunji, Y., et al. Role of fibrin coagulation in protection of murine tumor cells from destruction by cytotoxic cells. *Cancer Research,* 1988; 48: 5216.

Hagen, T.M., Jones, D.P. Transepithelial transport of glutathione in vascularly perfused small intestine of rat. *American Journal of Physiology,* 1987; 252(5 Pt 1): G607–G613.

Hagen, T.M., Wierzbicka, G.T., Sillau, A.H., et al. Bioavailability of dietary glutathione: effect on plasma concentration. *American Journal of Physiology,* 1990; 259(4 Pt 1):G524–G529.

Hamilton, P. J., et al. Disseminated intravascular coagulation: A review. *Journal of Clinical Pathology,* 1978; 31: 609.

Hanaoka, K. Antioxidant Effects of Reduced Water Produced by Electrolysis of Sodium Chloride Solutions (to be published in *Journal of Applied Electrochemistry,* 2001).

Hay, E. D., ed. *Cell Biology of Extracellular Matrix.* New York: Plenum Press, 1981.

Hayes, J.D., McLellan, L.I. Glutathione and glutathione-dependent enzymes represent a co-ordinately regulated defence against oxidative stress. *Free Radical Research,* 1999; 31:273–300.

Hayes, J.D., Strange, R.C. Glutathione S-transferase polymorphisms and their biological consequences. *Pharmacology,* 2000; 61:154–166.

Heinicke, R. M. The pharmacologically active ingredient of noni [a paper]. University of Hawaii, January 1996.

Hendler, S.S., Rorvik D.R., eds. *PDR for Nutritional Supplements.* 2nd ed. Montvale: Physicians' Desk Reference, Inc; 2008.

Hercbergs, A., Brok-Simoni, F., Holtzman, F., et al. Erythrocyte glutathione and tumor response to chemotherapy. *Lancet,* 1992; 339:1074–1076.

Hertog, M. G., Feskens, E. J., Hollmati, P. C., Katan, M. B., and Kromhout, D. Dietary antioxidants and risk of coronary disease. *Lancet,* 1993; 342: 32–34.

Hills, Christopher. *Nuclear Evolution.* Boulder Creek, Calif.: University of the Trees Press, 1977.

Holroyd, K.J., Buhl, R., Borok, Z., et al. Correction of glutathione deficiency in the lower respiratory tract of HIV seropositive individuals by glutathione aerosol treatment. *Thorax,* 1993; 48:985–989.

Hu, T., et al. Synthesis of tissue factor messenger RNA and procoagulant activity in breast cancer cells in response to serum stimulation. *Thrombosis Research,* 1993; 72: 155.

Hudson, David. Alchemical research: DNA alteration and the rediscovery of the light of life. Yelm, Wash.: *Leading Edge Research;* Article 79, February 1995.

Hume, E. Douglas. *Béchamp or Pasteur? A Lost Chapter in the History of Biology,* 1st ed. Ashingdon, Rochford, Essex, England: The C. W. Daniel Company, 1923; 2d. ed. (London: C. W. Daniel Company, 1932) reprinted by Health Research: Pomeroy, Wash., 1989.

Hunder, G., Schumann, K., Strugala, G., Gropp, J., Fichtl, B., and Forth, W. Influence of subchronic exposure to low dietary deoxynivalenol, a trichothecene mycotoxin, on intestinal absorption of nutrients in mice. *Food Chemistry Toxicology,* 1991; 29(12): 809–14.

Hwang, C., Sinskey, A.J., Lodish, H.F. Oxidized redox state of glutathione in the endoplasmic reticulum. *Science.* 1992; 257:1496–1502.

Ingram, D. M., Nottage, E., and Roberts, T. The role of *Saccharomyces cerevisiae*—baker's, or brewer's, yeast—in the development of breast cancer: A case-control study of patients with breast cancer, benign epithelial hyperplasia and fibrocystic disease of the breast. *British Journal of Cancer,* 1991; 64(1): 187–91.

Iwata, K., ed. *Yeasts and Yeast-Like Micro-Organisms in Medical Science.* Tokyo: University of Tokyo Press, 1976.

Janaky, R., Ogita, K., Pasqualotta, B.A., et al. Glutathione and signal transduction in the mammalian CNS. Journal of Neurochemistry, 1999; 73:889–902.

Jones, T. W. Observations on some points in the anatomy, physiology, and pathology of the blood. *British Foreign Medical Review,* 1842; 14: 585.

Jonsyn, Lahai. Aspergillus/aflatoxin contamination of dried fish. *International Journal of Cancer,* 1991; 4(1): 8–11.

Kalokerinos, A., and Dettman, G. *Second Thoughts About Disease: A Controversy and Béchamp Revisited.* Warburton, Victoria, Australia: Biological Research Institute [booklet published from an article in *Journal of the International Academy of Preventive Medicine,* July 1977; 4(1): 18].

Kamat, J.P., Boloor, K.K., Devasagayam, T.P. Chlorophyllin as an effective antioxidant against membrane damage in vitro and ex vivo. *Biochimica et Biophysica Acta,* 2000;1487(2–3):113–127.

Kensler, T.W., Groopman, J.D., Roebuck, B.D. Use of aflatoxin adducts as intermediate endpoints to assess the efficacy of chemopreventive interventions in animals and man. *Mutation Research,* 1998; 402(1–2):165–172.

Kephart, J.C. Chlorophyll derivatives—their chemistry, commercial preparation, and uses. *Economic Botany,* 1955;9:3–38.

Keys, A. The role of the diet in human atherosclerosis and its complications. In *Atherosclerosis and Its Origin* (Sandler, M., and Bourne, G. H., eds.). New York and London: Academic Press, 1963.

Kikuchi, S., Okamoto, N., Suzuki, T., Kawahara, S., Nagai, H., Sakiyama, T., Wada, O., and Inaba, Y. A case-control study of breast cancer/mammary cyst and dietary, drinking or smoking habits in Japan. *Japanese Journal of Cancer Clinics*, 1990; 24: 365–69.

Kleiner, S. Water: An Essential but Overlooked Nutrient, *Journal of the American Dietetic Association*, 99 (1999) 200.

Kono, S., Imanishi, K., Shinchi, K., Yanai, F. Relationship of diet to small and large adenomas of the sigmoid colon. *Japan Journal of Cancer Research*, 1993; 84(1): 9–13.

Kumar, S.S., Devasagayam, T.P., Bhushan, B., Verma, N.C. Scavenging of reactive oxygen species by chlorophyllin: an ESR study. *Free Radical Research*, 2001; 35(5):563–574.

Kumar, S.S., Shankar, B., Sainis, K.B. Effect of chlorophyllin against oxidative stress in splenic lymphocytes in vitro and in vivo. *Biochimica et Biophysica Acta*, 2004; 1672(2):100–111.

Kumon, K. What is Functional Water? *Artificial Organs*, 21 (1997) 2.

Kwon-Chung, K. J., and Bennet, John E. *Medical Mycology*. Malvern, Penn.: Lea and Febiger, 1992.

La Vecchia, C., Decarli, A., Negri, E., Parazzini, F., Gentile, A., Cecchetti, G., Fasoli, M., and Franceschi, S. Dietary factors and the risk of epithelial ovarian cancer. *Journal of the National Cancer Institute*, 1987; 79(4): 663–69.

La Vecchia, C., Negri, E., Decarli, A., D'Avanzo, B., and Franceschi, S. A case-control study of diet and gastric cancer in northern Italy. *International Journal of Cancer*, 1987; 40(4): 484–89.

Lancaster, M. C., Jenkins, F. P., and Philp, J. M. C. L. Toxicity associated with certain samples of broken or ground nuts. *Nature*, 1961; 192: 1095–96.

Larsson, S.C., Orsini, N. and Wolk, A. Processed Meat Consumption and Stomach Cancer Risk: A Meta-Analysis, *Journal of the National Cancer Institute*, August 2, 2006; 98(15): 1078–1087.

Lash, L.H., Hagen, T.M., Jones, D.P. Exogenous glutathione protects intestinal epithelial cells from oxidative injury. *Proceedings of the National Academy of Sciences*, 1986; 83:4641–4645.

Lenzi, A., Culasso, F., Gandini, L., et al. Placebo-controlled, double-blind, cross-over trial of glutathione therapy in male infertility. *Human Reproduction*, 1993; 8:1657–1662.

Lenzi, A., Picardo, M., Gandini, L., et al. Glutathione treatment of dyspermia: effect on the lipoperoxidation process. *Human Reproduction*, 1994; 9:2044–2050.

Levi, F., Franceschi, S., Negri, E., and La Vecchia, C. Dietary factors and the risk of endometrial cancer. *Cancer*, 1993; 71(11): 3575–81.

Levy, M. M. An evidence-based evaluation of the use of sodium bicarbonate during cardiopulmonary resuscitation. *Critical Care Clinic*, Jul, 1998;

14(3):457–83). Vukmir, R.B., Sodium bicarbonate in cardiac arrest: a reappraisal *American Journal of Emergency Medicine,* 1996 Mar; 14(2):192–206. Bar-Joseph, G., Clinical use of sodium bicarbonate during cardiopulmonary resuscitation—is it used sensibly? (*Resuscitation,* Jul, 2002; 54(1):47–55).

Linderfelser, L. A., Lillehoj, E. B., and Burnmeister, H. R. Aflatoxin and trichothecene toxins: Skin tumor induction and synergistic acute toxicity in white mice. *Journal of the National Cancer Institute,* 1974; 52: 113.

Livingston-Wheeler, Virginia, MD *The Conquest of Cancer.* New York: Franklin Watts, 1984.

Loguercio, C, Di Pierro, M. The role of glutathione in the gastrointestinal tract: a review. *Italian Journal of Gastroenterology and Hepatology,* 1999; 31:401–407.

Longenecker, Gesina L., PhD *How Drugs Work.* Emeryville, Calif.: Ziff-Davis Press, 1994.

Lorber, A., et al. Clinical application of heavy metal complexing of N-actyl cysteine. *Journal of Clinical Pharmacology,* 1973; 13: 332–36.

Lynes, Barry. *The Cancer Cure That Worked! Fifty Years of Suppression.* Queensville, Ontario, Canada: Marcus Books, 1987.

Lyons J., Rauh-Pfeiffer A., Yu Y.M., et al. Blood glutathione synthesis rates in healthy adults receiving a sulfur amino acid-free diet. *Proceedings of the National Academy of Sciences,* 2000; 97:5071–5076.

Mackman, et al. Lipopolysaccharides—mediated transcriptional activation of the human tissue factor gene in THP-1 monocytic cells requires both activator protein 1 and nuclear factor kappa B binding sites. *Journal of Experimental Medicine,* 1991; 174: 1517.

Maier-Kopf, P. Complexes of metals other than platinum as anti-tumor agents. *Journal of Clinical Pharmacology,* 1994; 47: 1–16.

Margolis, J. The interrelationship of coagulation of plasma and release of peptides. *Annals of the New York Academy of Sciences,* 1963; 104: 133.

Margulis, Lynn, and Sagan, Dorion. *Micro-Cosmos.* New York: Summit Books, 1986.

Mariano, F. Insufficient correction of blood bicarbonate levels in biguanide lactic acidosis treated with CVVH and bicarbonate replacement fluids. *Minerva Urologica e nefrologica,* Sept. 1997; 49(3): 133–6.

Martensson, J., Jain, A., Meister A. Glutathione is required for intestinal function. *Proceedings of the National Academy of Sciences,* 1990; 87:1715–1719.

Matthews, C.K., van Holde, K.E. *Biochemistry.* 2nd ed. Menlo Park: The Benjamin/Cummings Publishing Company; 1996.

Mattman, Lida H. *Cell Wall Deficient Forms—Stealth Pathogens.* Cleveland: CRC Press, 1974.

Meister A. On the antioxidant effects of ascorbic acid and glutathionine. *Biochemical Pharmacology*, 1992; 44:1905–1915.

Miles, M. R., Olsen, L., and Rogers, A. Recurrent vaginal candidiasis; importance of an intestinal reservoir. *Journal of the American Medical Association*, 1977; 238: 1836–37.

Morrison, D. C., et al. The effects of bacterial endotoxins on host mediation systems. *American Journal of Pathology*, 1978; 93: 526.

Motola, Lynne. Hidden in plain sight, the meaning of "grass" in Hebrew. *Western Wheatgrass Journal*, January–March 1995; 2(1): 3–4.

Mueller, H. E., et al. Increase of microbial neuraminidase activity by the hydrogen peroxide concentration. *Experientia*, 1972; 23: 397.

Muller-Berghaus, G., et al. The role of granulocytes in the activation of intravascular coagulation and the precipitation of soluble fibrin by endotoxin. *Blood*, 1975; 45: 631.

Murphy, M.E., Scholich, H., Sies, H. Protection by glutathione and other thiol compounds against the loss of protein thiols and tocopherol homologs during microsomal lipid peroxidation. *European Journal of Biochemistry*, 1992; 210:139–146.

Nachman, R. L., et al. Detection of intravascular coagulation by a serial-dilution protamine sulfate test. *Annals of Internal Medicine*, 1971; 75: 895.

———. Hypercoagulable states. *Annals of Internal Medicine*, 1993; 119: 819.

Nagasawa, H.T., Cohen, J.F., Holleschau, A.M., Rathbun, W.B. Augmentation of human and rat lenticular glutathione in vitro by prodrugs of gamma-L-glutamyl-L-cysteine. *Journal of Medicinal Chemistry*, 1996; 39:1676–1681.

Neuhauser, I., and Gustus, E. L. Successful treatment of intestinal moniliasis with fatty acid resin complex. *Archives of Internal Medicine*, 1954; 93: 53–60.

New Frontier Newsletter. Salt Lake City: New Frontiers, Inc., November 1994.

Norell, S. E., Ahlbom, A., Erwald, R., Jacobson, G., Lindberg-Navier, I., Olin, R., Tornberg, B., and Wiechel, K. L. Diet and pancreatic cancer: A case-control study. *American Journal of Epidemiology*, 1986; 124(6): 894–902.

Novi, A.M. Regression of aflatoxin B1-induced hepatocellular carcinomas by reduced glutathione. *Science*, 1981; 212: 541–542.

Ohinataab, Y., Yamasobac, T., Schachta, J., Millera, J.M. Glutathione limits noise-induced hearing loss. *Hearing Research*, 2000; 146:28–34.

Olson, Rick. *Ionized Alkaline Water Using Platinum Electrolysis, Micro-Water and Coral Calcium* [proprietary marketing pamphlet for Coral Calcium]. Olympia, Wash.: Vitality Press and Product Information, September 1995.

Orner, G.A., Roebuck, B.D., Dashwood, R.H., Bailey, G.S. Post-initiation chlorophyllin exposure does not modulate aflatoxin-induced foci in the liver and colon of rats. *Journal of Carcinogenesis*, 2006; 5:6.

Palamara, A.T., Perno, C-F, Ciriolo, M.R., et al. Evidence for antiviral activity of glutathione: in vitro inhibition of herpes simplex virus type 1 replication. *Antiviral Research*, 1995; 27:237–253.

Paolisso, G., Giugliano, D., Pizza, G., et al. Glutathione infusion potentiates glucose-induced insulin secretion in aged patients with impaired glucose tolerance. *Diabetes Care*, 1992; 15:1–7.

Park, K.K., Park, J.H., Jung, Y.J., Chung, W.Y. Inhibitory effects of chloro-phyllin, hemin and tetrakis(4-benzoic acid)porphyrin on oxidative DNA damage and mouse skin inflammation induced by 12-O-tetradecanoylphor-bol-13-acetate as a possible anti-tumor promoting mechanism. *Mutation Research*, 2003; 542(1–2):89–97

Pasquale, A. D., Monforte, M. T., Calabro, M. L. HPLC analysis of oleuro-pein and some flavonoids in leaf and bud of *Olea europaea*. *Il Farmaco*, 1991; 46(6): 803–15.

Pearson, R. B. *Pasteur: Plagiarist, Impostor! The Germ Theory Exploded* (1942). Reprinted Pomeroy, Wash.: National Health Research Association. (See Resources section for information on National Health Research Association.)

———. *The Dream and Lie of Louis Pasteur*. Collingwood, Australia: Sumeria Press, 1994.

Peck, S. M., and Rosenfeld, H. The effects of hydrogen ion concentration, fatty acids and vitamin C on the growth of fungi. *Journal of Investigative Dermatology*, 1938; 1: 237–65.

Perlman, H. H. Undecylenic acid given orally in psoriasis and neurodermatitis. *Journal of the American Medical Association*, 1949; 139: 444–47.

Peska, J. J., and Bondy, G. S. Alteration of immune function following dietary mycotoxin exposure. *Canadian Journal of Physiology and Pharmacology*, 1990; 68(7): 1009–16.

Qian, G.S., Ross, R.K., Yu, M.C., et al. A follow-up study of urinary markers of aflatoxin exposure and liver cancer risk in Shanghai, People's Republic of China. *Cancer Epidemiology, Biomarkers and Research*, 1994; 3(1):3–10.

Rapaport, S. I. Blood coagulation and its alterations in hemorrhagic and thrombotic disorders. *The Western Journal of Medicine*, 1993; 158: 153.

Ren, A., and Han, X. Dietary factors and esophageal cancer: A case-control study. *Chinese Journal of Epidemiology*, 1991; 12(4): 200–4.

Robey, I.F. et al. Bicarbonate increases tumor pH and inhibits spontaneous metastases. *Cancer Research*, 2009; 69(6): 2260–8.

Rodricks, J. B., Hessiltine, C. W., Mehlman, M. A., eds. *Mycotoxins in Human and Animal Health*. Park Forest South, Ill.: Pathotox Publishers, 1977.

Rosenberg, E. W., Belew, P. W., Skinner, R. B., and Crutcher, N. Response to Crohn's disease and psoriasis. *New England Journal of Medicine*, 1983; 308: 101.

Roum, J.H., Borok, Z., McElvaney, N.G., et al. Glutathione aerosol suppresses lung epithelial surface inflammatory cell-derived oxidants in cystic fibrosis. *Journal of Applied Physiology*, 1999; 87: 438–443.

Saleem, A., et al. Viscoelastic measurement of clot formation: A new test of platelet function. *Annals of Clinical and Laboratory Science*, 1983; 13: 115.

Samiec, P.S., Drews-Botsch, C., Flagg, E.W., et al. Glutathione in human plasma: decline in association with aging, age-related macular degeneration, and diabetes. *Free Radical Biology & Medicine*, 1998; 24:699–704.

Sander, F. F. *The Acid-Base Household of the Human Organism*. 1930

Sandler, M., and Bourne, G. H., eds. *Atherosclerosis and Its Origin*. New York and London: Academic Press, 1963.

Sava, G., Giraldi, T., Mestroni, G., and Zassinovich, G. Antitumor effects of rhodium, iridium, and ruthenium complexes in comparison with cisdichlorodiamino platinum in mice bearing Lewis lung carcinoma. *Chemico-Biological Interactions*, 1983; 45: 1–6.

Schmidinger, M., Budinsky, A.C., Wenzel, C., et al. Glutathione in the prevention of cisplatin induced toxicities. A prospectively randomized pilot trial in patients with head and neck cancer and non small cell lung cancer. *Wien Klin Wochenschr*, 2000; 112: 617–623.

Schwartz, G. J. et al. The lipid messenger OEA links dietary fat intake to satiety. *Cell Metabolism*, October 2008: 8(4):281–288.

Selig, M. S. Mechanisms by which antibiotics increase the incidence and severity of candidiasis and alter the immunological defense. *Bacteriological Review*, 1966; 30: 442–59.

Shaw, C.A., ed. *Glutathione in the Nervous System*. London: Taylor and Francis; 1998.

Shirahata, S., et al: Electrolyzed-Reduced Water Scavenges Active Oxygen Species and Protects DNA from Oxidative Damage, *Biochemical and Biophysical Research Communications*, 234 (1997): 269.

Shook, E. E. *Advanced Treatise in Herbology*. Banning, Calif.: Enos Publishing Co., 1992.

Siegel, L.H. The control of ileostomy and colostomy odors. *Gastroenterology*, 1960; 38: 634–636.

Sies, H. Glutathione and its role in cellular functions. *Free Radical Biology of Medicine*, 1999; 27: 916–921.

Silberberg, J. M., et al. Identification of tissue factor in two human pancreatic cancer cell lines. *Cancer Research*, 1989; 49: 5443.

Silomon, M. Effect of sodium bicarbonate infusion on hepatocyte Ca2+ overload during resuscitation from hemorrhagic shock. *Resuscitation*, April, 1998; 37 (1): 27–32.

Simonich, M.T. Egner, P.A., Roebuck, B.D., et al. Natural chlorophyll inhibits aflatoxin B1-induced multi-organ carcinogenesis in the rat. *Carcinogenesis*, 2007; 28(6): 1294–1302.

Smith, L.W.. The present status of topical chlorophyll therapy. *New York State Journal of Medicine*, 1955; 55(14): 2041–2050.

Smith, R.G.. Enzymatic debriding agents: an evaluation of the medical literature. *Ostomy Wound Management*, 2008; 54(8): 16–34.

Smyth, J.F., Bowman, A., Perren, T., et al. Glutathione reduces the toxicity and improves quality of life of women diagnosed with ovarian cancer treated with cisplatin: results of a double-blind, randomized trial. *Annals of Oncology*, 1997; 8: 569–573.

Spillert, C. R., et al. Altered coagulability: An aid to selective breast biopsy. *Journal of the National Medical Association*, 1993; 85: 273.

Sprince, H., et al. Protective action of ascorbic acid and sulfur compounds (including N-acetyl cysteine) against toxicity: Implications in alcoholism and smoking. *Agents and Actions*, 1975; 5: 164–73.

Steinmetz, K. A., and Potter, J. D. Food-group consumption and colon cancer in the Adelaide case-control study: Meat, poultry, seafood, dairy foods and eggs. *International Journal of Cancer*, 1993; 53(5): 720–27.

Stephens, D.J. The use of sodium chloride in the treatment of hypopituitarism. *The Journal of Clinical Endocrinology*, 1941; Vol. 1, No. 2 109–112.

Sternberg, P. Jr., Davidson, P.C., Jones, D.P., et al. Protection of retinal pigment epithelium from oxidative injury by glutathione and precursors. *Investigative Opthalmology & Visual Science*, 1993; 34:3661–3668.

Structure, Betina V. Activity relationships among mycotoxins. *Chemico-Biological Interactions*, 1989; 71(2–3): 105–46.

Sudakin, D.L. Dietary aflatoxin exposure and chemoprevention of cancer: a clinical review. *Journal of Toxicology—Clinical Toxicology*, 2003; 41(2): 195–204.

Sugiyama, S., et al. The role of leukotoxin (9, 10-epoxy-12-octadecenoate) in the genesis of coagulation abnormalities. *Life Sciences*, 1988; 43: 221.

Tachino, N., Guo, D., Dashwood, W.M., Yamane, S., Larsen, R., Dashwood, R. Mechanisms of the in vitro antimutagenic action of chlorophyllin against benzo[a]pyrene: studies of enzyme inhibition, molecular complex formation and degradation of the ultimate carcinogen. *Mutation Research*, 1994; 308(2):191–203.

Tallman, M. S., et al. New insights into the pathogenesis of coagulation dysfunction in acute promyelocytic leukemia. *Leukemia and Lymphoma*, 1993; 11: 27.

Topley and Wilson. *Principles of Bacteriology, Virology and Immunity*. Baltimore: Williams & Wilkins, 1984.

Toth, B., and Gannett, P. Carcinogenesis study in mice by 3-methylbutanol methylformylhydrazone of Gyromitra esculenta, in vivo. *Mycopathologia*, 1990; 4(5): 283–88.

Toth, B., Patil, K., Erickson, J., and Kupper, R. False morel mushroom Gyromitra esculenta toxin: N-methyl-N-formylhydrazone carcinogenesis in mice. *Mycopathologia*, 1979; 68(2): 121–28.

Toth, B., Patil, K., Pyssalo, H., Stessman, C., and Gannett, P. Cancer induction in mice by feeding the raw morel mushroom Gyromitra esculenta. *Cancer Research*, 1992; 52(8): 2279–84.

Toth, B., Taylor, J., and Gannett, P. Tumor induction with hexanol methylformylhydrazone of Gyromitra esculenta. *Mycopathologia*, 1991; 115(2): 65–71.

Tranter, H. S., Tassou, S., and Nychas, G. J. The effect of the olive phenolic compound, oleuropein, on growth and enterotoxin B production by Staphylococcus aureus. *Journal of Applied Microbiology*, 1993; 74: 253–59.

Trousseau, A. *Phlegmasia alba dolens Clinique Médicale de l'Hôtel-Dieu de Paris*. London: New Sydenham Society, 1865; 3: 94.

Truss, C. Orian, M.D. *The Missing Diagnosis*. Birmingham, Ala.: The Missing Diagnosis, Inc., 1983.

Uraguchi, K., and Yamazaki, M., eds. *Toxicology, Biochemistry, and Pathology of Mycotoxins*. New York: John Wiley & Son, 1978.

Van Deventer, S. J. H., et al. Intestinal endotoxemia. *Gastroenterology*, 1988; 94(3): 825–31.

Virchow, R. Hypercoagulability: A review of its development, clinical application, and recent progress. *Gesammelte Abhandlungen zur Wissenschäftlichen Medizin*, 1856; 26: 477.

Visioli, F., and Galli, C. Oleuropein protects low density lipoprotein from oxidation. *Life Sciences*, 1994; 55: 1965–71.

Vrijlandt, P. J., Sodium bicarbonate infusion for intoxication with tricyclic antidepressives: recommended in spite of lack of scientific evidence *Nederlands Tijdschrift voor Geneeskunde*, Sept., 2001;145(35): 1686–9). Knudsen, K., Epinephrine and sodium bicarbonate independently and additively increase survival in experimental amitriptyline poisoning. *Critical Care Medicine,* Apr 1997; 25(4): 669–74.

Wallach, Joel, BS, DVM, ND *Rare Earths.* Bonita, Calif.: Ma Lan and Double Happiness Publishing Co., 1994.

Weingarten, M., Payson, B. Deodorization of colostomies with chlorophyll. *Revista de Gastroenterologia,* 1951; 18(8): 602–604.

Weir, D., Farley, K.L.. Relative delivery efficiency and convenience of spray and ointment formulations of papain/urea/chlorophyllin enzymatic wound therapies. *Journal of Wound, Ostomy and Continence Nursing,* 2006; 33(5): 482–490.

Westhof, E. *Water and Biological Macromolecules,* CRC Press, Boca Raton, FL: 1993.

White, A., et al., eds. *Principles of Biochemistry.* New York: McGraw-Hill Book Co., 1964.

Wilson, C. L. The alternatively spliced V region contributes to the differential incorporation of plasma and cellular fibronectins into fibrin clots. *Journal of Cell Biology,* 1992; 119: 923.

Witschi, A., Reddy, S., Stofer, B., Lauterburg, B.H. The systemic availability of oral glutathione. *European Journal of Clinical Pharmacology,* 1992; 43:667–669.

Wray, B. B., and O'Steen, J. M. Mycotoxin-producing fungi from house associated with leukemia. *Archived Environmental Health,* 1975; 30: 571–73.

Wray, B. B., Rushing, E. J., Schindel, A., and Boyd, R. C. Suppression of response to phytohemagglutinin in guinea pigs by fungi from a leukemia-associated house. *Archived Environmental Health,* 1979; 22: 400.

Wylie, T. D., and Morehouse, L. G. *Mycotoxic Fungi, Mycotoxins, Mycotoxicoses: An Encyclopedia Handbook,* Vol. 3.

Yamada, O., et al. Deleterious effects of endotoxins on cultured endothelial cells: An in vitro model of vascular injury. *Inflammation,* 1981; 5: 115.

Yamazaki, H., Fujieda, M., Togashi, M., et al. Effects of the dietary supplements, activated charcoal and copper chlorophyllin, on urinary excretion of trimethylamine in Japanese trimethylaminuria patients. *Life Sciences,* 2004; 74(22): 2739–2747.

Yoshida, S., Kasuga, S. H., Hayashi, N., Ushiroguchi, T., Matsura, H., and Nakagawa, S. Anti-fungal activity of garlic. *Applied and Environmental Microbiology,* 1987; 53(3): 615–17.

Young, R.W., Beregi, J.S. Jr. Use of chlorophyllin in the care of geriatric patients. *Journal of the American Geriatrics Society,* 1980; 28(1): 46–47.

Young, Robert O. *Fermentology and oxidology.* The study of fungus-produced mycotoxic species and the activation of the immune system and release of reactive oxygen toxic species (ROTS) [Self-published]. Alpine, UT: Inner-Light Biological Research Foundation, 1994.

Yun, C.H., Jeong, H.G., Jhoun, J.W., Guengerich, F.P. Non-specific inhibition of cytochrome P450 activities by chlorophyllin in human and rat liver microsomes. *Carcinogenesis*, 1995; 16(6):1437–1440.

Zhang, L. Perhydrit and sodium bicarbonate improve maternal gases and acid-base status during the second stage of labor. Department of Obstetrics and Gynecology, Xiangya Hospital, Hunan Medical University, Changsha 410008. Maeda, Y., Perioperative administration of bicarbonate d solution to a patient with mitochondrial encephalomyopathy. *Masui*, Mar 2001; 50(3): 299-303.

Zieve, L., et al. Effect of hepatic failure toxins on liver thymidine kinase activity and ornithine decarboxylase activity after massive necrosis with acetaminophen in the rat. *Journal of Laboratory and Clinical Medicine*, 1985; 106(5): 583–88.

Zwicker, G. M., Carlton, W. W., and Tuite, J. Long-term administration of sterigmatocystin and *Penicillium viridicatum* to mice. *Food, Cosmetics and Toxicology*, 1974; 12: 491.

About the Authors

Dr. Robert O. Young and Shelley Redford Young are founders of the pH Miracle Retreat Center at the Rancho Del Sol in Valley Center, California, near San Diego. They are also coauthors of *The pH Miracle for Diabetes* and *The pH Miracle for Weight Loss*. Their books have been translated into more than twenty different languages.

Robert O. Young, PhD, DSc, is a nationally renowned cellular microbiologist and nutritionist who speaks to audiences around the world on health and wellness. He holds a degree in microbiology, nutrition, and naturopathic medicine. He has devoted his life to researching the causes of poor health and helping people reclaim their health and well-being. He is head of the pH Miracle Living Center and Foundation and has gained worldwide recognition for his research into diabetes, cancer, leukemia, and AIDS. He is a member of the American Society of Microbiologists and the American Naturopathic Medical Association, and he conducts classes in live and dried blood cell analysis, the New Biology, and the Science of Alkaline Living. Dr. Young is also the author of *Sick and Tired*; *One Sickness, One Disease, One Treatment*; *Profiles in Microbiology*; and *Herbal Nutritional Medications*.

Shelley Redford Young, LMT, is a licensed massage therapist specializing in lymphatic massage. Her passions include educating people on the healing effects of adopting an alkaline diet, and combining that with other effective healing modalities such as massage therapy and exercise. Her conviction is that healing should be simple, affordable, and available to all. Her heartfelt mission is to help the next generation, especially, learn about preventive and restorative health practices. She is also the author of *Back to the House of Health*, *Back to the House of Health 2*, and *Massage Therapy*, and the illustrator of *Doc Broc's Stone Hinge Cave Adventure*, a children's book teaching alkalizing principles.

Together, Robert and Shelley Young provide a dynamic dose of health and nutrition expertise that's designed to inform and enlighten.

Index

See also Recipe Index on page 255

acetaldehyde, 36–37, 101, 113
acidity (acidosis), 11–18; American diet and, 26; bacteria growth and, 19, 48; *Candida* and, 16–17; causes, 26–27; cycle of imbalance, 27; decomposition, death, and, 21–22; digestion and, 50–51, 133; disease and, 12, 13, 19, 30, 45, 47, 48–49; environmental toxins causing, 15; food causes, 6, 15, 31, 65, 101–16, 216; metabolic causes, 15; microforms and, 15–21, 26, 48; pH of blood and, 4, 5, 12–15, 17–18, 22–24; seven stages of, 14; symptoms of, 13, 14, 16–17, 29–49 (*see also specific disorders*); ten foods that cause symptoms, 35; tests for, 22–26; water and, 121–22
acupuncture or acupressure, 224
adrenal glands, 13, 16, 31, 36, 57, 186; supplements for, 186, 204–5
aging, 4, 9, 14, 42, 54, 75, 188
alcohol, 21, 37, 58, 65, 113, 116; supplements for damage, 186
alfalfa, 100; green drink/powder, 185, 262; seeds, 159, 160; sprouts, 90, 96, 163, 164, 165, 169–70, 290
algae, 35, 69, 112, 132, 182
alkalinity, 11, 145–46; Cleanse, 168–80; COWS, 65–85, 184; digestion and, 50–61; exercise and, 6, 27, 39, 41, 45, 215–29; 80–20 diet and, 5–6, 82, 179,

252; food combining with, 134–41; health and, 12, 15, 21, 27, 30, 42–43, 45–47; ideal, 23, 27; juices and, 128–31; mineral salts for, 22, 45, 77–80, 188–89; pH of blood/tissue, 5–6, 12–15, 21, 27; pH Miracle diet and lifestyle program for, 27–28; supplements for, 45, 172–73, 179, 188–89, 192; tests for, 22–26; tips and tricks, 166–67; transitioning and, 147–57; water and, 71–74, 120–28; what to eat, 6, 22, 27, 45, 65–71, 78, 82, 86–101
allergies, 6, 13, 17, 33–35, 42–43, 48, 70, 190; airborne (hay fever), 17, 33; food, 17, 33–35, 105; top ten foods that cause, 35
almond(s), 97, 106, 107, 151; pH, 101; recipes, 298, 302, 307, 311, 315, 316, 319, 351, 354, 378
almond milk, 24, 69, 105, 152, 156, 248; recipes, 268, 269
aloe vera juice, 56, 176
ALS (Lou Gehrig disease), 13
Alzheimer's disease, 75, 115
amaranth, 94, 159
amino acids 45, 88, 173; supplements, 194, 212, 213; what to eat, 90, 95, 96, 132
antibiotics, 57, 104, 108, 202, 211, 238
antifungals, 105, 182, 191, 193, 194, 198, 200, 201, 203, 211
antimycotoxics, 69, 173, 185, 193, 194
antioxidants, 67–68, 88, 89, 92, 195–96

anti-parasite formulas, 92, 179, 195, 211, 212
anti-yeast formulas, 179, 194, 198, 200, 201, 205, 207, 208
arthritis, 7, 9, 16, 26, 48, 70, 76, 85, 111, 115, 170, 204, 224; supplements for, 187, 195, 201
artichoke, 96, 100, 107
asparagus, 22, 87, 96, 107, 137, 153, 161; pH, 100; recipes, 272, 344
asthma, 16, 33, 37–38, 42–43, 48, 59, 70, 73
atherosclerosis, 13, 16, 26, 70, 186
avocado, 22, 65, 87–89, 96, 97, 106, 107, 160, 161, 185, 194, 247, 248, 249; for Cleanse, 171, 172, 178, 179; food combining, 139, 140; oil, 88–89, 160, 178, 179; pH, 100; recipes, 265, 266, 267, 273, 303–4, 305, 312, 315, 371; transitioning and, 153, 155

bacteria, 15, 16–21, 48, 109, 132; allergies and, 33–35; digestion and, 54, 58; supplements and, 201, 202
balance (pH balance), 3–8; acid foods, 6, 31, 216, 101–16; alkalizing foods, 6, 27, 82, 86–101; blood and, 5, 12–15, 74; Cleanse and, 168–80; supplements, 6, 45, 172–73, 179, 188–89, 192; tests 22–26; transitioning and, 151, 157; what to eat, 86–101. *See also* alkalinity
bamboo shoots, 96, 107
barley, 97, 107, 325; grass, 60, 69, 100, 169, 185
basil: pesto, 166, 249, 335; recipes, 299, 322, 353
beans (dried, all types), 7, 96, 97, 106, 107, 166, 167; canned, 93; Cleanse and, 177–78; pH of, 101; recipes, 288, 289, 329, 334, 339, 347, 365, 367; spouts, 87, 90, 163–65, 167; transitioning and, 149, 151; what to eat, 93–94, 159. *See also* edamame
beans, green, 69, 87, 100, 106, 129; recipes, 278, 367, 369
beans, lima, 97, 101, 107
Béchamp, Antoine, 20
beet, 100; greens, 87, 96, 107, 129; juice, 93, 128, 129; soup (borscht) 282
Bernard, Claude, 20
beta-carotene, 45
beverages: pH of common, 116; what not to drink, 66, 113; what to drink, 120–33. *See also* green drink; juices; water
bioflavonids, 85, 195–96

black currant, 187
black walnut hulls, 179, 212
bladder, 17; cancer, 74, 173
blood, 17–18, 27, 67, 74, 121; acidity, 5, 11, 13–15, 17, 23, 30, 50; Cleanse and, 169, 176; digestion and, 50, 53–54, 58; dried blood analysis, 25–26, 35; form changes of blood cells, 20, 53–54; live blood analysis, 24–25, 34, 35; microforms and, 15–18, 24–26; microwaved food and, 115; pH balance and, 5, 12–15, 17, 23, 27–28, 74; salt and, 75; supplements, 183, 191, 195, 202; testing pH, 22–26; in urine, 130; vegetable juice drink for, 264; what not to eat, 105, 108–9; what to eat, 67, 89
blood sugar, 6, 17, 38, 40–41, 94, 101, 136, 206, 237; stabilizing supplements, 188, 191, 202, 206; symptoms of acidity, 17, 31, 37, 38–39
body temperature, 59, 72, 74
bones, 14, 16, 41–52, 59, 74; calcium content of alkalizing foods, 107; supplements, 42, 188, 190, 205; what not to eat, 105, 111; what to eat, 105–6. *See also* osteoporosis
borage seed oil, 70, 101, 186, 187, 206
boron, colloidal, 208, 212, 213
brain, 6, 73, 109, 111, 113, 121, 115, 164, 209, 228, 239; supplements for, 70, 186, 200, 201, 202
Brazil nut, 97, 101, 107, 159
breads, 7, 8, 102, 111, 133, 136, 167; brands of, 159; food combining with, 138, 140; motivation tips, 235; pH, 116; recipes, 369; sprouted wheat, 370; transitioning and, 148, 153–54; yeast-free, 139, 153, 159, 379
breakfast, 8, 24, 82, 90, 113, 156, 162, 236; ideas for, 247–49, 358; transitioning, 148–49, 152–54
breast, 32, 33; cancer, 45–47, 73–74, 89, 97, 98, 108–9, 111
broccoli, 22, 87, 96, 107, 112, 129, 169, 185; pH, 100; recipes, 249, 270, 275, 277, 291, 328, 330
Brussels sprouts, 87, 96, 107, 328
buckwheat, 66, 94; cereal, 248; groats, 94, 100, 248; recipe, 363; sprouts, 91
burdock, 87
burns, 126, 197–98, 201
butyric acid, 200

cabbage, 87, 96, 100, 107, 129, 166, 169;
  Chinese, 96, 107; recipes, 286, 290, 292,
  293, 332, 338
caffeine, 32, 46, 113–14, 148, 199
calcium, 45, 74, 184, 192, 205, 208, 212,
  213; carbonate, 45, 98, 174, 175, 179,
  188, 189; cell salts, 192; content of
  alkalizing foods, 107 (chart); blood pH
  and, 14; bones and, 42, 74; elenolate,
  202; transitioning and, 151; what to eat,
  88, 105–6, 151
calories, 5, 61, 67, 70, 74, 96–97, 215, 247
cancer: artificial sweeteners and, 115;
  Cleanse for, 173–75; dehydration and,
  73; diet and lifestyle prevention, 45,
  85, 89, 97–98, 108–9; fungus and, 112;
  grains and, 111; lactic acid and, 59,
  104; mycotoxins and tumors, 21; pH
  balance and, 4, 6, 9 13, 14, 16, 26, 43,
  44–47; soup for, 277–78; supplements
  for, 45, 94, 187, 194, 201, 202, 205,
  207, 209, 211; yeast and, 111. *See also*
  specific types
Candida, 15–18, 188. *See also* yeast
caprylic acid, 105, 193–94, 198, 200, 202,
  203, 205, 207, 208, 211–12, 213
carbohydrates: Cleanse and, 178; complex,
  9, 93, 102, 103, 177–78; food combining
  with, 135; simple, 102, 111, 148 (*see
  also* sugar); transitioning and, 148–49,
  154–55; what not to eat, 101–2,
  103, 178; what to eat, 93–94 (*see also*
  vegetables)
carrot(s), 83, 84, 87, 100, 165; juice, 93,
  128, 129; recipes, 279, 302, 314, 319,
  354, 369, 378
cashews, 114, 116, 118
cauliflower, 87, 96, 100, 106, 107; recipes,
  249, 275, 276, 293, 311, 368
celery, 87, 96, 100, 106, 107, 129, 165, 169;
  recipes, 276, 279, 282, 319
cell salts, 75, 172, 192, 200
cereal, 111, 113, 137, 148, 152, 154, 248,
  326
chewing, 51, 84–85, 147
chia, 100, 159
chickpeas, 91, 97, 98, 106, 107; recipes, 313,
  334
chicory, 102, 115, 154
children and babies, 9, 10, 44, 95, 169, 201
chili peppers, 156, 159, 160; dried, 160;
  recipes, 304, 317, 359
chives, 96, 100, 107
chlorine, 65, 121, 125; dioxide, 126, 188

chlorophyll, 54, 66–70, 184, 185; liquid,
  173, 185. *See also* green powder
chocolate, 58, 66, 101, 113, 191
cholesterol, 24, 85, 88, 135–37, 170–71;
  blood acidity and high, 39–40; pH
  balance and, 5, 6, 7–8, 40, 85, 88,
  136–37, 171; supplements, 186, 188,
  200, 201, 202, 206
chromium, 172, 192, 203, 205, 206, 213
chronic fatigue syndrome, 16, 36, 115
cilantro, 69, 159, 161, 306, 322
cinnamon extract, 207
citron, 203, 214
Cleanse, 146, 168–80; after cleansing,
  177–78, 179–80; laxative effect, 175–76;
  supplements, additional alkalizing, 179;
  supplements, basic alkalizing,172–73;
  typical day, 174–75; what to look out for,
  176–77
coconut: milk, 101, 152; oil, 155; recipes,
  266, 270, 309, 310, 312
coffee, 58, 66, 116
colds, 13, 16, 19, 48, 57, 191, 209
colitis, 16, 58, 73
collards, 96, 107, 169
colon, 14, 52, 56, 121, 129; cancer of, 51,
  73, 109; Cleanse and, 169, 175–76;
  supplements and, 193
condiments, 113, 116, 155
congestion, 13, 48, 59, 190, 194, 205–6,
  209
constipation, 58, 73, 176, 189
cooking, 108, 150; cookware, 162–63;
  microwave, 114–15
copper, 65, 88, 89, 92, 173, 192
CoQ1 (NADH), 207–8
CoQ10, 207
corn and corn products, 114, 116, 154
COWS, 65–85, 86, 184; chewing, 84;
  chlorophyll (green vegetables), 67–70;
  80–20 diet, 5–6, 82, 179, 252; fresh,
  organic foods, 83–84, 129; meals, 82;
  oils (essential fats), 70–71; raw foods,
  82–83; salt, 74–80, 83; water, 71–74
Crohn's disease, 51, 176
cucumber, 22, 66, 87, 93, 96, 107, 129, 169,
  185; pH, 100; recipes, 270, 271, 273,
  284, 285, 293, 300
cysts, 14, 16, 32

daidzein, 97
dairy foods, 58, 59, 61, 65, 94, 95,
  104–6, 109; eliminating, 37; pH, 116;
  transitioning and, 148, 152

dandelion greens, 96, 100, 107
dehydrating foods, 90
dehydration, 71–73, 75, 165–66
depression, 16, 32, 37, 115
desserts, 236; recipes, 377–78;
    transitioning and, 150–51, 154
diabetes, 4, 6, 9, 13, 16, 26, 38–39,
    40–41, 115, 186; supplements for,
    202, 207
diarrhea, 16, 58, 92, 176
digestion, 50–61, 74, 110, 121, 131; chyme
    and, 52, 54; HCL, enzymes, probiotics
    warning, 54–56; microforms and, 51,
    54, 55, 56, 58, 59, 60; mucus and,
    57–59; poor (indigestion), acidity and,
    3, 16, 31, 50–51, 60, 133, 140, 233, 234;
    restoring health of, 59–61, 92, 168, 225;
    supplements, 60, 183, 188, 189, 194,
    206, 207; what not to eat, 110, 114, 135,
    140; what to eat, 60, 110, 133, 140, 177
disease: acidosis as cause, 12, 13, 19,
    30; Cleanse and "healing crisis," 176;
    confusing symptoms and, 29–49; germ
    theory and, 18–19; microforms and,
    16–18, 26; symptoms of acidity and, 13,
    29–49. *See also specific types*
diverticulitis, 58
DNA, 16, 20, 39, 102, 137, 183
docosahexanoic acid (DHA), 186
dog grass, 69, 100

ear/ear infections, 44, 207
eating out, 153, 236
edamame (soybeans), 93, 94, 97, 159, 178;
    recipes, 248, 249, 272, 308, 354
eggplant, 87, 96, 107
eggs, 35, 65, 94–95, 108–9, 116, 133;
    substitute, 379; transitioning and, 148, 154
eicosapentaenoic acid (EPA), 186
80–20 diet, 5–6, 82, 179, 252
Enderlein, Günther, 18
endometriosis, 16
energy, 16, 65; alkalizing diet and, 37, 66, 94,
    110; Cleanse and, 172; digestion and, 50,
    52, 54, 56, 60; EFAs and, 70; electron-
    charged water, 123–25; microforms and
    loss of, 36; mineral salts and, 77; pH
    balance and, 3, 6; raw foods and, 82–83,
    177; supplements and, 191, 200, 201, 202,
    207; symptoms of acidity and, 15, 31–32,
    35–37; transitioning and, 148
enzymes, 36, 38, 55, 152, 182, 193, 202;
    alkalizing foods and buffering, 66,
    98, 131; digestion and, 51, 54, 55–56;

juices and, 131, 132; supplement danger,
    54–55, 56
Epsom salts, 190, 220
equipment: blender, 162; cookware,
    stainless-steel, 162–63; dehydrator, 166;
    food processor, 161–62; juicer, 130;
    knives, 161; mandolin, 162; rice cooker,
    162, 167; saladacco, 162; salad spinner,
    162; Young pHorver Ionizer, 125
erectile dysfunction (ED), 191
esophageal cancer, 111, 114
essential fatty acids (EFAs), 70–71, 151;
    supplements and, 186–88
Essiac tea, 171, 211–12
evening primrose oil, 101, 187
exercise, 14, 27, 38, 47, 118; aerobic,
    221–22; aerobic vs. anaerobic, 217–18;
    alkaline, 6, 27, 215–29; amount of,
    218–20; lactic acid and, 218–19;
    lymphatic system and, 215–17, 223;
    passive, 223–29; pH balance and, 6, 27,
    39, 41, 45; static, 222–23
exotoxins, 15, 31, 33, 36, 38, 39
eyes, 4, 6, 16, 17, 33, 115; supplements,
    186, 207

fatigue, 3, 7–9, 13, 17, 32, 35–38, 60, 115,
    176
fats, dietary, 5, 9, 31, 70–71, 88, 99, 104,
    178; food combining with, 134, 139,
    140; pH of, 101, 116; supplements and,
    186–88, 207; transitioning and, 148,
    151; what not to eat, 104, 108; what to
    eat, 70–71, 108
fennel, 96, 107; seeds, 101
fermented foods, 66, 99, 104, 110, 113,
    116, 155
fertility, 48, 68–69
fevers, 17–18
fiber, 58, 67, 128, 131, 148
fibromyalgia, 13, 73, 115
fish, 96, 99, 139, 187, 326; oil capsules,
    187, 203, 210, 213; pH of, 101, 116
flavonoids, 194
flax, 275; seed oil, 70, 90, 101, 108, 206;
    seeds, 101; spouts, 96
flu, 13, 16, 19, 48, 176
folic acid, 88, 90, 91
food: allergies, 34–35; combining, 134–41;
    cooking, 83–84; cravings, 16, 79, 191;
    FDA food pyramid, 5, 82, 93, 136;
    fermented, 66, 99, 104, 110, 113, 116,
    155; fresh, organic, 83–84, 129; pH of,
    100–101, 104, 116; processed, 65, 83,

102–3, 108, 109, 169; raw, 66, 82–83, 149–50, 153, 167; what not to eat, 6, 15, 31, 65–66, 101–16, 216; what to eat, 6, 22, 27, 45, 82, 65–71, 86–101

fruits, 31, 61, 103; calcium content, 107; food combining, 134, 138, 139, 140; juice, 103, 116, 128; pH of, 104; transitioning and, 148, 151, 155; what not to eat, 66, 103, 91, 139, 140, 155, 235; what to eat, 27, 66, 71, 88–89, 91, 100, 104, 107, 139, 160, 172, 178, 195

fungus, 15–21, 22, 31, 33, 36, 43, 48, 54, 59, 94, 99, 112, 113, 148, 151; supplements for, 182, 191, 193, 194, 198, 200, 201, 203, 211

gallbladder, 111

gallium, 201

gamma-linolenic acid (GLA), 187

garcinia cambogia, 214

garlic, 87, 93, 96, 100, 107, 129, 155, 160; recipes, 296, 364

gas/bloating, 17, 58, 92

genistein, 97

germanium, 197, 200, 201

ginger, 129, 160, 167; recipes, 298, 316, 321, 354, 369

ginseng, 98

glandulars, 208–9

glutathione, 45, 88, 173, 179, 194

goat's milk, 105

gold, 201–2

gout, 9, 76, 92, 194

grains, 6, 87; calcium content, 107; for Cleanse, 177–78; food combining with, 138, 139, 140; for maintenance, 145; pH of, 116; stored, 94, 104, 110–11, 116; transitioning and, 148–49, 153–54; what not to eat, 66, 94; what to eat, 66, 94, 107, 159

grapefruit, 66, 91, 97, 103, 107, 160

grape seed oil, 108, 155

grasses, 60, 69–70, 106, 169–70; juices and, 128–31; supplements, 185

green drink, 69, 131–33, 182, 185; for Cleanse, 170, 171–72, 175; recipes, 261–63

green powder, 80, 81, 131, 171, 172, 175, 184, 185, 188, 247

greens, 87, 95, 96, 129, 132. *See also specific types*

halitosis (bad breath), 16

Hawkins, David R., 241

hazelnut (filbert), 97, 101, 106, 107, 151, 159

headaches and migraines, 17, 38, 73, 113, 115, 176

heartburn, 16, 58, 73, 188, 207

heart disease, 4, 6, 9, 13, 14, 70, 73, 92; supplements, 186–88, 201

hemorrhoids, 16

hemp, 151; seed oil, 70, 90, 101, 187; seeds, 101; sprouts, 91, 96, 185

herbs, 92, 115, 161; oil, 316; recipes, 300, 310, 326. *See also* tea

hiatal hernia, 17, 57

high blood pressure, 70, 75, 79–80, 92, 186–88

HIV/AIDS, 13, 16, 207

honey, 101, 116

hormones, 5, 13, 16, 36, 104, 190; what not to eat, 104, 108; what to eat, 97–98

horseradish, 100, 113, 159

hummus, 159, 166, 305

hydrochloric acid (HCL), 51–52, 54–55, 133

hyperactivity, 16, 44

hyperglycemia, 39, 206

hypoglycemia, 38, 136, 206, 237

IBS (irritable bowel syndrome), 13, 51, 57, 176

ice pops, 376

immune system, 14, 33, 44, 56, 58, 140, 216, 225; supplements for, 188, 194, 200; what to eat for, 70, 94, 124

infectious and degenerative symptoms, 207–8

inflammation, 13, 188

insulin, 6, 39, 40–41, 186; vegetable drink for, 263

intestines, 16, 17, 110. *See also* colon; small intestine

iodine, 65, 75–76, 192, 211, 213

iridium, 173, 196, 200, 203, 212

iron, 36, 65, 67, 74, 88, 89, 92, 106, 162, 192

irritability, 16, 115

isoflavones, 97

jicama, 129, 150, 167

joints. *See* muscles and joints

juices: for Cleanse, 169–70, 175; food combining with, 139, 141; recipes, 170, 261–64; supplements, 185; transitioning and, 148, 152; what not to drink, 103, 128; what to drink, 92–93, 128–31. *See also specific juices* junk food, 102–3

kale, 87, 96, 107, 161, 169, 185; recipes, 262, 294, 362, 364
kamut grass, 60, 69, 100, 159, 179, 185
kidneys, 14, 43, 57, 74, 106, 111, 130–31, 174–75, 186
kohlrabi, 100
Koop, C. Everett, 4

lactic acid, 21, 59, 104, 190, 217, 218, 219
Laurenzi, Rick, 117–19, 119n
laxatives, 145, 148, 175–76
lecithin, 98, 101, 150, 214
leek, 96, 100, 107
lemon(s), 66, 91, 97, 103, 139, 141, 160, 161, 167, 178, 248; for Cleanse and, 169, 175, 176; food combining with, 139, 141; juice, 97; pH, 100; recipes, 296, 299, 300, 303, 316; transitioning and, 155; with water, 91, 128, 132, 169, 175, 176
lemongrass, 69
lentils, 94, 97, 107, 159, 160, 178; pH, 100; recipes, 287; sprouts, 91, 163, 164, 165, 250
lettuce (all types), 96, 100, 107, 129, 169; salads, 286, 293
licorice root, 208, 209, 210, 212, 213
lime(s), 66, 91, 103, 139, 141, 160, 161, 167, 248; for Cleanse, 169, 175, 176; food combining with, 139, 141; pH, 100; recipes, 265, 267, 321; transitioning and, 155; with water, 91, 128, 132, 169, 175, 176, 178
lipoic acid, 202
liver, 13, 14, 31, 36, 37, 42, 58, 98, 110; supplements for, 187, 202, 208–9
Livingstone-Wheeler, Virginia, 18
l-taurine, 173, 195, 200, 205, 207, 208, 213
lung problems, 59, 190, 194, 209
lupus, 13, 16, 48–49, 115
lutein, 88
lycopene, 89, 90
Lyme disease, 13
lymphatic system, 14, 59, 215–17, 223, 224; formula, 210–11; massage, 219, 220, 225–26, 237; WBV and, 226

macadamia nuts, 101, 116, 159; recipes, 314, 338, 365
magnesium, 14, 37, 65, 74, 88, 106, 184, 189, 192, 193, 208; carbonate, 45, 179, 188, 189, 193; chloride, 205
maintenance, 82–85, 145, 250–51

malabsorption, 17
malted products, 113
massage, 211, 219, 220, 223, 225–27, 237
mayonnaise, 113, 155; pH, 116; recipes, 304, 311, 312
meat, 108–10; as acidifying, 6, 66, 106, 116; eliminating, 60, 108; food combining with, 149, 151; pH, 116; as protein source, 95, 106, 114; transitioning and, 148, 151
menopause, 42
menstrual disorders, 16, 48
mental clarity and memory, 3, 6, 17, 27, 38, 72, 115
microforms, 15–18, 26–27; death and, 21–22; digestion and, 51, 54, 55, 56, 58, 59, 60; form change and, 19–21; stages of growth, 17–18; symptoms of disease and, 29–49; tests for, 24–26
microwave, 114–15
microzymas, 19–21, 44, 98, 129
millet, 66, 94, 97, 107, 137, 154, 159, 179; pH, 66, 94, 100; recipes, 356, 358, 361, 363
minerals, 65, 91–92, 114, 128, 132, 139, 163, 184, 187, 206, 225; alkalizing, 88–89, 121, 123; blood acidity and, 14, 36; cooking and, 162; digestion and, 51–52; supplements, 172–73, 184, 192, 196, 213. *See also specific minerals*
mineral salts, 22, 60, 67, 74, 77–78, 128, 132, 138, 141, 145, 151, 155, 165, 166, 167, 172, 174, 175, 179, 188, 248, 267; brands recommended, 77–78, 159, 188–89; liquid colloidal, 78, 172, 190; salt therapy, 189–92, 206; solution, how to make, 78, 189
mint, 185, 207
Mittleman, Stu, 80
mold, 15, 16–21, 22, 24, 27, 101, 103, 104, 114, 122, 125, 152, 187, 201, 224, 230; symptoms of acidity and, 31, 36, 39
mood disorders, 16, 38, 198–200
motivation, 230–42
mouth, 16, 50, 51, 53, 55. *See also* chewing
MS (multiple sclerosis), 13, 17, 38, 115, 187
mucopolysaccharides, 94
mucus, 13, 48, 57–59; foods and, 94, 99, 104, 113, 135, 138
mugwort, 154
mung bean sprouts, 90
muscles and joints, 6, 14, 20, 16, 17, 36, 38, 41, 42, 53, 72, 73, 74, 80, 115, 119;

supplements for, 190, 194, 208; what not
to eat, 115; what to eat for, 70, 74, 75, 96
mushrooms, 69, 112, 154
mustard greens, 96, 107
Mycotoxic/Oxidative Stress Test (M/
OST), 25
mycotoxins, 15, 21, 24, 31, 33, 36, 38, 39,
65, 67, 91, 94, 98, 99, 103–4, 108, 109,
110, 111, 112–13, 114, 173, 184, 185,
186, 187, 195, 196, 200, 202, 213. *See
also* antimyotoxin formulas; toxic stress

n-acetyl cysteine, 173, 179, 194–95
Naessens, Gaston, 18
nail (finger and toe) fungus, 16, 48
nervous system, 36–38, 58, 59;
supplements for, 186, 187
New Biology (of health), 3–10, 158
niacin, 91
noni fruit concentrate, 195, 207
nori, 87, 160; recipes, 331, 371
nuts and seeds, 96, 97, 114, 151, 159, 177,
178, 204, 248, 249; calcium content,
107; dehydrating, 165–66; milks from,
160; oils and fats, 70, 88, 139; peanut
warning, 35, 114, 151, 161; pH of, 101,
116; recipes, 248, 319, 325, 349, 356;
soaking of, 21, 90, 152, 166; sprouts, 21,
66, 90–91; storing, 167; transitioning
and, 151; what to eat, 66, 159. *See also
specific types*

oat grass, 69
OEA (oleoylethanolamide), 88
oils, 82, 99, 109, 118, 137, 160, 177, 178,
186–88, 206; brands of, 70–71, 108,
155, 160; Cleanse and, 177–78, 179;
COWS and, 66, 70–71, 184; dressings
with, 155, 289, 290, 293, 295–303;
food combining with, 138, 139, 140,
141; heating, avoidance of, 71, 114,
150; pantry stocking, 160; peanut oil
warning, 35; pH of, 101, 116; processed
foods and, 103; recommended, 70–71,
108, 160, 178; saturated/unhealthy, 103,
108; storing, 167; supplements, 187, 206,
208, 210, 213; transitioning, 137, 155,
149–50, 155
okra, 87, 96, 106, 107, 169, 366
olive: leaf extract, 202; oil, 88, 90, 101,
108, 109, 114, 137, 155
omega-3 oils, 99, 151, 186–87, 188, 200,
203
omega-5 CLA oils, 71, 92, 187

omega-6 oils, 187, 188
onions, 87, 93, 100, 106, 160, 165; green,
96, 107, 303
osmium, 203, 207
osteoporosis, 16, 41–43, 85, 105, 106, 205

palladium, 203, 207
pancreas, 14, 36, 39, 52, 60, 73, 90, 135,
204, 224; cancer, 109, 114; supplements
for, 206–7. *See also* diabetes
pantry stocking, 158–61
parasites, 59, 60, 110, 125, 148, 199;
supplements for, 92, 179, 195, 211, 212
parsley, 69, 87, 96, 107, 129, 159, 161, 206,
210, 212, 213; juicing, 129, 169–70,
261–64; recipes, 296, 306
parsnips, 87
pasta, 102, 159, 162; food combining
with, 138, 140; recipes, 321, 350, 353;
transitioning and, 149, 154
Pasteur, Louis, 18–19, 20–21, 29
peanuts, 35, 114, 116, 135, 151, 161
peas, 87, 93, 94, 100, 179
pecan(s), 151, 159; recipes, 307, 309, 374
peppers, bell, 66, 69, 84, 87, 96, 107, 137,
139, 150, 157, 160, 161; dehydrating,
165; juicing, 128, 129; recipes, 283, 317,
338
peppers, hot, 96, 100, 107
pH: alkaline water, 71, 120–23; balancing
of, 6, 8–10; of common foods (charts),
100–101, 104, 116; definition, 12, 66;
drops, 47, 81, 84, 126–28, 129, 131, 132,
136, 169, 170, 171, 172, 176, 184, 219,
225; ideal, 23, 27; mineral salts for, 22;
self-testing, 23–24
physic acid, 98
phytonutrients, 67, 84–85, 110, 195
pine bark extract, 195–96, 205, 206, 207,
208, 209, 211, 213
pine nuts, 159, 166, 285; recipes, 268, 362
platinum, 203
pleomorphism, 20
PMS (premenstrual syndrome), 16, 70, 186
polyps, 14
pomegranates, 91–92, 187; seed oil, 71, 92,
101, 179
potassium, 14, 37, 65, 74, 88, 91, 192–93,
263, 290; bicarbonate, 39, 42, 45, 60, 78,
126, 179; chloride, 205
potatoes, 93, 111, 116, 138, 139, 140, 153,
178, 179
poultry, 108, 116; transitioning, 151. *See
also* meat

probiotics, 54–55, 132, 182
prostaglandins, 70, 186
prostate, 32, 48, 89, 97, 98, 108, 111
protease inhibitors, 98
protein, 9, 16, 56, 134; average American intake daily, 95; Cleanse and, 176; daily requirement, 94–95; fish, 96; food combining with, 134, 139, 140; meat vs. vegetable, 95; non-animal, 94–96; percentage of calories from protein in alkalizing foods, 96–97; supplements and, 185; transitioning and, 148–49, 151; what not to eat, 65, 106, 109–10; what to eat, 94–99. *See also* meat
pumpkin, 93; recipes, 309, 378; seed oil, 155, 160; seeds, 97, 101, 107, 137, 151, 159, 187, 212

quinoa, 94, 154, 159, 179

radish, 87, 96, 100, 107, 137, 161, 166, 258; juicing, 129; sprouts, 100, 164, 165
recipes, 245–378; anytime, 249–6; Cleanse, 246–47; 80 or 20, 252; healthy snacks, 252–53; Index, 255; maintenance, 250–51; substitutions, 379. *See also specific ingredients*
R-lipoic and R-dihydrolipoic, 174
reproductive disorders, 36, 212, 191
respiratory system/disorders, 16, 17, 19, 36, 48, 111, 115; supplements for, 205–6, 209
rhodium, 173, 196, 200, 203, 212
rhubarb, 97, 100, 107
rice (white and brown), 94, 97, 102, 107, 136, 137, 139, 149, 150, 153, 154, 159, 179; cooker, 162, 167; milk, 152, 160; pH of, 100; recipes, 339, 340, 347, 358, 360; syrup, 98, 116, 152
rutabagas, 87, 100
ruthenium, 203, 207

salad dressings, 113, 166; recipes, 295–303; transitioning and, 152, 155
salads, 83, 94, 165, 248; food combining with, 139, 141; recipes, 285–94; spinners, 162; transitioning and, 148–49, 153
saliva, 12, 51, 78; testing, 22, 34
salivary glands, 51, 187
salsify, 87
salt(s), 74–80, 92; good salt, 77; liquid colloidal mineral salts, 78; mineral salts, 77–78; processed, 75, 108; salt test, 76;

sea salt and rock salt, 77, 82, 90; sodium bicarbonate, 79; using, 79–80. *See also specific types of mineral salts*
sandwiches, 135, 139, 153, 165, 248; recipes, 346, 359
saponins, 98
sauna, infrared, 224–25
scallions, 87
seasonings. *See* spices
sea vegetables, 87, 97, 107, 160
seeds. *See* nuts and seeds
selenium, 45
sesame: oil, 160, 299; seeds, 101, 106, 107, 151, 159; sprouts, 91. *See also* tahini
70–30 diet, 149
sex drive (libido), 16, 191
shave grass, 69, 100
shellfish, 99
silver, 65; colloidal, 173, 196–98, 203, 206, 207, 209, 211, 213
sinus problems, 13, 136, 190, 205–6
skin, 4, 6, 14, 16, 17, 33, 45, 48, 176; supplements for, 187, 190, 191, 200, 201; vegetable juice drink for, 264; water for, 73; what to eat, 70
sleep, 15, 37, 47, 73, 91, 171, 203, 204; apnea, 117, 190; problems, 17, 45, 48, 115; supplements for, 190
small intestine, 52, 53–54, 84, 134; acid damage to, 53, 55; Cleanse and, 175–76; pH of, 53; supplements for, 198, 200
snacks, 165, 167; recipes, 252–53, 371–76; transitioning and, 149
sodium/sodium bicarbonate, 45, 74, 78, 79, 89, 126, 179, 188–89, 192, 206; blood pH and, 14, 39, 42, 79; digestion and, 51–52, 56, 60, 133
sodium chloride, 74, 76, 77, 79, 192
sodium chlorite, 126, 206
soups, 165; for Cleanse, 171, 172, 175, 178; recipes, 270–84; transitioning and, 148, 149, 153
soy, 97–99, 107, 145, 156, 159; fermented products, 99, 113, 116, 155; milk, 105, 152, 156, 160; oil, 187; pH, 100, 101, 116; recipes, 299, 300, 321, 377; sprouts, 91, 97, 98, 100, 107, 164, 165, 177, 212, 213; sprouts powder, 247, 265, 266. *See also* edamame; tofu
spelt, 66, 94, 100, 154, 159, 179
spices, 92, 155–56, 159, 166, 248; basic seasoning, 316; recipes, 357, 367;

Spice Hunter, 155–56, 159, 248, 384; transitioning and, 155–56

spinach, 69, 87, 95, 97, 137, 160, 161, 166, 185; calcium content, 107; juicing, 169, 261, 263–64; pH, 100; recipes, 265, 266, 267, 273, 288, 306, 318, 348, 358

spirulina, 112

sports and athletes, 37–38, 80–81, 191–92

sprouts, 90–91, 96, 97, 100, 107, 137, 160, 165, 166, 167, 170, 200, 248, 249; juicing, 129; recipes, 262–63, 288, 290, 291, 326, 329, 367; sprouting directions, 163–64. *See also specific types*

squash, summer, 84, 87. *See also* zucchini

squash, winter, 93, 128, 165, 179; recipes, 282, 332, 340, 357

stevia, 102, 115, 154–55

stomach, 31, 51; cancer, 108–9, 111, 114; supplements for, 200. *See also* digestion

stools, 52, 56, 58

stress, 6, 13, 25, 27, 33, 47, 59, 60, 83, 200, 225, 227, 237, 241; digestion and, 56, 58, 131, 134; exercise for, 215, 216, 219, 222; supplements for, 194, 203, 201–12; toxic, 213

stroke, 13, 40, 70, 108, 186

sugar, 31, 33, 39, 75, 88, 90, 95, 105, 111, 113, 128, 132, 148–49, 216, 231; as acidifying, 7, 8, 9, 31, 32, 36, 39, 60, 66, 82, 90, 91, 101–2, 103; allergic reaction and, 35; cravings, 72, 79, 155, 157, 167, 231, 252; eliminating, 36, 37, 45, 47, 82, 90, 101–2, 115, 136, 153, 154, 169, 187, 232, 235, 236; exercise and, 218–19, 221; fat vs., 218–19; food combining with, 135, 138–39, 140; forms of, 101; fruits high in, 91, 139, 140, 155, 235; pH of, 116; supplements and, 181, 185, 195, 207; transitioning and, 148–49, 150, 152, 153, 154–55; vegetable high in, 86, 93, 129, 170

suicidal tendencies, 17

sulfur, 37, 65, 173, 195, 205, 207, 208, 213

sunflower: oil, 101, 187; seeds, 97, 101, 107, 151, 159, 309; spouts, 91, 97

supplements, 6, 181–214; addressing symptoms with, 204–14; alkaline stars, daily use, 184–93; alkalizing (for Cleanse), 172–73, 179; brands, 182; cameos (to regain pH balance), 200–203; chlorophyll and concentrated green powder, 185; dosing, 182–83; liquid colloids, 78, 172, 190, 183; multivitamin and mineral, 192–93;

omega-3 and -6 oils, 186–88; salts and sodium bicarbonate, 188–89; salt therapy, 189–92; starting with the right products, 181–82; supporting (expanded use), 193–98; using, 183–84. *See also* green drink; *specific minerals, vitamins*

surgery, 8, 26, 43, 135–36, 153, 183

sweeteners, 115, 116, 154–55; artificial, 66, 102, 115, 116, 154. *See also* sugar

sweet potatoes, 93, 128, 179

Swiss chard, 96, 107

tahini, 152, 159; recipes, 268, 301, 302, 314, 320

tamari, 113

tea: black or green, 66, 113, 116; herbal, 92, 167, 171, 211–12

thioctic acid, 202

thrush, 15, 16

thyroid gland, 13, 16, 42, 57, 115, 121, 237; cancer, 109; supplements for, 189, 213; weight and, 31, 189

titanium, 173

tofu, 96, 97, 98, 101, 106, 135, 137, 149, 151, 156, 159, 160, 166, 167, 178; recipes, 305, 308, 327, 329, 337, 343, 348, 359

tomato(es), 66, 83, 89–90, 97, 107, 129, 160, 161, 248, 249; for Cleanse, 172, 178; dehydrating, 165; food combining with, 135, 138, 139; pH, 100; recipes, 264, 281–82, 321–24, 367, 371; transitioning and, 148, 153, 155

tortillas, 160, 167, 248, 249, 252; recipes, 346, 370, 376

toxic stress, 213

transitioning, 145, 147–57; breakfast, 148–49; condiments, 155–56; dairy, 152; dessert, 150–51; fruit, 155; meat, 151; raw foods, 149–50; 70–30 diet, 149; sugar, 154–55; white flour, 154; white rice, 154; yeast, 153–54

tumors, 14, 16, 21, 32, 48, 98, 115

turnip, 87, 100; greens, 97, 107

ulcers, 13, 16, 58, 59, 133, 201

undecylenic acid, 198, 200, 202, 203, 205, 207, 208, 211, 213

urine/urination; blood in, 130; pH of, 12, 17, 78, 79; testing, 22–24, 35

urinary tract infections, 48

vanadium, 203, 205, 206, 213
varicose veins, 191
vegans, 95, 106, 153
vegetable(s), 42, 58, 66, 80, 110, 160–61;
   broths, 93, 160; calcium content,
   106, 107 (chart); chlorophyll and
   green, 67–70; for Cleanse, 169–71,
   177–78; dehydrating, 90, 165–66; food
   combining with, 134–35, 138–41;
   juice, 8, 37, 45, 128–32; pH, 100–101
   (chart), 116 (chart); protein content
   of alkalizing, 96–97 (chart); raw, 66,
   82–83, 149–50, 153, 167, 177; recipes,
   261–64, 325, 331, 336, 338, 341, 342,
   343–44, 356, 372; snacks, 371, 372;
   sprouts and, 90–91, 194; stocking the
   pantry, 160; transitioning and, 148–50,
   153; washes for, 84; water content, 128,
   167; what to eat (low-carb), 6, 27, 37,
   45, 66, 67–70, 71, 82, 83, 86–87(chart),
   93–94; what to eat in moderation (high-
   carb), 86, 93, 116, 154. *See also specific
   types*
vegetarianism, 5, 9, 70, 81, 93, 95, 109,
   110, 149, 153, 236; COWS and, 65–80;
   transitioning and, 98, 99, 149, 151
vinegar, 35, 113, 116, 161; substitute, 167,
   369; transitioning and, 153, 155
Virchow, Rudolph, 16
vitamins: A, 69, 83, 88; B-complex, 36, 69,
   88, 106, 114, 186; B$_1$, 70, 91; B$_2$, 90, 91;
   B$_5$, 90, 203, 205; B$_6$, 90, 91, 212, 213;
   B$_{12}$, 90, 112, 199; B$_{17}$, 94; C, 45, 69, 70,
   85, 88, 91, 130; for Cleanse, 172–73; D$_3$,
   42, 179, 193, 205; E, 45, 69, 88, 91,114;
   H, 88; K, 69, 88; multivitamin, 172,
   184, 192, 200, 213; vegetable juice drink
   (high C & E), 263; what to eat, 69–70,
   106

walnut, 101, 159,
water, 71–74, 120–28, 160, 167, 188;
   alkaline, 122–23; amount needed daily,
   127, 132; dangers of dehydration, 71–73;
   digestion and, 56, 57, 133; distilled, 127;
   electron-charged, 123–24; filtering, 121;
   health benefits, 73–74; how to make
   good water, 125–28; hydration schedule,
   132; molecularly structured, 124–25;
   pH, 71, 101, 122, 125; pH drops,
   126–27; pure, 121–22; reverse-osmosis,
   126; the right water, 120–21
water chestnuts, 87
watercress, 97, 100, 107, 169
weight issues, 7–8; acidity and, 5, 14, 17,
   31–33; aging and, 42–43; American
   and popular diets, 5, 8, 26; exercise and
   loss, 118; microforms and, 31; obesity,
   4, 9, 29, 73, 92, 119, 202; pH balance
   and loss, 3–4, 7–8, 9, 27, 34, 37–38, 43,
   48–49, 92, 117–19; supplements for, 186,
   213; water and, 73, 74
wheat, 94, 97, 100, 101, 107, 136, 159, 179;
   bran, 107; bread (Nature's Path Manna),
   159; white flour, transitioning from, 154
wheat, sprouted, 91, 137, 153, 159, 160,
   167, 249, 252; recipes, 291, 326, 369,
   370; sprouting, 163–65
wheatgrass, 60, 69, 97, 185, 197; juice
   powder, 129, 185; juicing, 130, 169; pH,
   100; recipes, 261, 262
Whole-Body Vibration (WBV), 226–29
wraps, 137, 153, 148, 160, 165, 166, 249,
   305, 335

yam(s), 69, 93, 139, 154; dehydrating,
   165; recipes, 361, 362; wild, root,
   supplement, 208, 212, 213
yeast, 15–21, 31, 33, 39, 48, 66, 111, 233;
   digestion and, 50, 54, 59, 60; health
   risks of, 111; supplements for, 179,
   194, 198, 200, 201, 205, 207, 208;
   transitioning and, 148, 153–54; vaginal
   infection, 16, 48, 184
yogurt, 148, 150

zinc, 65, 192, 208, 212, 213; soup for, 207
zucchini, 87, 97, 129, 161, 162; pH, 100;
   recipes, 292, 354, 358, 366